APPLICATIONS MANUAL FOR

Health & Physical Assessment in Nursing

Second Edition

Donita D'Amico, MEd, RN
Associate Professor
William Paterson University
Wayne, New Jersey

Colleen Barbarito, EdD, RN
Associate Professor
William Paterson University
Wayne, New Jersey

Grace Maria Carcich, MSN, RN
Instructor
William Paterson University
Wayne, New Jersey

Contributing Editor
Lizy Mathew, EdD, RN, CCRN
Assistant Professor
William Paterson University
Wayne, New Jersey

Pearson
Boston   Columbus   Indianapolis   New York   San Francisco   Upper Saddle River
Amsterdam   Cape Town   Dubai   London   Madrid   Milan   Munich   Paris   Montreal   Toronto
Delhi   Mexico City   São Paulo   Sydney   Hong Kong   Seoul   Singapore   Taipei   Tokyo

Publisher: Julie Levin Alexander
Publisher's Assistant: Regina Bruno
Executive Acquisitions Editor: Pamela Fuller
Development Editor: Melisa Leong
Editorial Assistant: Cynthia Gates
Managing Production Editor: Patrick Walsh
Production Liaison: Cathy O'Connell
Production Editor: Roxanne Klaas, S4Carlisle Publishing Services
Manufacturing Manager: Ilene Sanford
Art Director: Christopher Weigand
Cover Designer: Robert Siani
Art Editor: Patricia Gutierrez
Director of Marketing: David Gesell
Marketing Manager: Phoenix Harvery
Marketing Specialist: Michael Sirinides
Composition: S4Carlisle Publishing Services
Printer/Binder: Bind-Rite Graphics/Robbinsville
Cover Printer: Bind-Rite Graphics/Robbinsville
Cover Image: Shutterstock

Notice: Care has been taken to confirm the accuracy of information presented in this book. The authors, editors, and the publisher, however, cannot accept any responsibility for errors or omissions or for consequences from application of the information in this book and make no warranty, express or implied, with respect to its contents.

The authors and publisher have exerted every effort to ensure that drug selections and dosages set forth in this text are in accord with current recommendations and practice at time of publication. However, in view of ongoing research, changes in government regulations, and the constant flow of information relating to drug therapy and drug reactions, the reader is urged to check the package inserts of all drugs for any change in indications of dosage and for added warnings and precautions. This is particularly important when the recommended agent is a new and/or infrequently employed drug.

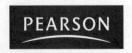

www.pearsonhighered.com

ISBN-10: 0-13-237609-1
ISBN-13: 978-0-13-237609-9

Preface

The nursing profession evolves to meet the needs of clients in a continuously changing health care environment. The nurse must acquire knowledge and skills and use all available resources and evidence to meet client needs. The nursing process has always guided nurses to practice in an organized and competent manner. Assessment is the first part of this process, and it is the foundation for nursing practice. This Applications Manual is designed to accompany the *Health & Physical Assessment in Nursing* (2nd edition) textbook by Donita D'Amico and Colleen Barbarito. It provides the student with opportunities to review the content in the text, reinforce what has been learned, and apply the new knowledge to clinical scenarios and various activities that support critical thinking. It furthers the development of knowledge and skills required in application of nursing process in clinical practice. The workbook is designed to be used independently, with a laboratory partner, in class, or in study groups. The exercises allow the student to fully engage in each experience.

Each chapter of the workbook coincides with the same numbered chapter of the text. In each chapter you will find:

- The use of puzzles to review key terminology and abbreviations.
- A variety of exercises to reinforce key concepts of the chapter.
- Critical thinking exercises that will continuously build on what was learned in previous chapters.
- NCLEX®-style review questions.

The Assessment chapters also include:

- Anatomy and Physiology Review.
- Health history and focused interview exercises.
- Scenarios for various age levels that put emphasis on interpretation of findings as normal and abnormal.
- Documentation worksheets.
- Case studies.

When a student leaves the classroom or lab, he or she should feel confident that this workbook is a resource to continue to practice health assessment skills and evaluate his or her own progress. Recognizing one's own strengths and weaknesses can be a motivating force for students to push themselves to the next level. I personally challenge each student to be a better nurse than they ever imagined they could be.

Remember the Native American saying that inspired me when writing this workbook: *"Tell me, and I'll forget. Show me, and I may not remember. Involve me, and I'll understand."*

Grace M. Carcich, MSN, RN
William Paterson University

Contents

Health Assessment 1

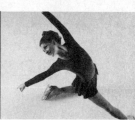

A journey of a thousand miles must begin with a single step.
—Lao Tzu

This chapter addresses introductory concepts for health assessment. The exercises are intended to assist learning and may be assigned for completion by the individual, or as part of classroom activities.

OBJECTIVES

At the completion of these exercises you will be able to:

1. Define key terminology regarding health assessment.
2. Develop a personal definition of health.
3. Formulate methods to operationalize topic areas of *Healthy People 2020*.
4. Differentiate between and among the various components of the health history.
5. Identify problems with confidentiality in simulated situations.
6. Utilize various documentation methods.
7. Apply critical thinking in analysis of case studies.
8. Differentiate between and among the various roles of the professional nurse.
9. Apply principles of teaching and learning.
10. Complete NCLEX®-style review questions related to the health assessment.

RESOURCES

Pearson Nursing Student Resources
Find additional review materials at
nursing.pearsonhighered.com

Prepare for success with additional NCLEX®-style practice questions, interactive assignments and activities, Web links, animations and videos, and more!

Additional resources: *www.healthypeople.gov*

CROSSWORD PUZZLE FOR KEY TERMS

Read each definition below and fill in the correct term on the puzzle grid. If the answer requires two words do not leave a blank space between the words. Use a pencil so you can erase easily.

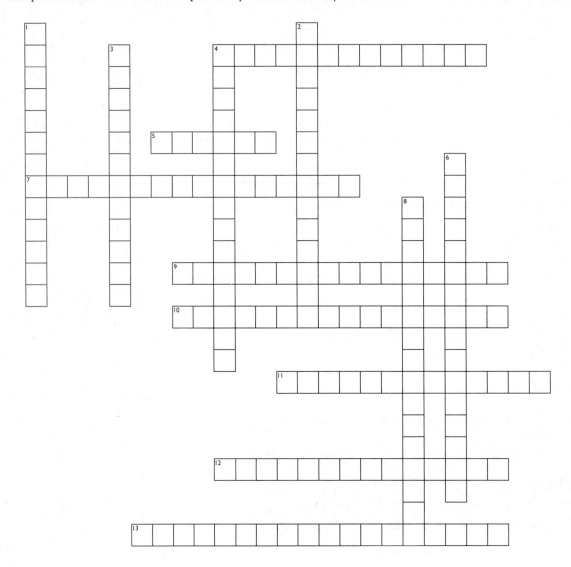

CLUES

Across

4. Exchange of information, thoughts, and ideas
5. Considering more than the physiological health status of a client
7. Occurs as a natural part of a client encounter, may provide instructions, explain a question or procedure, or reduce anxiety (**two words**)
9. A systematic method of collecting data about a client for the purpose of determining the client's current and ongoing health status (**two words**)
10. A process of purposeful and creative thinking about resolutions of problems or the development of new ways to manage situations (**two words**)
11. Data observed or measured by the professional nurse (**two words**)
12. A systematic, rational, dynamic, and cyclic process used by the nurse for planning and providing care for the client (**two words**)
13. Hands-on examination of the client (**two words**)

Down

1. Information about the client's health in his or her own words and based on the client's own perceptions (**two words**)
2. Information that the client experiences and communicates to the nurse (**two words**)
3. A legal document used to plan care, to communicate information between and among healthcare providers, and to monitor quality care (**two words**)
4. Protecting information, sharing with only those directly involved in client care
6. An interview that enables the nurse to clarify points, to obtain missing information, and to follow up on verbal and nonverbal cues identified in the health history (**two words**)
8. The second step of the nursing process (**two words**)

DEFINING HEALTH

1. Read each sentence. Using the numbers 1 through 6, rank the following clients according to health status. (1 = the highest level of health and 6 = the lowest level of health)

_____ 25-year-old female who smokes ½ pack of cigarettes per day

_____ 17-year-old male who just had his appendix removed

_____ 48-year-old female with diabetes

_____ 75-year-old male who has been treated for prostate cancer 15 years ago

_____ 56-year-old female who suffers from depression

_____ 90-year-old male with no health issues but lives in a long-term care facility

2. How did you do? Did you find it difficult to determine who is the healthiest? This exercise was designed to challenge your idea of "health." You may find that your classmates do not have the same answers. Provide a rationale for the ranking of each client.

Client 1

Client 2

Client 3

Client 4

Client 5

Client 6

3. What model, guidelines, or factors influenced your decisions for the above ranking in part 1?

4. Many factors contribute to one's personal definition of health. Consider each of the following factors and circle the response that indicates your beliefs.

   1. Age   YES   NO   NOT SURE
   2. Gender   YES   NO   NOT SURE

3. Culture	YES	NO	NOT SURE
4. Family	YES	NO	NOT SURE
5. Spirituality	YES	NO	NOT SURE
6. Financial status	YES	NO	NOT SURE
7. Environment	YES	NO	NOT SURE

5. Write your own definition of health.

6. Compare and contrast your definition of health with your peers and the definitions provided in your text (chapter 1).

HEALTHY PEOPLE 2020

Healthy People 2020 focuses on improving the health of people living in the United States of America.

1. Search newspapers or electronic news websites to find a current article that relates to any one of the *Healthy People 2020* topic areas.

Name the news or web source _____

Identify the selected focus area _____

2. Log on to a healthcare agency website (e.g., a local hospital or your local health department). Does the agency offer any programs that relate to or support *Healthy People 2020*'s topic areas? Identify:

Name the agency _____

Name the program _____

Explain how the program supports *Healthy People 2020*.

_____

_____

3. Consider the students who attend your college or university. Name at least five health issues that affect college students on your campus.

  1.

  2.

  3.

  4.

  5.

4. Identify your top three health concerns on campus.

   1.

   2.

   3.

PROGRAM DEVELOPMENT

1. Using the above list of health concerns, describe a program that you would develop to improve the health of your campus community.

2. Present your idea to your class, and ask your peers if they would participate in your proposed program if it was "actually" offered. What is the rationale for their decision?

3. Did more than 50% of your class choose to participate? If not, why not?

HEALTH ASSESSMENT

HEALTH HISTORY

Match each piece of assessment data in Column A with the appropriate Health History Component in Column B.

Column A

_____ 1. Father died of cancer

_____ 2. "I'm as strong as an ox"

_____ 3. Denies bloating

_____ 4. Widowed for 10 years

_____ 5. Walks 3 miles, 3 times per week

_____ 6. Hypertension for 2 years

_____ 7. Felt a pop in the left knee when playing tennis today

_____ 8. Allergic to sulfa-based medications

_____ 9. Smokes 1 ppd (pack per day) × 3 yr

_____ 10. Last BM (bowel movement) 2 days ago

Column B

A. Biographical Data
B. Perceptions About Health
C. Past History of Illness and Injury
D. Present History of Illness and Injury
E. Family History
F. Review of Systems
G. Health Practices

DATA

For each piece of data collected, determine the following: Is it subjective or objective? Is it collected during the health history or the physical assessment? Write the appropriate letters on the lines provided to label each piece of information.

S = Subjective   HH = Health History   O = Objective   PA = Physical Assessment

1. _____ & _____ Blood pressure 136/80 in an adult

2. _____ & _____ Client states "I had a fever last night"

3. _____ & _____ Abdomen is soft and nondistended

4. _____ & _____ Lung sounds are clear

5. _____ & _____ Client states "I have so much pain in my right knee"

6. _____ & _____ Client's mother had breast cancer

7. _____ & _____ Heart rate 72 beats per minute (bpm)

8. _____ & _____ Weight 175 lb

9. _____ & _____ Client states "I think I vomited three times last night"

10. _____ & _____ Saliva present in oral cavity

CONFIDENTIALITY

Put a check next to each scenario where a breech in confidentiality has occurred. Identify the actual breech on the line provided.

_____ 1. A nurse is discussing her client's status with a nurse from another unit during lunch in the cafeteria.

Breech _____

_____ 2. A nurse is discussing his client's status with an Advanced Practice Nurse in order to improve wound care.

Breech _____

_____ 3. A nurse leaves a client's chart open on the desk at the nurses' station while he goes to medicate the client for pain.

Breech _____

_____ 4. A nurse looks into the hospital computer system to see if her neighbor has delivered her baby.

Breech _____

_____ 5. A nurse pulls up a computerized chart to see why his old girlfriend was admitted through the emergency department.

Breech _____

_____ 6. A nurse uses a computerized documentation system and leaves the screen open to a client's medication administration record while she goes to answer a call light.

Breech _____

_____ 7. A nurse is contacting the state services for suspected child abuse.

Breech _____

_____ 8. A nurse is contacting the sharing network (an organ donation network) about a client who expired.

Breech _____

_____ 9. The client in Room 201A asks the nurse about the health condition of his roommate in Room 201B. The nurse explains to him that the roommate is no longer contagious from an infection he had 2 weeks ago.

Breech _____

_____ 10. A mother calls the hospital looking for her 23-year-old daughter. The nurse explains to the mother that she was discharged 2 hours ago with her boyfriend.

Breech _____

DOCUMENTATION

Write the term represented by each standard abbreviation listed.

Example: RUQ = Right Upper Quadrant

1. Dx = _____

2. Hx = _____

3. HIPAA = _____

4. NANDA = _____

5. BP = _____

6. CBC = _____

7. ABD = _____

8. LMP = _____

9. CVA = _____

10. VS = _____

11. WBC = _____

12. CNS = _____

13. Ht = _____

14. ADL = _____

15. Wt = _____

CHARTING

Read the following scenario and document the findings and events using the stated documentation methods.

On a hot summer day Sister Mary Katherine (a 63-year-old female) presents to the Emergency Department with weakness and a rapid heartbeat. She states she was gardening all day in the church courtyard and never took a break to eat or drink. Her blood pressure (BP) is 86/40 and her heart rate (HR) is 119 beats per minute (bpm). Her mucous membranes are dry and she cannot recall the last time she urinated. You begin to infuse intravenous fluids as ordered by the healthcare provider. After 2 hours she has received 1 liter of fluid. Her BP is now 109/62 and her HR is 88 bpm. She was also able to provide a urine sample of 475 ml (clear amber) during this time, which was sent to the lab for a urinalysis test.

1. Using the APIE method of documentation, sort out the information provided to chart the events.

    A

    P

    I

    E

2. Using the same scenario, try to document the events using the SOAP method.

    S

    O

    A

    P

3. Read the following narrative note for the above scenario.

    IV fluids were started on client because she showed signs of dehydration. Pt improved upon completion of infusion. Vital signs are stable.

    Is this nurse's note written correctly? If yes, provide rationale. If not, write the note correctly.

THE NURSING PROCESS AND CRITICAL THINKING

In the following scenario, identify information that corresponds to steps in the nursing process.

1. Percy Chan, RN, is a staff nurse on a busy medical-surgical unit. Her client is a 25-year-old female who has had her uterus removed (hysterectomy). The client complains of intermittent sharp pains in the lower abdomen scaled as an 8 on a scale of 0–10. After careful questioning, Nurse Chan interprets her findings as "pain related to the surgical incision" and plans to administer 4 mg of morphine to the client. After administering the medication via subcutaneous injection, she returns in 30 minutes to reassess her client's pain status. The client states her pain has decreased and rates it a 2 on a scale of 0–10.

    Assessment

    Diagnosis

Planning

Implementation

Evaluation

Read the following scenario and answer the questions.

2. Sally Johnson is a 21-year-old female who has been treated for depression as an outpatient at her county's mental health clinic. She has been taking an antidepressant medication for 6 weeks and has come to the clinic today for a follow-up visit. During the assessment, Sally states she has been feeling more energetic and has more of an appetite than she did on her first visit. However, she has been experiencing dry mouth and frequent headaches.

   A. As the nurse assessing Sally, determine which findings are normal and which findings are abnormal.

   B. Develop a nursing diagnosis based upon your findings.

   C. Explain the difference between planning and implementation.

CRITICAL THINKING

ELEMENTS OF CRITICAL THINKING

Place the following essential elements of critical thinking in the correct order. (1 being the first step and 5 being the last)

_____   Selection of alternatives

_____   Analysis of the situation

_____   Collection of information

_____   Evaluation

_____   Generation of alternatives

APPLICATION OF THE CRITICAL THINKING PROCESS

Read the following scenario and answer the questions as you go along.

You are in a gourmet chocolate shop at the mall when you suddenly hear shouts for help and see a crowd of people forming at the entranceway to the shop. You run over to find a young woman on the ground who appears to be unconscious. As a student nurse who is certified in Basic Life Support you offer to help. A bystander tells you they have already called Emergency Medical Services (EMS).

THE CRITICAL THINKING PROCESS BEGINS

Collection of Information

1. What information do you need to collect? (identify the information as subjective or objective)

2. How will you obtain this information?

You gather the following information:

The woman is Caucasian and approximately 25 years old. She was shopping with a friend. The friend tells you that the woman has no medical history but is severely allergic to peanuts. Last, she noted her friend was sampling chocolates the store provided. After completing the airway, breathing, circulation assessment, you find the woman is not breathing and has no pulse.

Analysis of the Situation

1. What normal and abnormal data have you collected?

2. Cluster the data that you have collected and identify any patterns that are forming.

3. List any information that is missing.

4. What are your conclusions?

As you quickly determine that her cardiopulmonary assessment is alarmingly abnormal, you begin the process for cardiopulmonary resuscitation (CPR). However, you then find out important missing information. Another bystander informs you that the woman never ate any chocolate because she witnessed the woman trip and hit her head on a metal display and then fall to the ground hitting her head again. Are your conclusions starting to change based on the additional data collected?

Generation of Alternatives

1. What are your priorities for this woman?

2. Are there any alternate options for her current treatment?

You decide that your priority remains maintaining her airway, breathing, and circulation. You feel you are tiring and may not be providing CPR as well as you were when you started. You quickly ask if anyone else is capable of performing two-rescuer CPR with you. Another bystander assists you.

Selection of Alternatives

1. What is your continued plan of care?

2. What are your expected outcomes?

Your plan of care is to continue two-rescuer CPR until EMS arrives. At that point you will communicate to the EMS team the information that you have already collected. Your anticipated outcome is that the CPR that has been provided to the woman allowed for adequate oxygenation and circulation in order to survive the incident with minimal or no deficits.

Evaluation

1. How can you evaluate the outcome of this scenario?

2. Would you change any of the steps you followed?

It may be difficult for you to truly evaluate if the expected outcome will be achieved in this particular kind of scenario given the environment you are in. The next day it is printed in the newspaper how a shopper saved a woman's life in the mall.

ROLE OF THE PROFESSIONAL NURSE IN HEALTH ASSESSMENT

Match the role in Column B with the task in Column A. A role may be used more than once.

Column A

_____ 1. Planning a budget to accommodate Medicare reimbursement cutbacks

_____ 2. Orienting staff to new equipment and technology

_____ 3. Conducting a study on the relationship between postpartum depression and spirituality

_____ 4. Educating a community about community acquired *methicillin-resistant Staphylococcus aureus (MRSA)*

_____ 5. Monitoring the urine output of a postoperative client

_____ 6. Gathering data to prevent ventilator-acquired pneumonia

_____ 7. Repositioning a client in bed to prevent skin breakdown

_____ 8. Reviewing wound care products from vendors to determine which would be the best for the hospital to purchase

Column B

A. Nurse Caregiver
B. Clinical Nurse Specialist
C. Nurse Researcher
D. Nurse Administrator
E. Nurse Educator

TEACHING PLANS

OBJECTIVES

Read each objective. Determine the domain of the objective and circle the appropriate letter
(C = Cognitive, A = Affective, P = Psychomotor)

1. At the completion of this learning session, the student will be able to differentiate among isotonic, hypertonic, and hypotonic solutions.

   C   A   P

2. At the completion of this learning session, the client will be able to demonstrate safe crutch walking.

   C   A   P

3. At the completion of this learning session, the client will be able to avoid foods high in cholesterol.

   C   A   P

4. At the completion of this learning session, the student will be able to calibrate the glucometer.

   C   A   P

5. At the completion of this learning session, the client will be able to assume responsibility for his alcohol consumption.

   C   A   P

6. At the completion of this learning session, the client will be able to name five foods high in trans-fat.

   C   A   P

7. At the completion of this learning session, the client will be able to state the risk factors for stroke.

   C   A   P

8. At the completion of this learning session, the student will be able to differentiate among the three domains of educational objectives.

   C   A   P

TEACHING METHODS

Read each learning need and circle the best teaching method to present the content.

1. A community needs to learn about protective measures against West Nile Virus:

   Role Play   OR   Lecture

2. A client needs to learn how to apply a smoking cessation patch:

   Demonstration   OR   Case Study

3. A mother needs to learn how to breastfeed her baby:

   Practice   OR   Lecture

4. A husband needs to learn how to change a dressing on his wife's foot:

   Audiovisual Presentation   OR   Demonstration

5. A client needs to learn what to expect when they go for a nuclear stress test:

   Group Discussion   OR   Printed Material

6. A mother's group needs to learn about stress management techniques after delivering twins:

   Group Discussion   OR   Lecture

7. A mother needs to learn how to suction her son's tracheostomy at home:

   Role Play   OR   Demonstration

8. A client needs to learn about the side effects of her chemotherapy:

   Explanation   OR   Practice

TEACHING SCENARIO

Read the following scenario and answer the questions.

You have been caring for a client with an exacerbation of asthma for 3 days. The client admits to smoking two packs of cigarettes per day for 35 years. You have identified a learning need for this client to stop smoking.

1. Develop a short-term and long-term goal. Explain your response.

2. State the goal(s) for this client.

3. Write three objectives to support one of the goals:

   a.

   b.

   c.

4. Name three specific resources you would use to seek out information when formulating the content for your plan: (e.g., scholarly journals, textbooks, websites)

   a.

   b.

   c.

5. One of the teaching methods you have selected is to demonstrate how to apply the nicotine patch. What is the best method to evaluate that learning has taken place? Why?

NCLEX®-STYLE REVIEW QUESTIONS

Read each question carefully. Choose the best answer for each question.

1. The nurse identifies the letters in SOAP charting as:
   1. S- subjective, O- objective, A- analysis, P- prioritizing.
   2. S- subjective, O- orders, A- assessment, P- prioritizing.
   3. S- signs & symptoms, O- organization of data, A- analysis, P- planning.
   4. S- subjective, O- objective, A- assessment, P- planning.

2. The nurse understands that charting by exception is a documentation method that is based on: (Select all that apply)
   1. preestablished norms.
   2. the elimination of repetition.
   3. the use of phrases and sentences.
   4. the frequent use of scales.
   5. a computer program.

3. The nurse understands the importance of the health history because it:
   1. eliminates the need for a full physical assessment.
   2. provides cues and guides further data collection.
   3. saves the nurse time by focusing only on verbal cues.
   4. is the basis of formulating the nursing diagnosis.

4. The nurse identifies which component(s) in the following statement as variable data?

   A 55-year-old African American male has a blood pressure of 156/80.

   1. Age and BP
   2. Ethnicity and sex
   3. Age and sex
   4. Ethnicity and BP

5. Which of the following activities are the responsibility of the nurse educator? (Select all that apply)
   1. Teaching a new graduate how to use an IV pump
   2. Coordinating a workshop for critical care nurses
   3. Providing staff nurses with information about a new medication
   4. Writing a grant for funds to conduct research
   5. Assessing the client's daily intake of food

6. The nurse is obtaining a health history from a 67-year-old male with a history of hypertension and diabetes. After obtaining the history of past illness, the next step would be to:
   1. obtain a BP and a finger stick glucose level.
   2. continue with a family history and review of systems.
   3. educate the client about a low-sodium, sugar-controlled diet.
   4. discuss referring the client to a cardiologist.

7. The nurse has developed a teaching plan for a senior center that has requested information on weight-bearing exercises to prevent osteoporosis. The nurse has identified the objectives are in the psychomotor domain. Which teaching method would be the **least** appropriate choice?
   1. Practice
   2. Demonstration
   3. Case Study
   4. Computer Assisted Instruction

8. The nurse has completed a comprehensive health assessment on a middle-aged female client. When analyzing the data, the nurse is able to develop clusters. Which cluster has the poorest relationship?
   1. Cough, chest pain, green sputum
   2. Weight loss, poor appetite, "my father passed away 2 weeks ago"
   3. Diarrhea, swelling of the ankles, exercises three times per week
   4. Frequent urination, nocturia, drinks five cups of coffee per day

9. The nurse has just completed a comprehensive health assessment on a 76-year-old female who recently lost her husband of 48 years to stomach cancer 3 months ago. She currently lives alone in the single-family colonial style home she shared with her husband throughout their marriage. She admits to skipping meals and states, "what's the point of cooking a full meal if I am the only one who will eat it?" She has lost 16 pounds from her already petite 110-pound frame (height 4′11″). She attends church service every Sunday and has recently started to attend a widows' support group on Thursday evenings. Which behaviors should the nurse interpret as abnormal?
   1. Skipping meals and the widows' support group
   2. Weight loss and living alone
   3. Skipping meals and weight loss
   4. Church services and widows' support group

10. A male client arrives at a preadmission testing center for laboratory work and a chest x-ray 5 days prior to his scheduled back surgery (lumbar laminectomy). He tells the nurse that he is very anxious about his upcoming surgery. The nurse's next step would be to:
   1. take the client on a tour of the perioperative area.
   2. ask the client if he has ever had surgery before.
   3. instruct the client to obtain a prescription for antianxiety medication.
   4. tell the client that he has a great surgeon and has nothing to worry about.

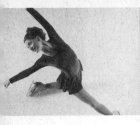

2   Wellness and Health Promotion

It is not the mountain we conquer but ourselves.
—Edmund Hillary

Wellness and health promotion are important areas of focus for today's nurse. Promoting the best possible health is not only cost effective but will increase the quality years of life for our clients and communities. This chapter will assist the student in using theories, models, and frameworks in order to promote the health of clients, families, and communities.

OBJECTIVES

At the completion of these exercises you will be able to:

1. Define key terminology regarding wellness and health promotion.
2. Apply wellness theory and health promotion models to client scenarios.
3. Relate *Healthy People 2020* topic areas to various roles of the nurse.
4. Identify immunizations that are appropriate for clients across the life span.
5. Apply critical thinking in analysis of a case study related to wellness and health promotion.
6. Complete NCLEX®-style review questions related to wellness and health promotion.

RESOURCES

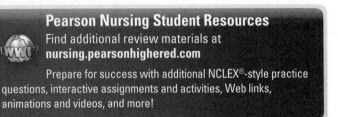

Pearson Nursing Student Resources
Find additional review materials at
nursing.pearsonhighered.com

Prepare for success with additional NCLEX®-style practice questions, interactive assignments and activities, Web links, animations and videos, and more!

Additional resources: *www.healthypeople.gov*

WORD SEARCH

Find and circle the correct term in the word search puzzle for each of the definitions listed below. The word may be horizontal, vertical, or diagonal.

```
N K H F P C T S K K A A A G E D B Y R U I O I K U U N
U Y Y L X J S Y Y E N F T S Q F I L O N H W O S V O Y
S D T L T E B T N L D P I O G F W P U B H E R R O G P
T F J P N T O J K Z W C B I O I G H F J L O K S D N P
C N Q L Z L C Z A Q R G F Y E V H B N T T W F Z O Q N
N K L J J Z I S I E Y O J V V Y T O I A O X L I I L P
F E G B K J E Q X E Z X Z H Y Y I M C O I F T E P A F
W R S J U F Y E Y R U D W K B T T I N K L N S V Y J D
A L G S P M C R D H M D I J N B D X T B E O J A E R X
A M U N R I H M A T R X K E N N N N F V Q K G N Y O M
G N O A B Z B A B X E G V B I O E Q E L Q V O Y D E Q
Z K S O G B P U U T S E Y H B M U R Z W O I K B Z M J
T N R C T Q N D J J R R T N N I P D F C T N D P J Z H
H E J V Z F A N U P R L V O S Y B R I N Q Q T D C F E
A R F I P L B H Y V A H R Q R S V B E J N M E I F A A
V U O B P N I R E E K I V A R A J V P Z J H V W C T L
S F X S W G A Q H A V O M D R Y E Y M F H G Q P A K T
T T L S I D N G B N L I G H A R E N D V W T V T M P H
C U A Q N T N V E C R T L R P A U N L T H V Q S L T P
K N F O G I V L H P D V H Y D D N Y U N P G A L G D R
G Q C T D B A T A Y G E R Y I E Y V A G L A Z Z Y R O
G E T A W C J A C M S A Z C P G T B Y H C I L K B I M
S C E Q I K D J W W I F P F B E K Q L K R J S P J Y O
D L Q S R D S S B T K S X A K F O F O S W M A X Y O T
L J Y U Y C N Y R O M H L F Q Z W P N B A K S Y Q U I
N H X Q A A E E V O F U Q U N F Z V L S H S G V W Z O
P P C S Y L T Y X R C T X J K L F X P E R G T G C G N
```

CLUES

Read the phrases below and identify the term described.

1. A state of life that is balanced, personally satisfying, and characterized by the ability to adapt and to participate in activities that enhance quality of life _____

2. Genetic background, gender, race and ethnicity, family history, and problems occurring throughout life

   _____

3. Interventions that occur to promote health and well-being before a problem occurs **(two words)** _____

   _____

4. Activity in which oxygen is metabolized to produce energy **(two words)** _____ _____

5. Consists of all the things that are experienced through the individual's senses and some harmful elements such as radiation, ozone, and radon **(two words)** _____ _____

6. Behavior motivated by the desire to increase well-being and actualize human potential **(two words)** _____

   _____

7. A report and program sponsored by the United States Department of Health and Human Services, focusing on health promotion of individuals, families, and communities **(two words)** _____ _____

8. Factors that impact individual and community health and wellness **(three words)** _____ _____ _____

9. Focus on early diagnosis of health problems and prompt treatment with the restoration of health **(two words)** _____ _____

10. Activity aimed at restoring the individual to the highest possible level of health and functioning **(two words)** _____ _____

WELLNESS THEORY

1. Identify the theory represented in the grid provided below _____

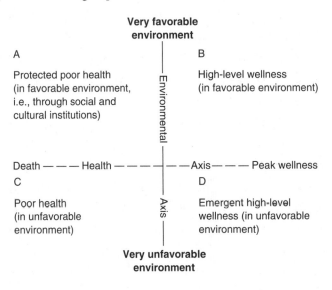

2. Read each scenario. Apply the above theory to each of the following situations. In the space provided, write the letter (A, B, C, or D) that represents the level of wellness each client is experiencing.

_____ 1. Victoria is a 45-year-old account executive for a large advertising agency. She has excellent health benefits that include well visit checkups for general health, vision, and dental health. She runs 3 miles every day after work at her company's fitness center.

_____ 2. Gerald is a 9-year-old asthmatic who lives in a homeless shelter with his father. He uses his maintenance inhaler every other day to "make the medicine last" as his father told him to do. He often is seen in the emergency department for upper respiratory infections and has been hospitalized with pneumonia twice in the past the 2 years.

_____ 3. Kavita is a 22-year-old mother of twin girls (age 15 months). Her husband is currently unemployed and is searching for work. They live in a subsidized housing development in an old urban neighborhood. Kavita walks her daughters in their stroller every day for over an hour. She is using government assistance to make sure she can prepare healthy meals for herself and her family.

_____ 4. Floyd is a 55-year-old retired semiprofessional baseball player. He lives in an upscale private beach community on the West Coast. He has had a personal trainer for the past 20 years that has kept him physically fit. Recently, Floyd was diagnosed with pancreatic cancer that has metastasized to the bone and brain. He is scheduled to have a feeding tube inserted into his stomach in 2 days.

_____ 5. Simon is an 81-year-old man who has just auditioned for a reality television show. He lives in an active adult retirement community where he swims daily and likes to participate in various clubs. He has been singing and dancing in his town's holiday pageant every year for the past 10 years.

_____ 6. Claudia is a 14-year-old girl who has just found out that she is pregnant. She lives in a small two-bedroom apartment with her mother and three other sisters. She smokes marijuana "once in a while" and enjoys drinking alcoholic beverages on the weekends. She is not sure what her plan will be in regard to her pregnancy. She indicates the first step is probably to determine who the father might be.

LEVELS OF PREVENTION

1. Identify the level of prevention (primary, secondary, or tertiary) described in each of the following actions below by circling your answer.

   1. Having an annual mammogram

      Primary **Secondary** **Tertiary**

   2. Getting a flu shot every Fall

      Primary **Secondary** **Tertiary**

   3. Running 3 miles per day to stay fit

      Primary **Secondary** **Tertiary**

   4. Going for physical therapy after knee surgery

      Primary **Secondary** **Tertiary**

   5. Taking antibiotics for a sinus infection

      Primary **Secondary** **Tertiary**

   6. Wearing a seat belt

      Primary **Secondary** **Tertiary**

   7. Following a diabetic diet

      Primary **Secondary** **Tertiary**

   8. Using a maintenance inhaler for asthma

      Primary **Secondary** **Tertiary**

   9. Applying sunscreen

      Primary **Secondary** **Tertiary**

   10. Handwashing

      Primary **Secondary** **Tertiary**

   11. Having a colonoscopy

      Primary **Secondary** **Tertiary**

   12. Attending a support group meeting for alcoholics

      Primary **Secondary** **Tertiary**

2. Identify an example of a health-related activity or action that you or a family member has undertaken in the past year, and place it under the appropriate level of prevention.

   1. Primary

   2. Secondary

   3. Tertiary

THE ILLNESS/WELLNESS CONTINUUM

Using the figure below, answer the following questions in the space provided.

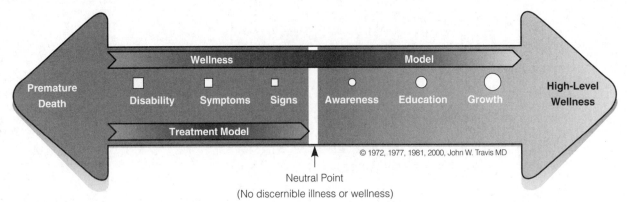

Neutral Point
(No discernible illness or wellness)

Source: The Illness/Wellness continuum. From: Travis, J., and Ryan, R. *Wellness Workbook.* Berkley, CA. Tan Speed Press. Retrieved from Wellness Associates Website at www.thewellspring.com. Reprinted with permission.

1. Draw an X on the continuum to determine your personal level of wellness.

   Provide a rationale for your position.

2. List three measures that you could take to move closer to a higher level of wellness on the continuum.

   1.

   2.

   3.

HEALTH PROMOTION

Read the following scenario and answer the following questions.

Richard is a 28-year-old African American who suffers from hypertension. He is obese (weight 349 lb and height 5'11"). His mother is an obese type 2 diabetic female. His father died 5 years ago at the age of 52 from complications of diabetes. As a child, Richard did not participate in sports or outdoor activities; rather, he enjoyed his computer and video games. Richard works 10-hour days as an Information Technology Consultant for a software company. His job is very sedentary, and he enjoys going outside for frequent smoke breaks. He has smoked 1.5 packs of cigarettes per day since he was 19. He lives alone and often grabs quick meals at his company's coffee shop or orders "take out meals." Whenever anyone suggests that Richard lose some weight he replies, "I was born a big boy and I will die a big boy. It's in my genes." Richard did lose 25 lb once when a group of colleagues in his department ran a weight loss contest. With the support of his peers, he found the willpower. Soon after the contest, he regained all of the weight. His company has a fitness center that he does not use. Richard states he is too embarrassed to exercise in the center because his colleagues have made remarks like "Do you think those machines can handle you?" and "Are you trying to fit into your skinny jeans?" Richard also states that it is really hard to lose weight, and he is not really sure how much better his life would be if he did. His mother pushes him to lose weight so he doesn't die young like his father, but this just leads Richard to avoid her.

1. Write your own definition of health promotion.

2. What risk factors for heart disease does Richard have?

3. Which factors can be controlled and which factors cannot? Explain.

4. Use Pender's Health Promotion Model to analyze the information provided in the above scenario. Develop health promoting behaviors for Richard. Refer to the textbook for model application assistance.

Individual Characteristics and Experiences	Behavior-Specific Cognitions and Affect	Behavioral Outcome

HEALTHY PEOPLE 2020

Nurses represent the largest group of healthcare professionals. It is the responsibility of the nurse to promote health and wellness to all clients. Becoming familiar with *Healthy People 2020* (HP2020) is an excellent way to comprehend the health issues of the United States and what can be done to make improvements.

Answer each of the following questions in the space provided.

1. What do you think are the three most important health issues facing the United States today?

    1.

    2.

    3.

2. Log on to the HP2020 website (*www.healthypeople.gov*) and review topics and objectives. Identify an objective that relates to each of the health issues you have listed in Question 1 and write it in the space provided below.

    1.

    2.

    3.

3. Explain the importance of each health issue.

   1.

   2.

   3.

4. Search the Internet, newspapers, or magazines for programs, educational offerings, government-sponsored funding, and so on that support one of your objectives.

   Source:

   Offering:

   Rationale of how it supports the objective:

5. HP2020 does not focus on one specific age group. It promotes health and wellness across the age span. Identify an HP2020 topic and an objective that supports each age group provided.

   1. Infants

   2. Toddlers

   3. Preschoolers

   4. School-aged children

   5. Adolescents

   6. Young adults

   7. Middle-aged adults

   8. Older adults

6. Select an HP2020 objective from one of the age groups above. For each of the nursing roles listed, provide an example of how the nurse can intervene to assist in attainment of the objective.

   Selected Objective _____

   1. Caregiver

   2. Counselor

3. Nurse educator

4. Nurse researcher

5. Nurse administrator

IMMUNIZATIONS

Circle the immunization that the nurse may prepare for each client who enters the clinic. Draw an X over any immunization that would absolutely NOT be considered for this client.

1. 4-month-old female (no medical history)

   Hep A   Hib   MCV

2. 15-month-old male (history of gastroesophageal reflux)

   PCV   DTaP   Zoster

3. 4-year-old male (no medical history)

   Hep B   RV   MMR

4. 8-year-old female (history of fractured humerus)

   DTaP   Influenza   HPV

5. 15-year-old female (history of chicken pox—age 4)

   IPV   Hep B booster   HPV

6. 22-year-old female (4 months pregnant)

   Influenza   Varicella   Zoster

7. 42-year-old male (history of asthma)

   HPV   RV   Pneumococcal

8. 60-year-old female (history of HIV)

   Influenza   IPV   MMR

APPLICATION OF THE CRITICAL THINKING PROCESS

Read the following scenario and answer the questions.

Congratulations, the SmithVille Township Board of Education has just offered you a position as a school nurse in their high school (grades 9–12). SmithVille Township is a rural area. There are 350 students enrolled in your school for the new academic year.

1. List two primary prevention strategies appropriate for this age group.

   1.
   2.

2. List two secondary prevention strategies appropriate for this age group.

   1.
   2.

In order to explore the needs of the student body, you decide to have students fill out questionnaires during the first week of school. After analyzing the data, you note the following:

- 35% of the students are sexually active
- 20% of the students who are sexually active report not using a method of birth control
- 58% of the students report experimentation with recreational drugs or alcohol
- 18% of the students report smoking more than 1 cigarette per day
- 82% of the students receive fewer than the recommended hours of sleep per night
- 38% of the students report experiencing anxiety or depression in the past 12 months
- 5% of the students report having thought about suicide in the past 12 months

3. Identify an HP2020 topic and objective for two of the questionnaire findings above.

   1. Finding-

      Topic-

      Objective-

   2. Finding-

      Topic-

      Objective-

4. Discuss your role as the school nurse. Identify interventions you could implement to promote the health of your students in relation to your selected objectives.

   1.

   2.

5. What other disciplines or organizations would you collaborate with in order to promote the health of these students? Explain.

6. Discuss any barriers you may face (social, financial, administrative, parental, developmental, etc.).

NCLEX®-STYLE REVIEW QUESTIONS

Read each question carefully. Choose the best answer for each question.

1. The nurse defines early identification of illness or disease as:
   1. primary prevention.
   2. secondary prevention.
   3. tertiary prevention.
   4. health promotion.

2. The nurse understands tertiary prevention is related to:
   1. prepathology.
   2. pathology.
   3. rehabilitation.
   4. screenings.

3. A young adult new mother, states "I just don't think I will be able to breastfeed. It is very complicated and I don't know that I can do it." The nurse interprets this statement as:
   1. low self-efficacy.
   2. high self-efficacy.
   3. situational influences.
   4. interpersonal influences.

4. An adult client decides to lose 25 lb She states "I joined a gym and signed up at a weight loss center." The nurse can interpret this as:
   1. a commitment without a strategy.
   2. a commitment with a strategy.
   3. competing demands.
   4. behavior-specific cognition.

5. A middle-aged adult client smokes two packs of cigarettes per day. When the nurse mentions the health benefits of quitting, the client responds "My mother never smoked a cigarette in her life and died of lung cancer at the age of 48, so what difference does it make?" The nurse interprets this as:
   1. the client is influenced by mother's decision not to smoke.
   2. the health promotion behavior should focus on the client's coping with the loss of a parent.
   3. the client is experiencing competing demands.
   4. the client is unable to perceive a benefit to a health promoting action.

6. The nurse understands that *Healthy People 2020* is a report by:
   1. the office of Medicare and Medicaid.
   2. the Centers for Disease Control and Prevention.
   3. the United States Department of Health and Human Services.
   4. the Joint Commission.

7. The nurse is explaining different types of exercise to a group of middle-aged adults. The nurse uses the term _____ to describe exercise that includes short periods of high intensity activity.
   1. Aerobic
   2. Anaerobic
   3. Metabolic equivalent
   4. Isometric

8. What topic would the nurse be assessing if using the CAGE questionnaire?
   1. Mental health
   2. Substance abuse
   3. Sexual behavior
   4. Injury and violence

9. A young teenager goes to bed at 11:30 p.m. and awakens at 6:30 a.m. for school. The nurse determines that this amount of sleep is:
   1. adequate for his age.
   2. inadequate for his age.
   3. adequate if a 30-minute nap is included.
   4. adequate if a 60-minute nap is included.

10. A new mother brings her recently adopted 3-week-old infant to the healthcare provider's office for a well visit. The nurse anticipates that the baby has received which of the following immunizations at birth?
    1. Hib and Hep A
    2. Hep A only
    3. Hep B only
    4. RV and Hep B

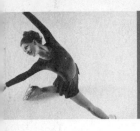

3 Health Assessment Across the Life Span

. . . focus on the journey, not the destination. Joy is found not in finishing an activity but in doing it.

—Greg Anderson

This chapter addresses ways in which a variety of factors related to growth and development influence an individual's health. It provides a foundation for assessment and planning nursing intervention appropriate for the age and developmental level of the client.

OBJECTIVES

At the completion of these exercises you will be able to:

1. Define key terminology regarding growth and development.
2. Categorize developmental tasks for various stages of development.
3. Differentiate among the stages of psychosocial theory.
4. Interpret health assessment findings according to growth and development principles.
5. Apply the critical thinking process to case studies.
6. Complete NCLEX®-style review questions related to health assessment across the life span.

RESOURCES

Pearson Nursing Student Resources

Find additional review materials at
nursing.pearsonhighered.com

Prepare for success with additional NCLEX®-style practice questions, interactive assignments and activities, Web links, animations and videos, and more!

CROSSWORD PUZZLE FOR KEY TERMS

Read each definition below and fill in the correct term on the puzzle grid. If the answer requires two words, do not leave a blank space between the words. Use a pencil so you can erase easily.

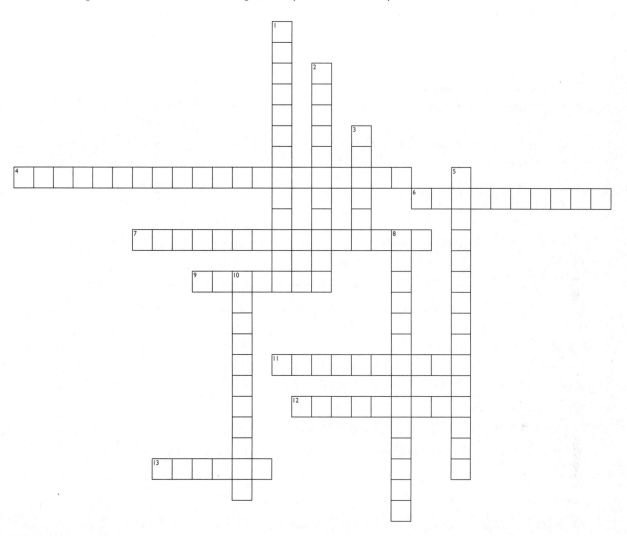

CLUES

Across

4. Defines the structure of personality as consisting of three parts: the id, the ego, and the superego **(two words)**
6. The period between 11 and 21 years of age
7. The period of a person's life when 40 to 65 years of age **(two words)**
9. Child who is at least 1 year old but who has not yet reached 3 years old
11. The period of a person's life between 20 and 40 years of age **(two words)**
12. A child between 6 and 10 years old **(two words)**
13. A child from 1 month of age through 11 months of age

Down

1. Head to toe, direction
2. A child between 3 and 5 years of age
3. Measurable physical change and increase in size
5. How people learn to think, reason, and use language **(two words)**
8. The period of a person's life when over 65 years of age **(two words)**
10. An orderly, progressive increase in the complexity of the total person

STAGES OF DEVELOPMENT

Read each developmental task and place the letter representing the appropriate stage of development on each line.

I = Infancy   **P** = Preschool-Age   **A** = Adolescents   **M** = Middle-Age

T = Toddler   **S** = School-Age   **Y** = Young Adults   **O** = Older Adults

_____ **1.** Controls body functions

_____ **2.** Conducting a life review

_____ **3.** Coping with children leaving home

_____ **4.** Developing a meaningful philosophy of life

_____ **5.** Developing hobbies and leisure activities

_____ **6.** Preparing for death

_____ **7.** Mastering physical skills

_____ **8.** Developing a conscience

_____ **9.** Differentiating self from others

_____ **10.** Interacting with the environment

_____ **11.** Forming close relationships with primary caregivers

_____ **12.** Developing logical reasoning

_____ **13.** Identifying sex role

_____ **14.** Searching for identity

_____ **15.** Tolerates separation from primary caregivers

_____ **16.** Learns to use language for social interaction

_____ **17.** Fitting into a peer group

_____ **18.** Forming a value system

_____ **19.** Beginning a parenting role

_____ **20.** Adjusting to aging parents

PSYCHOSOCIAL THEORY

Read each scenario. Write the crisis each person is facing in the space provided. Circle whether or not the nurse would need to intervene. Provide a rationale for your decision.

Crisis Bank

Trust vs. Mistrust   Autonomy vs. Shame and Doubt

Initiative vs. Guilt   Industry vs. Inferiority

Identity vs. Role Confusion   Intimacy vs. Isolation

Generativity vs. Stagnation   Integrity vs. Despair

1. A 5-month-old girl cries when a neighbor holds her, yet coos when returned to her mother's arms.

   Crisis: _____

   Intervention required: Yes or No

   Rationale: _____

2. An 85-year-old man lost his wife of 65 years to cancer 3 months ago. Since her death, he has not attended his Elk's Club meetings and has lost interest in chatting in the evening with his neighbors.

   Crisis: _____

   Intervention required: Yes or No

   Rationale: _____

3. A 35-year-old female is celebrating her tenth wedding anniversary. She is planning a surprise romantic weekend for her husband.

   Crisis: _____

   Intervention required: Yes or No

   Rationale: _____

4. A 55-year-old female has sent her last child off to college. With the free time she will now have, she has decided to start an environmentalist group in her community to encourage people to "Go Green."

   Crisis: _____

   Intervention required: Yes or No

   Rationale: _____

5. A 4-year-old boy wants to help his father paint the garage. He puts on his overalls, grabs a paintbrush, and exclaims "I'm just like Daddy."

   Crisis: _____

   Intervention required: Yes or No

   Rationale: _____

6. An 18-month-old girl wants to feed and dress herself.

   Crisis: _____

   Intervention required: Yes or No

   Rationale: _____

7. A 17-year-old has decided to apply to college after high school graduation and pursue a career in trauma nursing.

   Crisis: _____

   Intervention required: Yes or No

   Rationale: _____

8. An 8-year-old boy wants to quit the soccer team after attending only four practices. He states "I'll never be any good at sports."

   Crisis: _____

   Intervention required: Yes or No

   Rationale: _____

ASSESSMENT FINDINGS

Items 1 through 10 include health assessment data collected for various age groups. Identify each as normal or abnormal by circling the correct response.

1. Weight at birth is 7.2 lb on July 26, weighs 6.8 lb on July 28
   Normal   or   **Abnormal**

2. A 56-year-old is sad because her only child is getting married
   Normal   or   **Abnormal**

3. Height at birth is 21 inches, one year later height is 27 inches
   Normal   or   **Abnormal**

4. At 9 months is unable to sit briefly without support
   Normal   or   **Abnormal**

5. A 10-month-old imitates sounds
   Normal   or   **Abnormal**

6. A 2½-year-old wants to touch everything in the examination room
   Normal   or   **Abnormal**

7. A 4-year-old loves to play dress up

   Normal   **or**   **Abnormal**

8. A 75-year-old writes his living will

   Normal   **or**   **Abnormal**

9. An 8-year-old begins to have voice changes

   Normal   **or**   **Abnormal**

10. A 15-year-old prefers to spend his weekends with his grandparents instead of his peers

    Normal   **or**   **Abnormal**

APPLICATION OF THE CRITICAL THINKING PROCESS

Read the following scenario and answer the questions as you go along.

Janie Perkins is a 68-year-old female who arrives at your clinic for an annual physical. She retired 2 weeks ago from her postal job after 40 years of service. She states, "I want to make sure I enjoy a long and healthy retirement with my husband."

1. According to Erikson's Psychosocial Theory, Janie is facing which maturational crisis?

2. Write three questions you would ask Janie to assess how she is dealing with the developmental tasks she is facing.

   1.

   2.

   3.

> *Did you ask questions related to Janie's plans for her retirement? What will she be doing with her free time? How does she feel about entering this stage of her life?*

After further questioning, Janie tells you she has signed up as a volunteer for the Women's Auxiliary at the local hospital. She has also joined a health club with an interest in starting yoga or Pilates.

3. Which developmental task does this information relate to?

4. Is this a positive or negative response?

> *Janie is developing post-retirement activities that will help her maintain her self-worth and usefulness. This is a positive response for her developmental tasks.*

In the health history, you learn that Janie is lactose intolerant and hasn't had her cholesterol checked in 10 years.

5. Why is this information important for Janie at this stage of her life?

Women over the age of 65 have a decrease in skeletal mass. The decreased density in the bones can lead to brittle bones that may fracture easily. People with lactose intolerance may not be taking in an adequate amount of calcium, which is needed during this time. Heart disease is the leading cause of death among women of this age group. A cholesterol screening is an important part of the care of this client. The nurse should consider a complete nutritional assessment.

Continuing the health history, you learn that Janie's 88-year-old father lives with her and her husband. Through the years he has been becoming less and less independent and is requiring more supervision. Janie shares this responsibility with her sister, who lives 5 miles away. She is becoming a bit concerned about this situation because her sister is having a total hip replacement in 3 weeks and will require months of rehabilitation.

6. List two questions you would ask Janie to further assess this situation.

   1.

   2.

7. Imagine that Janie lives in your town. Search websites for resources in your community (local hospital, local health department, etc.) and find two resources that would help Janie with this situation.

   1. Name the website.

   2. Describe the resource or program.

   3. Is there a cost or fee that is required?

NCLEX®-STYLE REVIEW QUESTIONS

Read each question carefully. Choose the best answer for each question.

1. When conducting a physical assessment on a 72-year-old client, the nurse must consider which changes in physiological development?
   1. Increased vital capacity
   2. Increased filling and emptying ability of the heart valves
   3. Increase in peripheral vascular resistance
   4. Increased filtering abilities of the kidneys

2. Which teaching topic would be most appropriate for a nurse to plan for an adolescent?
   1. Seat belt safety
   2. Prostate screening
   3. Importance of influenza vaccinations
   4. Adjusting to aging parents

3. The nurse understands that myelinization in the spinal cord is almost complete by _____ years of age.
   1. 1
   2. 2
   3. 3
   4. 4

4. The nurse is aware that children of low socioeconomic status:
   1. have been found to have higher heights and weights than those in other economic groups.
   2. are more likely to include fresh fruits, vegetables, and lean meats in their diet.
   3. may have an impaired ability to meet their nutritional needs.
   4. are less likely to be exposed to environmental elements that influence physical health and well-being.

5. The nurse is aware that an appropriate age to give a child a tricycle for his birthday would be:
   1. 15 months.
   2. 1 year.
   3. 3 years.
   4. 5 years.

6. Which sentence would be age appropriate for the language development of a 3-year-old?
   1. "Mama, Mama"
   2. "Juice please"
   3. "Can I color now?"
   4. "Will we be going to the movies today?"

7. A new mother refuses to offer a pacifier to her newborn baby. The nurse is aware that according to Freud's Stages of Psychosexual Development, this affects the:
   1. phallic phase.
   2. latency phase.
   3. oral phase.
   4. anal phase.

8. A fifth-grade male student visits the school nurse's office of a large urban elementary school each day complaining of various ailments. The nurse speaks with the student's teacher and learns that his grades have been poor and he doesn't interact with the other children in his class. The nurse's next action should be:
   1. sit down and speak with the student to obtain more information about his home situation.
   2. refer the student to the school counselor.
   3. call the student's parents to discuss his school performance.
   4. instruct the student to discuss with his parents the possibility of starting antidepressants.

9. A 3-year-old child enters the clinic with her mother for her annual physical examination. When attempting to assess her blood pressure, the nurse should state:
   1. "Let me take your blood pressure."
   2. "I'm going to assess your blood pressure."
   3. "I will be putting this cuff on your arm, and it will start to give your arm a small squeeze."
   4. Try to distract the child and then quickly put the cuff on without saying anything.

10. Which clients require further assessment by the nurse? (Select all that apply)
    1. a 43-year-old male who lives in the same home he grew up in as a child with his elderly parents and can't keep a job
    2. a 15-year-old female who is unsure of how many sexual partners she has had
    3. a 48-year-old female who has undergone more than 20 cosmetic procedures in the past 5 years and has scheduled a liposuction and abdominoplasty next month
    4. a 30-year-old female who is unable to maintain an intimate relationship with anyone for longer than 1 month
    5. a 45-year-old female who leaves the business world and goes back to college to pursue a career in education

Cultural Considerations 4

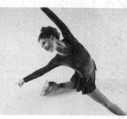

*What we need to do is learn to respect and embrace our differences
until our differences don't make a difference in how we are treated.*
—Yolanda King

The United States is historically known as the "Melting Pot," a multicultural mix of people living together as one society. Nurses are the largest group of healthcare professionals in the United States and have the most direct and continuous contact with clients of all ethnic and cultural backgrounds.

Nurses must include attention to the values, beliefs, and customs of clients from diverse cultures in order to plan, provide, and evaluate individualized care. This chapter will review the basic phenomena related to cultural care. It will also help you to develop and utilize a cultural assessment tool.

OBJECTIVES

At the completion of these exercises you will be able to:

1. Define key terminology regarding culture.
2. Identify beliefs and values associated with various cultures.
3. Explain the ways in which culture can impact nursing care.
4. Develop a cultural assessment tool.
5. Perform a cultural assessment.
6. Complete NCLEX®-style review questions related to the cultural assessment.

RESOURCES

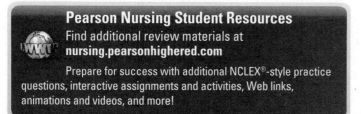

Pearson Nursing Student Resources

Find additional review materials at
nursing.pearsonhighered.com

Prepare for success with additional NCLEX®-style practice questions, interactive assignments and activities, Web links, animations and videos, and more!

Additional resources: *www.jointcommission.org*

CROSSWORD PUZZLE FOR KEY TERMS

Read each definition below and fill in the correct term on the puzzle grid. If the answer requires two words do not leave a blank space between the words. Use a pencil so you can erase easily.

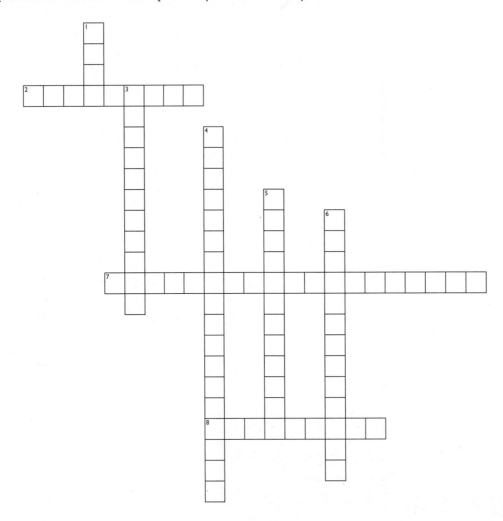

CLUES

Across

2. The state of being different
7. Spoken language to share information and ideas **(two words)**
8. The awareness of belonging to a group in which certain characteristics or aspects such as culture and biology differentiate the members of one group from another

Down

1. The identification of an individual or group by shared genetic heritage and biological or physical characteristics
3. Groups that exist within larger culture
4. The capacity of nurses or health service delivery systems to effectively understand and plan for the needs of a culturally diverse client or group **(two words)**
5. The adoption and incorporation of characteristics, customs, and values of the dominant culture by those new to that culture
6. The tendency to believe one's way of life, values, beliefs, and customs are superior to those of others

BELIEFS AND VALUES

Read each statement. Recall the descriptions of cultural characteristics in the literature. Determine if the statement agrees (A) or disagrees (D) with the textbook. If it does not, rewrite the statement to reflect the textbook.

1. Mexican Americans do not believe in fatalism.

   A   D   _____

2. Cuban Americans speak very slowly and softly.

   A   D   _____

3. Rice and vegetables are main ingredients in the Filipino diet.

   A   D   _____

4. Native Americans are future oriented.

   A   D   _____

5. Mexican Americans find it impolite to not make direct eye contact when speaking to someone.

   A   D   _____

6. Filipino Americans have a great deal of respect for their elderly.

   A   D   _____

7. Medicine men are no longer used to provide care to Native Americans.

   A   D   _____

8. Chinese Americans may say they understand a concept when they do not in order to avoid "loss of face."

   A   D   _____

9. European Americans are past oriented.

   A   D   _____

10. Cuban Americans use family as their primary source of healthcare advice.

   A   D   _____

APPLICATION OF THE CRITICAL THINKING PROCESS

Read each client scenario and answer the following questions in the space provided.

Nana Gaya is a 67-year-old African male from Kenya, Africa, who moved to the United States 15 years ago after his daughter married an American soldier from North Carolina. He is fluent in Swahili and is able to speak English very well.

1. List five questions you would ask Mr. Gaya during a cultural assessment.

   1.

   2.

   3.

   4.

   5.

Bernice Grosenstein is an 82-year-old Jewish female who has lived in Brooklyn, New York, her entire life. She claims to be "very strict" with her religion and follows a kosher diet.

1. List two ways Ms. Grosenstein's culture will affect the care that you will provide her.

   1.

   2.

2. Place a check mark next to each menu item that would be appropriate for Ms. Grosenstein to eat.

   _____ 1. Buttered bagel

   _____ 2. Ham & cheese omelet

   _____ 3. Pepperoni pizza

   _____ 4. Pasta with tomato sauce

   _____ 5. Roast beef & cheddar cheese wrap

Rachelle is an RN taking care of a 37-year-old female who has large uterine fibroids. The client had heavy vaginal bleeding for over a week before she sought medical attention. Lab values reveal a hemoglobin (Hgb) of 6.2 g/dl and a hematocrit (Hct) of 19.8%. The doctor ordered 2 units of packed red blood cells (PRBC) to be transfused. The client states she is a Jehovah Witness and refuses the blood transfusions. Rachelle remarks in the hallway, "Well, if she bleeds to death it's her own fault! If I was her I would just take the blood and save everyone the trouble."

Use the spaces provided to write your response to the following:

1. Rachelle's comment can be labeled as:

2. When a client's cultural beliefs and values differ from one's own personal beliefs and values, it is important for the nurse to:

DEVELOPMENT OF THE CULTURAL ASSESSMENT TOOL

Define each component of a cultural assessment and review the sample question for each. (Find questions in Table 4.2, page 74 of the textbook.) Use the space provided to write two questions that pertain to each component. Once completed, answer your questions to help you to assess your own cultural beliefs and values.

Ethnicity

Define _____

   1.

   2.

Communication

Define _____

   1.

   2.

Space

Define _____

   1.

   2.

Social Organization

Define _____

   1.

   2.

Time

Define _____

   1.

   2.

Environment Control

Define _____

   1.

   2.

Biological Variations

Define _____

   1.

   2.

PERFORMING THE CULTURAL ASSESSMENT

On a separate sheet of paper, use the cultural assessment tool you developed in the preceding section to assess the cultural beliefs and values of a classmate from a cultural background that is different from your own. Then answer the following questions.

Use the space provided to answer the following:

1. Describe the nonverbal communication observed during the assessment.

2. How would the use of nonverbal communication by you or your classmate reflect ethnic, cultural, or other factors that may influence the collection of data, analysis of the data, or client care?

3. Compare and contrast your cultural values and beliefs with that of the classmate you interviewed.

NCLEX®-STYLE REVIEW QUESTIONS

Read each question carefully. Choose the best answer for each question.

1. A nurse can become culturally competent by:
    1. acquiring knowledge and experience.
    2. taking a course on cultural diversity.
    3. researching his or her own culture.
    4. disregarding a client's culture and treating all clients the same.

2. The nurse is aware that material culture refers to:
    1. nonverbal language.
    2. art and clothing.
    3. social structure.
    4. customs.

3. According to the World Health Organization (WHO), childhood obesity in the United States has:
    1. decreased since 1980.
    2. remained the same since 1980.
    3. doubled since 1980.
    4. tripled since 1980.

4. The nurse is aware that black Americans who are overweight are more likely to report that:
    1. they are overweight.
    2. they are an average weight.
    3. they are underweight.
    4. being overweight is very unattractive.

5. A 68-year-old female who speaks only Italian was hospitalized 2 days ago with abdominal pain. She is scheduled to go to the operating room (OR) for a small bowel resection. The surgeon is attempting to have the client sign a consent for surgery. He does not speak Italian. The nurse knows in this situation that the client:
    1. has an excellent surgeon and will be just fine.
    2. can sign the consent now and ask questions later when her family comes in.
    3. has the right to a translator to provide her information regarding her care.
    4. is willing to sign the consent; it is her own fault if she does not understand what she is signing.

6. A 31-year-old, Spanish-speaking female is visiting America from Spain. She twisted her ankle while running on the beach and is being treated in the emergency department. Her injury is a minor sprain and she is ready to be discharged home. When the nurse provides the client with her discharge instructions, it is important to:
    1. have the client's 6-year-old daughter translate the instructions because she is able to speak English.
    2. use another, English-speaking client who is waiting to be seen to translate.
    3. provide her with discharge instructions written in Spanish so there is no need to translate anything.
    4. use a bilingual staff member who has been trained in interpretation for clinical purposes.

7. Which of the following statements is true about cultural competence education?
    1. Cultural competency is incorporated into the curriculum in nursing education; therefore, it is unnecessary for healthcare agencies to train employees.
    2. The U.S. Department of Health & Human Resources has developed a mandatory course that all nurses must complete in order to renew their nursing licenses.
    3. All healthcare delivery agencies must develop structures and procedures to address cross-cultural ethical and legal conflicts in healthcare delivery.
    4. Only healthcare delivery agencies that serve communities with a large culturally diverse population are required to provide employee training on cultural competence.

8. A 21-year-old Muslim girl, whose family has moved to the United States, has enrolled at a community college near her home. She has received permission from her family not to wear her burqa (face veil) to her classes or when she goes out with friends. This can be viewed as:
    1. cultural diversity.
    2. ethnocentrism.
    3. assimilation.
    4. ethnic adoption.

9. A 45-year-old Vietnamese woman is escorted to the emergency department by her husband when she experiences vaginal bleeding 9 weeks into her pregnancy. There are two emergency healthcare providers available, a male and a female. The male healthcare provider enters the room, and the client's husband kindly requests that his wife be examined by the female healthcare provider. The nurse understands that this request is most likely due to:
   1. a very jealous husband.
   2. a bad experience with the male healthcare provider in the past.
   3. clients of the Vietnamese culture having a preference for healthcare providers of the same sex.
   4. None of the above.

10. A 67-year-old Filipino American is learning to care for his Foley catheter and leg bag at home. While the nurse is explaining how to change the drainage bag, she notices the client continues to nod his head. The nurse can interpret this as:
   1. reassurance that he understands what is being taught.
   2. he hears what she is saying, but may not understand.
   3. a sign that he probably has done this before.
   4. an abnormal response of the central nervous system.

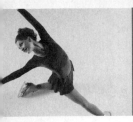

5   Psychosocial Assessment

It is confidence in our bodies, mind and spirits that allow us to keep looking for new adventure, new directions to grow in, and new lessons to learn—which is what life is all about.

—Oprah Winfrey

The psychosocial assessment provides the nurse with the information needed to develop an individualized plan of care. It encompasses mental, emotional, social, and spiritual health, which can affect the client's physical well-being.

This chapter will allow you to explore factors that can influence psychosocial health and tools that can be used to conduct the assessment.

OBJECTIVES

At the completion of these exercises you will be able to:

1. Define key terminology regarding the psychosocial assessment.
2. Differentiate between internal and external factors that influence psychosocial health.
3. Utilize various psychosocial assessment tools.
4. Interpret psychosocial assessment findings.
5. Develop questions for a psychosocial assessment tool.
6. Complete NCLEX®-style review questions related to the psychosocial assessment.

RESOURCES

Pearson Nursing Student Resources
Find additional review materials at
nursing.pearsonhighered.com

Prepare for success with additional NCLEX®-style practice questions, interactive assignments and activities, Web links, animations and videos, and more!

WORD SEARCH

Find and circle the correct term in the word search puzzle for each of the definitions listed below. The word(s) may be horizontal, vertical, or diagonal.

```
P  S  Y  Z  X  P  K  Z  Y  B  W  Q  P  W  X  H  C  D  N  K  V  N  L
R  T  F  U  F  Q  N  H  Z  J  R  L  Q  B  D  K  C  H  P  E  G  E  F
Z  X  B  V  F  B  M  U  T  T  I  Q  S  C  K  I  E  N  W  E  H  Z  M
N  K  F  V  B  A  N  J  R  B  E  O  Z  K  N  S  O  W  X  M  M  C  M
T  X  Z  P  S  Y  C  H  O  S  O  C  I  A  L  H  E  A  L  T  H  F  M
P  O  P  T  P  J  G  L  V  H  I  L  Z  R  V  G  V  H  U  U  I  E  M
Z  R  R  M  H  M  K  Y  L  N  X  M  G  Z  Q  N  F  X  C  P  S  F  F
J  L  U  R  O  N  O  N  C  U  T  X  L  H  P  O  B  J  W  R  W  J  S
J  B  N  O  B  T  G  Q  X  P  B  B  L  K  C  V  H  M  F  R  I  J  N
A  K  C  P  X  P  Y  N  E  G  Q  D  X  A  J  P  T  D  S  X  O  Y  G
I  V  H  A  G  B  J  C  H  Y  G  X  N  K  N  R  J  H  T  V  A  T  X
B  R  L  U  H  N  N  N  Z  W  U  K  V  A  H  B  F  Q  T  G  G  C  V
G  K  Q  T  R  O  L  E  D  E  V  E  L  O  P  M  E  N  T  V  C  E  J
K  H  Z  Z  C  G  V  Q  S  K  P  I  T  O  T  R  F  Q  J  E  Z  K  G
V  G  T  F  S  M  C  W  U  Z  X  H  Q  K  A  F  Y  C  A  R  O  S  S
W  Y  L  M  L  B  P  X  U  F  G  I  U  K  U  S  R  V  W  L  I  K  B
B  E  Y  H  M  T  G  S  A  C  A  Q  L  B  I  Y  N  C  C  F  J  W  Q
S  D  B  N  L  G  X  F  Z  T  D  E  D  Z  Z  N  J  L  C  J  X  E  B
P  Q  Z  D  G  G  K  B  R  W  E  W  X  I  V  I  M  T  D  W  B  K  L
E  L  G  A  W  D  I  A  F  V  V  Q  Y  B  Z  P  W  A  V  G  L  R  Z
P  S  Y  C  H  O  S  O  C  I  A  L  F  U  N  C  T  I  O  N  I  N  G
K  E  A  B  F  Q  J  T  N  Y  P  Z  C  S  T  R  E  S  S  G  U  G  W
C  Z  Y  I  W  Q  H  E  O  G  V  K  B  H  Y  Z  G  A  A  Q  L  A  R
```

CLUES

1. Being mentally, emotionally, socially, and spiritually well _____
2. The way a person thinks, feels, acts, and relates to self and others _____
3. Perceived or physical response to environmental factors _____
4. The beliefs and feelings one holds about oneself _____
5. The individual's capacity to identify and fulfill the social expectations related to the variety of roles assumed in a lifetime _____

FACTORS THAT INFLUENCE PSYCHOSOCIAL HEALTH

Identify each piece of data as either an internal factor or external factor to be considered during a psychosocial assessment. Write an "I" for internal or "E" for external on each line provided.

_____ 1. Client is living in an urban housing development

_____ 2. Client's mother suffers from schizophrenia

_____ **3.** Client teaches cardio kickboxing 5 days per week

_____ **4.** Client uses county welfare assistance and has applied for food stamps

_____ **5.** Client's closest relative lives in Australia

_____ **6.** Client is living on a farm 50 miles away from the closest hospital

_____ **7.** Client received a promotion at work and will be receiving a six-figure salary

_____ **8.** Client's father is an alcoholic

_____ **9.** Client is morbidly obese

_____ **10.** Client states "I have been under a tremendous amount of stress lately"

_____ **11.** Client smokes two packs of cigarettes per day

_____ **12.** Client practices yoga and meditation

_____ **13.** Client has a large extended family involved in her care

_____ **14.** Client attends a prayer group 3 days per week

INTERPRETATION OF ASSESSMENT FINDINGS

Items 1 through 10 include psychosocial health assessment data collected for various age groups. Identify each as normal or abnormal by circling the correct response. Provide a rationale on the line provided for all abnormal findings.

1. A 24-year-old female who states she has had approximately 50 sexual partners.

Normal or **Abnormal**

Rationale: _____

2. A 56-year-old male who looks down to the ground when responding to your questions.

Normal or **Abnormal**

Rationale: _____

3. A 17-year-old female who forces herself to vomit after every meal so she does not gain weight.

Normal or **Abnormal**

Rationale: _____

4. A 30-year-old mother of four, who will not take her children to the beach because she admits she does not want to wear a bathing suit in public.

Normal or **Abnormal**

Rationale: _____

5. A 75-year-old male who joins a social group for widows.

Normal or **Abnormal**

Rationale: _____

6. A 45-year-old divorced female who refuses to date because she believes all relationships end in disaster.

Normal or **Abnormal**

Rationale: _____

7. A 48-year-old male who works 80 hours per week and doesn't have much time for his family.

Normal or **Abnormal**

Rationale: _____

8. A 16-year-old male who becomes angry and verbally abusive with others very quickly.

Normal or **Abnormal**

Rationale: _____

9. A 22-year-old female who starts a volunteer group in her neighborhood to provide underprivileged children recycled sports and dance equipment.

   Normal   **or**   **Abnormal**

   Rationale: _____

10. A 62-year-old female who will not leave the house unless her husband is with her.

    Normal   **or**   **Abnormal**

    Rationale: _____

PSYCHOSOCIAL ASSESSMENT TOOLS

SPIRITUAL ASSESSMENT

Read each question listed for the HOPE Approach to Spiritual Assessment. In the space provided, write an additional question related to spirituality for each component. When you complete the questions, utilize them to assess the spirituality of your lab partner or a family member.

HOPE APPROACH TO SPIRITUAL ASSESSMENT

H (Spiritual Resources)

  1. What are your sources of hope or comfort?

  2. What helps you during difficult times?

  3. _____

Data collected: _____

_____

O (Organized Religion)

  1. Are you a member of an organized religion?

  2. What religious practices are important to you?

  3. _____

Data collected: _____

_____

P (Personal Spirituality)

  1. Do you have spiritual beliefs, separate from organized religion?

  2. What spiritual practices are most helpful to you?

  3. _____

Data collected: _____

_____

E (Effect on Care)

  1. Is there any conflict between your beliefs and the care you will be receiving?

  2. Do you hold beliefs or follow practices that you believe may affect your care?

  3. _____

Data collected: _____

SUICIDE ASSESSMENT

Read the scenario and answer the following questions.

Steven is a 23-year-old Native American who spends most evenings at the local bar. He has recently moved back home with his mother Sasha. Sasha has suffered from anxiety and depression ever since her husband, Steven's father, committed suicide 5 years ago. Steven is a college graduate who majored in finance. Out of college he received a great job with a financial planning firm where he worked for 2 years before he was fired 8 months ago. His long-term girlfriend has decided to leave him because she claims he has lost focus and has no direction since he has been laid off. While ordering his fifth beer for the night, he confides to the bartender "what the hell do I have left to live for?"

1. List four characteristics that Steven has that increase his risk for suicide.

   a.

   b.

   c.

   d.

2. Develop three assessment questions the nurse should ask Steven to further explore his risk for suicide.

   a.

   b.

   c.

STRESS ASSESSMENT

Read the scenario and complete the following questions.

Madison is a 42-year-old female that you (the nurse) will assist to complete the Holmes Social Readjustment Scale. She reveals the following information. Her husband recently passed away from pancreatic cancer. She is very worried about how she will support her two small children (Isabel: 3 years old and Harry: 4 months old). Her husband had always supported her, and she has minimal working skills. She can no longer keep up paying for the medical bills and has not paid the mortgage in months. She fears her home will go into foreclosure next month. Her husband's parents have decided to come and stay with her during this difficult time, especially with Christmas approaching. Although their gesture is sincere, Madison does not get along well with her mother-in-law. She has been so busy caring for her children and trying to find work that she has not been able to attend her junior women's club meetings or play tennis with her friends. To make matters worse, she received a ticket and had her car towed for parking in a handicapped parking spot at the supermarket. She has not had a good night's sleep in months.

1. Circle each "Event Value" for each stressor on the Holmes Social Readjustment Scale (provided on page 44) that Madison is experiencing. What is Madison's total score?

   Score: _____

2. Name five physical signs that Madison may experience related to her stress level.

   a.

   b.

   c.

   d.

   e.

3. List two questions you would ask Madison to further assess her stress level.

   a.

   b.

4. Imagine that Madison comes to you for help managing her stress. Using available resources (web, community publications, etc.), find a stress management program in your community that she would be able to attend.

   a. Program information
      i. Title:

      ii. Sponsor:

      iii. Location:

      iv. Cost:

Holmes Social Readjustment Scale

EVENT	EVENT VALUE
1. Death of a spouse	100
2. Divorce	73
3. Marital separation	65
4. Jail term	63
5. Death of a close family member	63
6. Personal injury or illness	53
7. Marriage	50
8. Fired at work	47
9. Marital reconciliation	45
10. Retirement	45
11. Change in health of family member	44
12. Pregnancy	40
13. Sex difficulties	39
14. Gain of a new family member	39
15. Business readjustment	39
16. Change in financial state	38
17. Death of a close friend	37
18. Change to different line of work	36
19. Change in number of arguments	35
20. Mortgage or loan over $10,000	31
21. Foreclosure of mortgage or loan	30
22. Change in responsibilities at work	29
23. Son or daughter leaving home	29
24. Trouble with in-laws	29
25. Outstanding personal achievement	28
26. Spouse begins or stops work	26
27. Begin or end school	26
28. Change in living conditions	25
29. Revision of personal habits	24
30. Trouble with boss	23
31. Change in work hours or conditions	20
32. Change in residence	20
33. Change in schools	20
34. Change in recreation	19
35. Change in church activities	19
36. Change in social activities	19
37. Change in sleeping habits	16
38. Change in number of family get-togethers	15
39. Vacation	13
40. Christmas	12
41. Minor violations of the law	11
Total Points	

Directions for completion: Add up the point values for each of the events that you have experienced during the past 12 months.

Scoring

Below 150 points:

The amount of stress you are experiencing as a result of changes in your life is normal and manageable. There is only a 1 in 3 chance that you might develop a serious illness over the next 2 years based on stress alone. Consider practicing a daily relaxation technique to reduce your chance of illness even more.

150 to 300 points:

The amount of stress you are experiencing as a result of changes in your life is moderate. Based on stress alone, you have a 50/50 chance of developing a serious illness over the next 2 years. You can reduce these odds by practicing stress management and relaxation techniques on a daily basis.

Over 300 points:

The amount of stress you are experiencing as a result of changes in your life is high. Based on stress alone, your chances of developing a serious illness during the next 2 years approaches 90%, unless you are already practicing good coping skills and regular relaxation techniques. You can reduce the chance of illness by practicing coping strategies and relaxation techniques daily.

Source: Reprinted from Holmes, T., & Rahe, R. J. (1967). Social Readjusting Rating Scale. *Journal of Psychosomatic Research*, 11, 213–218. Copyright 1967, with permission from Elsevier.

THE PSYCHOSOCIAL ASSESSMENT

Recall the information in the textbook regarding psychosocial assessment. Formulate two of your own questions for each component of the psychosocial assessment. When complete, use the questions to assess the psychosocial health of your lab partner.

Physical Fitness

1.

2.

Data Collected: _____

_____

Self-Concept

1.

2.

Data Collected: _____

_____

Family History

1.

2.

Data Collected: _____

_____

Culture

1.

2.

Data Collected: _____

_____

Geography

1.

2.

Data Collected: _____

_____

Economic Status

1.

2.

Data Collected: _____

_____

Roles and Relationships

1.

2.

Data Collected: _____

_____

Stress and Coping

1.

2.

Data Collected: _____

_____

Spirituality and Beliefs

1.

2.

Data Collected: _____

_____

Sort the data collected in your psychosocial assessment of your lab partner by placing it in the categories listed below:

Client Strengths   **Client Weaknesses**

NCLEX®-STYLE REVIEW QUESTIONS

Read each question carefully. Choose the best answer for each question.

1. When a nurse gathers data about the mental, emotional, social, and spiritual well-being of a client, she is performing a:
   1. psychosocial assessment.
   2. psychological screening.
   3. mental health assessment.
   4. cultural assessment.

2. The nurse is about to begin an assessment on a 57-year-old female, who has been hospitalized for depression. The nurse greets her by saying "Hello Mrs. Rodriguez." She responds by rocking back and forth in her chair repeating "Hello, Hello, Hello, Hello." She does not stop until the nurse instructs her to stop. This abnormal speech pattern associated with an altered thought process is called:
   1. word salad.
   2. flight of ideas.
   3. circumlocution.
   4. echolalia.

3. A 38-year-old homeless man has been frequently experiencing chest pain and palpitations. He has gone to the local Emergency Department three times in the past month. His medical workups have been negative. Which intervention would be most appropriate for this client at this time?
   1. Further assessment of his psychosocial status
   2. A prescription for an analgesic due to his chest pain
   3. Education for a caffeine-free diet
   4. Education on stroke prevention

4. The nurse recognizes which of the following as physical signs of stress? (Select all that apply)
   1. Decreased blood clotting time
   2. Dilated bronchi
   3. Elevated blood pressure
   4. Decreased blood supply to vital organs
   5. Constricted pupils

5. The nurse is aware that the two components of Self-Concept are:
   1. body image and interdependence.
   2. role function and self-esteem.
   3. body image and self-esteem.
   4. role function and interdependence.

6. A 45-year-old woman has recently lost her only daughter to an aggressive form of brain cancer. Her husband has brought her to the emergency department because he is concerned for her well-being. He states that on multiple occasions he has witnessed his wife talking to the air as if she was talking to their daughter. Which questions would be appropriate to help assess if this client is in touch with reality?
   1. Do you know where you are right now?
   2. Do you feel well today?
   3. What is your husband's name?
   4. Do you miss your daughter?

7. A 6-year-old boy is frequently in trouble at school. He screams and hits the other children and is very disrespectful to the teachers. The school nurse is concerned about this behavior because: (Select all that apply)
   1. the child's home environment may influence how he copes with stress at school.
   2. the child may have witnessed or may be the victim of some form of abuse in the home.
   3. the child obviously does not like his teacher.
   4. the child does not know how to make friends.
   5. the child is demonstrating a developmental delay.

8. After a nurse collects data for a psychosocial assessment, the next step would be:
   1. make referrals to community resources.
   2. determine the nursing diagnosis.
   3. sort, group, and categorize the data.
   4. evaluate the plan of care.

9. A 23-year-old female states "The voices in my head are telling me to kill people." This is an example of a (an):
   1. command hallucination.
   2. illusion.
   3. delusion.
   4. somatic hallucination.

10. A 34-year-old female is a successful financial analyst. She is very attractive and outgoing. She has high self-esteem and is confident that she will achieve her goal of writing a book by the time she is forty. She is most likely to seek a relationship with:
    1. a 38-year-old Harvard Law graduate.
    2. a 20-year-old who lives at home with his parents while he works on writing a comic book series.
    3. an unemployed 54-year-old.
    4. a 42-year-old married man with three children.

Techniques and Equipment

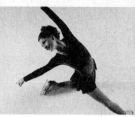

Some men succeed because they are destined to, but most men succeed because they are determined to.

—Greame Clegg

Physical assessment is a process in which the nurse gathers objective and measurable data in order to evaluate a client's overall health status. A systematic approach will assist the nurse in performing an organized assessment. This approach includes four basic techniques: inspection, palpation, percussion, and auscultation. These techniques are used in a repetitive sequence throughout assessment except during abdominal assessment, where the sequence is altered. In order to enhance the nurse's ability to perform these techniques, various types of equipment may be used. This chapter will also review safety and comfort measures that should be considered when performing the physical assessment.

OBJECTIVES

At the completion of these exercises you will be able to:

1. Define key terminology regarding techniques and equipment used during the physical assessment.
2. Differentiate between and among the various assessment techniques.
3. Review the purpose of equipment used in the physical assessment.
4. Apply critical thinking in analysis of a case study related to physical assessment.
5. Complete NCLEX®-style review questions related to assessment techniques and equipment.

RESOURCES

Pearson Nursing Student Resources

Find additional review materials at
nursing.pearsonhighered.com

Prepare for success with additional NCLEX®-style practice questions, interactive assignments and activities, Web links, animations and videos, and more!

CROSSWORD PUZZLE FOR KEY TERMS

Read each definition below and fill in the correct term on the puzzle grid. If the answer requires two words, do not leave a blank space between the words. Use a pencil so you can erase easily.

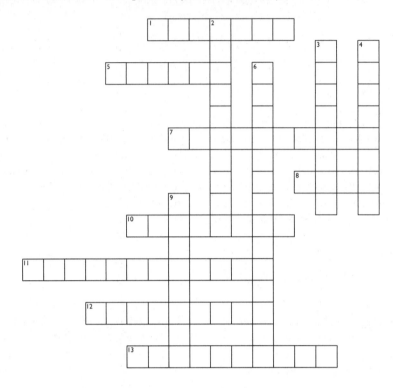

CLUES

Across

1. A loud, high-pitched, drumlike tone of a medium duration characteristic of an organ that is filled with air
5. A hammer or tapping finger used to strike an object
7. The skill of observing the client in a deliberate, systematic manner
8. Bits of information that hint at the possibility of a health problem
10. A dull percussion tone that is soft and has a short duration
11. Using a stethoscope to listen to the sounds produced by the body
12. The skill of assessing the client through the sense of touch to determine specific characteristics of the body
13. The device that accepts the tap or blow from a hammer

Down

2. "Striking through" a body part with an object, fingers, or reflex hammer, ultimately producing a measurable sound
3. The palpable vibration on the chest wall when the client speaks
4. A flat percussion tone that is soft and of short duration
6. Abnormally loud auscultatory tone that is low and of long duration
9. An electronic storage unit that contains subjective and objective data gathered about a client's medical history and physical examination findings

ASSESSMENT TECHNIQUES

INSPECTION

Read the following statements regarding the physical assessment technique of inspection. Place a check mark next to each **true** statement. If the statement is not true, rewrite the statement in the space provided so that it accurately reflects the assessment technique of inspection.

_____ 1. Inspection is the first and last technique used in physical assessment.

_____

_____ 2. Inspection begins the moment the nurse meets the client.

_____

_____ 3. Inspection moves from specific details to the general.

_____

_____ 4. Inspection requires bright lighting.

_____

_____ 5. Inspection includes the sense of smell.

_____

_____ 6. Inspection does not require critical thinking skills.

_____

_____ 7. Inspection may determine symmetry.

_____

_____ 8. Inspection should be combined with palpation.

_____

_____ 9. Novice nurses usually feel very comfortable with inspection.

_____

_____ 10. Inspection may require specialty equipment.

_____

PALPATION

The following exercise pertains to the assessment technique of palpation. Circle the type of palpation the nurse should use in the assessments identified, then identify which part of the hand the nurse should use to perform the assessment.

1. Lymph nodes

   Light   Moderate   Deep

   Hand surface _____

2. Liver

   Light   Moderate   Deep

   Hand surface _____

3. Skin texture

   Light   Moderate   Deep

   Hand surface _____

4. Skin temperature

   Light   Moderate   Deep

   Hand surface _____

5. Pulses

Light	Moderate	Deep

Hand surface _____

6. Fremitus

Light	Moderate	Deep

Hand surface _____

PERCUSSION

Part I

The following statements refer to the physical assessment technique of percussion. Using the percussion sounds below, match the appropriate sound to the following statements. Place the letter on the line provided.

T = Tympany   **H** = Hyperresonance   **F** = Flatness

R = Resonance   **D** = Dullness

_____ 1. High-pitched, soft tone of short duration

_____ 2. Low-pitched, loud, hollow tone of long duration

_____ 3. Sound heard when percussing over solid body organs

_____ 4. Sound heard when percussing over air-filled intestines

_____ 5. Sound heard when percussing hyperinflated lungs

_____ 6. High-pitched, loud, drumlike tone of medium duration

_____ 7. Abnormally loud tone of long duration

_____ 8. Sound heard when percussing over bone

_____ 9. Sound heard when percussing over air-filled lungs (normal inflation)

_____ 10. High-pitched, soft tone of short duration

Part II

Label each figure with the correct percussion method (direct, indirect, blunt) and describe the technique in the space provided.

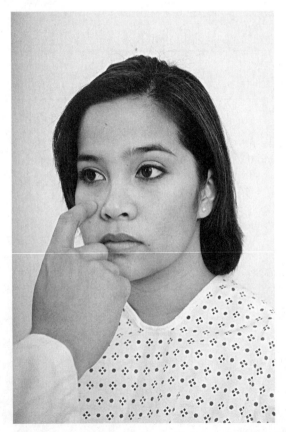

A. _____

_____

_____

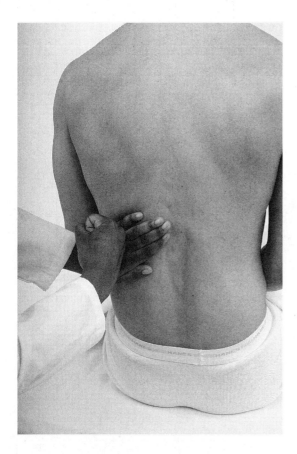

B. _____

_____

_____

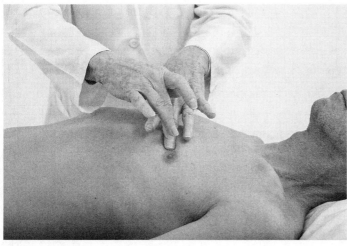

C. _____

_____

_____

Part III

Identify the appropriate method of percussion (direct, indirect, blunt) for the following physical assessments.

_____   **1.** Maxillary sinuses of a 26-year-old with sinusitis

_____   **2.** Posterior thorax to determine diaphragmatic excursion on a 45-year-old

_____   **3.** Costovertebral tenderness on a 68-year-old

_____   **4.** Borders of the liver on a 19-year-old

_____   **5.** Gallbladder tenderness on a 54-year-old

_____   **6.** Anterior thorax on a 6-month-old

_____   **7.** Frontal sinuses of a 9-year-old

_____   **8.** Bladder of a 34-year-old

AUSCULTATION

Part I

The following statements pertain to auscultation. Read each statement, determine if the statement is correct or incorrect, then circle your response. If the statement is incorrect, rewrite the statement correctly.

1. The binaurals of the stethoscope should fit snugly but comfortably.

    Correct   **Incorrect**

    Correction: _____

2. Long stethoscope tubing produces a clearer sound than short tubing.

    Correct   **Incorrect**

    Correction: _____

3. The diaphragm or bell of the stethoscope should be held between the fourth and fifth fingers and placed on the client's chest.

    Correct   **Incorrect**

    Correction: _____

4. The diaphragm should be used to auscultate low-pitched sounds.

    Correct   **Incorrect**

    Correction: _____

5. When auscultating body sounds it is acceptable to place the stethoscope over a client's gown or clothing as long as it is a thin, flat material.

    Correct   **Incorrect**

    Correction: _____

6. The bell should be used to auscultate heart sounds only.

    Correct   **Incorrect**

    Correction: _____

7. Lung sounds obtained by placing the stethoscope on a hair-covered chest require no further assessment.

    Correct   **Incorrect**

    Correction: _____

8. It is best to use a smaller diaphragm and bell when auscultating the body sounds of a child.

    Correct   **Incorrect**

    Correction: _____

9. Heavy pressure should be applied to the skin when using a Doppler ultrasonic stethoscope to obtain pulses.

    Correct   **Incorrect**

    Correction: _____

10. A water-soluble transmission gel should be used with the Doppler ultrasonic stethoscope.

    Correct   **Incorrect**

    Correction: _____

Part II

Identify the sounds below that are detected with a stethoscope. Place a D for diaphragm or a B for bell on the line provided to indicate which part of the stethoscope the nurse would use in order to best assess the sound. If the sound does not require the use of a stethoscope to be detected, leave the blank empty.

_____ 1. Dry hacking cough

_____ 2. Faint expiratory wheeze

_____ 3. Dorsalis pedis pulse

_____ 4. Bowel sounds

_____ 5. Tympany of the abdomen

_____ 6. Hoarseness of the voice

_____ 7. Heart murmur

_____ 8. Carotid bruit

_____ 9. Clicking of the temporomandibular joint

_____ 10. Apical pulse

_____ 11. Pleural friction rub

_____ 12. Resonance

EQUIPMENT

Match each piece of equipment in Column A with its appropriate use from Column B. Items in column B are to be used only once.

Column A

_____ 1. Cotton-tipped swab

_____ 2. Gloves

_____ 3. Goggles

_____ 4. Goniometer

_____ 5. Nasal speculum

_____ 6. Ophthalmoscope

_____ 7. Otoscope

_____ 8. Penlight

_____ 9. Reflex hammer

_____ 10. Bell of the stethoscope

_____ 11. Sphygmomanometer

_____ 12. Diaphragm of the stethoscope

_____ 13. Thermometer

_____ 14. Tongue blade

_____ 15. Tuning fork

_____ 16. Vision chart

Column B

A. Provides a direct light source and tests pupillary reaction

B. May be used to obtain specimens

C. Tests deep tendon reflexes

D. Measures body temperature

E. Inspection of the external ear and tympanic membrane

F. Facilitates examination of the oropharyngeal cavity

G. Measures the degree of joint flexion and extension

H. Offers eye protection from splashing of body fluids

I. Auscultation of heart murmur

J. Dilates nares

K. Auscultation of lung sounds

L. Inspection of the interior structures of the eye

M. Assessment of sensation and auditory function

N. Protects the client and nurse from contamination

O. Screening near and distant vision

P. Measures systolic and diastolic blood pressure

APPLICATION OF THE CRITICAL THINKING PROCESS

Read the following scenario and answer the questions as you go along.

Sarah is a registered nurse who works in a women's health clinic. This morning, Gloria, a 26-year-old female, is scheduled for a physical assessment.

1. Name three ways Sarah can prepare a safe and comfortable environment for the client during the physical assessment:

   a.

   b.

   c.

When Sarah first walks into the examination room, she notices that Gloria does not make eye contact with her. Gloria is wearing the examination gown and a pair of dirty mismatched socks. As Sarah begins to interview the client, she notes that Gloria only provides one- to two-word responses.

2. Identify three observations in this scenario that the nurse should investigate further.

   a.

   b.

   c.

The first thing that Sarah does when she begins the physical assessment is place her stethoscope on Gloria's posterior thorax in order to auscultate her lung sounds. She then has Gloria lay flat in order to palpate and percuss her abdomen. When percussing the abdomen she pays close attention to ensure her motion is coming from the forearm and not the wrist. Sarah uses two strikes before repositioning the pleximeter to avoid muffled sounds. Upon completing the assessment, Sarah washes her hands and informs Gloria that there are some areas in the assessment she feels are abnormal.

3. Name at least three mistakes that Sarah made during this physical assessment. For each mistake, write how she can improve her technique.

   a. Mistake-

      Correction-

   b. Mistake-

      Correction-

   c. Mistake-

      Correction-

NCLEX®-STYLE REVIEW QUESTIONS

Read each question carefully. Choose the best answer for each question.

1. Which of the following sequences used during physical assessment reflects the proper order for the nurse to assess a client?
   1. Auscultation, percussion, palpation, inspection
   2. Inspection, percussion, palpation, auscultation
   3. Inspection, palpation, percussion, auscultation
   4. Palpation, inspection, percussion, auscultation

2. A young adult is involved in a motorcycle crash and sustains injuries to the right leg. As the nurse inspects the client's injured leg, it is best to proceed from:
   1. distal to proximal and then to the entire leg.
   2. proximal to distal and then to the entire leg.
   3. the entire leg and then distal to proximal.
   4. the entire leg and then proximal to distal.

3. The nurse uses _____ percussion when assessing the thorax of an infant.
   1. indirect
   2. blunt
   3. direct
   4. deep

4. When using the ophthalmoscope to inspect the interior structures of the eye, the nurse identifies an abnormal finding. The best aperture to use to further assess a lesion would be:
   1. small aperture.
   2. slit.
   3. grid.
   4. red-free filter.

5. Two agencies that help to establish protocols to protect both nurses and clients from the spread of disease are:
   1. the Centers for Disease Control and the Occupational Safety and Health Administration.
   2. the American Nurses Association and the American Medical Association.
   3. the Centers for Disease Control and the American Nurses Association.
   4. the American Medical Association and the Occupational Safety and Health Administration.

6. A nursing student is performing a physical assessment in the clinical setting. The nursing instructor provides further teaching when the student:
   1. performs hand hygiene only at the beginning of the assessment.
   2. cleanses the bell and diaphragm of the stethoscope with disinfectant prior to applying it on a client.
   3. carefully inspects a body part before palpating the area.
   4. wears gloves if there is any potential for exposure to blood or body fluids.

7. The nurse is preparing to assess the fetal heart rate of a client who is 5 months pregnant using a Doppler ultrasonic stethoscope. The nurse understands in order to accurately obtain the fetal heart rate, it is important to:
   1. use a transducer gel.
   2. use heavy pressure.
   3. cool the transducer before touching the client's skin.
   4. have the client exhale and then hold her breath.

8. The nurse is palpating the peripheral pulses of an older adult client. Important factors for the nurse to consider when performing this type of assessment are: (Select all that apply)
   1. making certain fingernails are short and smooth.
   2. not wearing jewelry.
   3. assessing the client for a latex allergy.
   4. hand hygiene before and after assessment.
   5. putting on sterile gloves for the assessment.

9. The nurse is assessing the abdomen of a client who may be infected with hepatitis B. In order to assess for hepatomegaly, the nurse will palpate:
   1. less than 1 cm deep over the left upper quadrant.
   2. 2–4 cm deep over the left upper quadrant.
   3. less than 1 cm deep over the right upper quadrant.
   4. 2–4 cm deep over the right upper quadrant.

10. The nurse identifies which of the following assessment findings as cues that might indicate child abuse?
    1. Welts and small burns on the skin
    2. Skin rash
    3. A 3-year-old who hides behind her parents
    4. An infant who cries when held by a stranger

General Survey 7

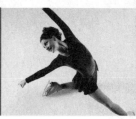

The undertaking of a new action brings new strength.
—Richard L. Evans

The General Survey begins when the nurse first sees the client. This "first impression" requires education, skillful use of the senses to recognize clues and gather information, and knowledge to quickly analyze the data to determine the appropriate approach for the physical assessment. Some may call the ability to create a first impression a sixth sense; however, with education and practice you will learn how to focus on important observations during the first few minutes spent with the client. This chapter will review and apply the knowledge learned about the general survey and the measurement of vital signs.

OBJECTIVES

At the completion of these exercises you will be able to:

1. Define key terminology regarding the general survey and vital signs.
2. Categorize observations as part of the general survey.
3. Select the appropriate routes for measuring body temperatures.
4. Identify the location of peripheral pulses.
5. Review the proper sequence for obtaining a blood pressure.
6. Recognize factors that influence vital signs.
7. Perform a general survey.
8. Obtain a full set of vital signs.
9. Prioritize scenarios based on general survey observations.
10. Document data collected during a general survey.
11. Apply the critical thinking process to case studies related to the general survey.
12. Complete NCLEX®-style review questions related to the general survey.

RESOURCES

Pearson Nursing Student Resources
Find additional review materials at
nursing.pearsonhighered.com

Prepare for success with additional NCLEX®-style practice questions, interactive assignments and activities, Web links, animations and videos, and more!

WORD SEARCH

Find and circle the correct term in the word search puzzle for each of the definitions listed below. The word may be horizontal, vertical, or diagonal.

```
G J X N O A P F J D D S D Z U S F R P B W Y O B S B R
C U K W S H V U P R L N I H O V L Z F G K L K K B B B
S F Z F Y W M N R K B H U Q Z U M V F G E D J D M F B
U V U X S Z F C D E T M R H V B O V G P A G X G L T E
J O L Y T I L T Q L S Q R K C T P J W F B R Z N E C L
Q Q N W O V I I D J S P B J E H O I E G A U H R Y Z I
W F V X L E E O M H Z W I S D E K H F B Z I O X P T I
S O K I I H Y N J V Y H M R D V I T A L S I G N S U O
U D M Z C E W A Q O B P X Z A S Y A X A Y R T Y I A A
G H C S P H K L Z A T Y O B X T N Q I H B I O H F Z X
A J B P R X B A Q G P X Q T Q T O M A Y L V B D P F E
J T P H E R L S O W F Y N R H H R X D E F Y I L P N
V B X Y S Q W S O M Y W E F R E R J Y K L N Q A C O X
V Q X G S M W E K Y K A F S H C R I E R U V O S I M B
E Y H M U A K S A A S A E T V S I M O A A O G T G F W
S U Y O R O Y S W X F V R U R X E W I C Q T A O E A Q
F D E M E B T M P Y T E M Z X B K S H A E R E L N L V
N H T A O Y B E O W P G T C B J J X R R U M E I E E N
H W F N L C S N L Y G R M O A P T O U T K V A C R B U
V N V O H D E T H E O P C V V T Z T A A Z P K P A H G
Y F C M S F J H H B X U R Y W S A S A B U C H R L U O
G T W E Z A R L L Q R L U W M R N A V I F S A E S T B
T E C T C V T I P E E S S P E E C G H B I A T S U S H
P Z S E S J U O U D B E I P G F B V J P W G D S R A L
T G E R P D U U X C B N M Y X B S M W N X L A U V B V
R V R M L F U M S Z X E X B F L T X B Y B S T R E M E
O H A L V X X N J A T O L V Y L Z J Q W K J X E Y A J
```

CLUES

1. Body temperature that is less than expected _____
2. A highly unpleasant sensation that affects a person's physical health, emotional health, and well-being

   _____
3. Observations made to gather data while the client is performing common or routine activities **(two words)**

   _____ _____
4. The systematic measurement of temperature, pulse, respirations, blood pressure, and pain status **(two words)**

   _____ _____
5. Impressions based on what is seen, heard, or smelled during the initial interview phase of assessment **(two words)**

   _____ _____
6. Wave of pressure felt at various points in the body due to the force of the blood against the walls of the arteries

   _____
7. The pressure between ventricular contractions when the heart is at rest **(two words)** _____

   _____

8. An instrument used to measure arterial blood pressure _____
9. Body temperature that is greater than expected _____
10. The pressure of the blood at the height of the wave when the left ventricle contracts (**two words**) _____ _____
11. The percentage of saturated oxygen in the blood (**two words**) _____ _____
12. The intensity of pain is most accurately assessed through the use of (**three words**) _____ _____ _____
13. The degree of hotness or coldness within the body as measured by a thermometer _____
14. The number of times the individual inhales and exhales during a one-minute period of time (**two words**) _____ _____

CLASSIFICATION OF OBSERVATIONS

Read each observation noted during the general survey. Place the letter for the appropriate component next to each observation.

P = Physical Appearance   **B** = Behavior of Client   **N/A** = Not Assessed During the General Survey
MS = Mental Status   **M** = Mobility

_____ 1. Wearing ripped dirty clothes
_____ 2. Alcohol odor to breath
_____ 3. Petite frame
_____ 4. Hyperactive bowel sounds
_____ 5. Does not make eye contact
_____ 6. Right leg lags behind
_____ 7. Clean and smells like soap
_____ 8. Unilateral facial paralysis

_____ 9. Oriented to person, place, and time
_____ 10. Inability to stand erect
_____ 11. Cheerful and laughing
_____ 12. Head bobbing
_____ 13. Pallor
_____ 14. Speaks rapidly and fidgets with hands
_____ 15. Unresponsive
_____ 16. Lymphadenopathy

ROUTES FOR MEASURING TEMPERATURE

Read each clinical presentation. On each line provided write the name of the most appropriate method for measuring body temperature (oral, tympanic, axillary, rectal, and temporal artery). Some may have more than one answer. Write the rationale for your answer on the line provided.

_____ 1. An older adult female who presents with shortness of breath

Rationale: _____

_____ 2. A school-aged child who presents with a laceration on his head

Rationale: _____

_____ 3. A newborn who presents with jaundice

Rationale: _____

_____ 4. An older adult who is unresponsive and hot to touch

Rationale: _____

_____ 5. A young adult who complains of fever and fatigue

Rationale: _____

_____ 6. A middle-aged adult who had an appendectomy 9 hours ago

Rationale: _____

_____ 7. A toddler who presents to the emergency department with possible febrile seizures

Rationale: _____

_____ 8. A young adult who injured his shoulder playing tennis

Rationale: _____

PULSE LOCATIONS

On the line provided write the name of the pulse described in each of the statements. Locate the pulse on the diagram by placing the number on the line matching the anatomical position of the pulse.

1. Pulse Locations

    1. Located between the eye and the top of the ear _____

    2. Located halfway between the anterior superior iliac spine and the symphysis pubis _____

    3. Located behind and slightly inferior to the medial malleolus _____

    4. Located in the popliteal fossa lateral to the midline _____

    5. Located on the thumb side of the anterior wrist _____

    6. Located in the medial aspect of the antecubital fossa _____

    7. Located in the groove between the trachea and the sternocleidomastoid _____

    8. Located on the medial side of the dorsum of the foot _____

2. Explain the steps the nurse may take if she is unable to palpate a pedal pulse.

    _____

    _____

    _____

RESPIRATIONS

Read each statement and decide whether it is true or false. Circle your answer. If the answer is false, rewrite the statement to make it true.

1. Each inspiration should be counted independently of each expiration.

    True   **False**

    _____

2. A respiratory rate of 52 respirations per minute for a newborn is a normal finding.

    True   **False**

    _____

3. The nurse should count a respiratory rate for one full minute at all times.

    True   **False**

    _____

4. To obtain accurate data the nurse should not inform the client that he is counting respirations.

    True   **False**

    _____

5. A respiratory rate of 26 respirations per minute for a 6-year-old is an abnormal finding.

   True   **False**

   _____

6. Medications may alter a client's respiratory rate.

   True   **False**

   _____

7. A full respiratory cycle contains one inspiration and one expiration.

   True   **False**

   _____

8. A respiratory rate of 8 is considered a normal finding in the older adult.

   True   **False**

   _____

BLOOD PRESSURE

Place the following steps for measuring a client's blood pressure in the correct order from 1 (the first step) through 15 (the last step).

_____ Palpate the brachial pulse.

_____ Place the client in a comfortable position.

_____ Deflate the cuff rapidly and completely.

_____ Place the diaphragm of the stethoscope over the brachial pulse.

_____ Palpate the radial pulse.

_____ Remove any clothing from the client's arm.

_____ Confirm that the blood pressure cuff is the appropriate size for the client's arm.

_____ Note the manometer reading at each of the five Korotkoff phases.

_____ Close the release valve on the pump.

_____ Remove the cuff from the client's arm.

_____ Slightly flex the arm and hold it at the level of the heart with the palm upward.

_____ Pump up the cuff until the sphygmomanometer registers 30 mmHg above the palpatory systolic blood pressure.

_____ Place the cuff on the arm with the lower border 1 inch above the antecubital area making sure that the cuff is smooth and snug.

_____ Inflate the cuff until the radial pulse is no longer palpable and note the reading on the sphygmomanometer.

_____ Release the valve on the cuff carefully so that the pressure decreases at the rate of 2 to 3 mmHg per second.

FACTORS THAT INFLUENCE VITAL SIGNS

Read each statement. Circle the anticipated change for the stated vital sign discussed in the statement.

1. A male who has stepped off the treadmill after running 7 miles

    Temperature   Lower   No Change   Higher

2. A preschool child who has a fever of 103.6°F

    Respirations   Lower   No Change   Higher

3. An adolescent 14 days into her 28-day menstrual cycle

    Temperature   Lower   No Change   Higher

4. A middle-aged adult who was on bedrest for 3 days and is getting out of bed for the first time

    Blood Pressure   Lower   No Change   Higher

5. A school-aged child who has a fever of 104.2°F

    Pulse   Lower   No Change   Higher

6. A young adult who has climbed to the top of Mount Everest

    Respirations   Lower   No Change   Higher

7. An older adult who has just returned to his hospital room after a physical therapy session

    Pulse   Lower   No Change   Higher

8. A client who has just received an injection of morphine to relieve her postoperative pain

    Blood Pressure   Lower   No Change   Higher

9. A young adult who is giving a presentation to 1,000 people at work that he just finished preparing 1 hour ago

    Temperature   Lower   No Change   Higher

10. An adolescent client who has lost 400 ml of blood from her abdominal incision reopening

    Pulse   Lower   No Change   Higher

11. A middle-aged adult who is anxious about his upcoming colonoscopy

    Respirations   Lower   No Change   Higher

12. An older adult who is meditating

    Blood Pressure   Lower   No Change   Higher

13. A middle-aged adult who has gained 100 lb in the past 10 years

    Blood Pressure   Lower   No Change   Higher

14. An adolescent who is shoveling snow

    Respirations   Lower   No Change   Higher

PERFORMANCE OF THE GENERAL SURVEY AND MEASUREMENT OF VITAL SIGNS

Perform a general survey and obtain a full set of vital signs on your lab partner and record the data in the space provided.

Client Initials: _____ DOB: _____ Gender: _____ Today's Date: _____

General Survey:

Physical Appearance:

Mental Status:

Mobility:

Behavior of Client:

Height: _____ Weight: _____

Vital Signs: BP _____ HR _____ RR _____ Temp _____ O₂ Saturation _____

APPLICATION OF THE CRITICAL THINKING PROCESS

Read each general survey scenario. List the clients in the order that they should be evaluated based on your observations. Provide a rationale for your first and last priority in the space provided.

_____ A 75-year-old male who is sitting in a wheelchair, skin color pale. Client is in no apparent distress. Client is wearing clean, warm clothing.

Vital signs: BP 168/102 – HR 112 – RR 16 – Temp 98.2

_____ A 26-year-old female who is sitting with her head leaning over into her lap, skin color is pink. She is dressed appropriately for the weather. Her body frame is large and she appears overweight.

Vital Signs: BP 122/84 – HR 110 – RR 18 – Temp 102.4

_____ A 56-year-old male who is unresponsive with agonal breathing, skin color pallor with bluish undertones.

Vital Signs: BP 68/42 – HR 42 – RR 4 – Temp 96.2

_____ A 15-year-old female who limps in the doorway wearing a cheerleading uniform, skin color pink. She sits down slowly and moves a chair to raise her left leg and places an ice pack to her ankle. She is laughing with the people who accompanied her in and is eating a bag of chips.

Vital Signs: BP 110/62 – HR 76 – RR 16 – Temp 98.1

_____ A 66-year-old male grabbing at his chest and moaning in pain. His skin color is pink. He is morbidly obese and wearing pajama pants and a T-shirt that appears to have vomit on it.

Vital Signs: BP 168/92 – HR 86 – RR 24 – Temp 99.7

First Priority

Rationale: _____

_____

_____

Least Priority

Rationale: _____

_____

_____

Read the following scenario and answer the following questions.

Allison is a 32-year-old female who arrives at an urgent care center stating "my stomach has been killing me since last night." She is sitting in a chair using her arms to hold her abdomen as she rocks back and forth. She is dressed in a long, blue velvet gown with a tiara on her head. As you move closer to her, you note the smell of cigarette smoke. She is about 5′2″ and 120 lbs. When you speak to her, she replies with short answers and makes facial grimaces.

1. Identify at least four observations made regarding the general survey.

   1.

   2.

   3.

   4.

You begin to gather more data and decide to continue by measuring her vital signs. You decide to measure an oral temperature. The temperature reading is 101.2°F. Her blood pressure reading is 116/72. Her right radial pulse is 122 bpm and feels weak. Next you obtain the respiratory rate, which is 18 respirations per minute. The oxygen saturation is 99% on room air.

2. Sort the data identified as normal or abnormal finding.

   Normal   **Abnormal**

Allison reveals that her pain is located in the right lower quadrant of her abdomen, rated a 7 on a numerical scale of 0 to 10. She describes it as a constant stabbing pain that increases when she moves. She tried taking Tylenol last night but she stated "it didn't do a darn thing." She said she knew it was really a problem when she tried to go to her theatre practice this morning and had trouble even putting her costume on. She said she took 10 minutes to go backstage and meditate hoping to complete rehearsal, but it was difficult. She claims "I'm really scared and anxious I might need my appendix out because I'm the lead actress in my theatre group, and opening night is in 3 days."

3. Pain is the fifth vital sign. List the components of the pain assessment using the acronyms below.

   O-   R-

   L-   T-

   D-   I-

   C-   C-

   A-   E-

4. Sort the information provided in the scenario above into the pain assessment acronym.

   O-   R-

   L-   T-

   D-   I-

   C-   C-

   A-   E-

5. Were the data collected in the scenario sufficient to complete the pain assessment? If not, explain.

6. How does the information you have revealed affect your conclusions made earlier from the general survey?

NCLEX®-STYLE REVIEW QUESTIONS

Read each question carefully. Choose the best answer for each question.

1. The nurse is aware that the four major categories of the general survey are:
   1. physical appearance, mental status, mobility, and behavior.
   2. physical appearance, mental status, cognitive function, and vital signs.
   3. physical appearance, cognitive function, ht vs. wt ratio, and vital signs.
   4. mental status, cognitive function, mobility, and behavior.

2. The nurse assessing the heart rate of a 5-month-old baby knows the most appropriate place to assess is:
   1. radial pulse.
   2. carotid pulse.
   3. apical pulse.
   4. brachial pulse.

3. The nurse is counting the respiratory rate of a client experiencing an acute asthma attack. The nurse knows in order to obtain an accurate count he should:
   1. count each inspiration and expiration separately.
   2. count the number of breaths for 30 seconds and then multiply by 2.
   3. not inform the client that he is counting a respiratory rate.
   4. estimate the rate and document tachypnea in the client record.

4. A 32-year-old female, with a large frame, has a height of 5'8" and a weight of 175 lb. The nurse concludes that:
   1. this is an appropriate weight for her height and large frame.
   2. this is underweight for her height and large frame.
   3. this is overweight for her height and large frame.
   4. the client is morbidly obese.

5. The nurse obtains an oxygen saturation level on an adult client as 97%. The nurse concludes that this reading is:
   1. within a normal range.
   2. less than expected.
   3. life threatening.
   4. The oxygen saturation level is not measured in percentages.

6. A young adult client has been monitoring her body temperature to determine when she is ovulating. She measures her oral temperature every morning when she awakens at 6:30 a.m. Each day the thermometer reads 98.2°F, what reading would indicate ovulation?
   1. 97.2°F
   2. 96°F
   3. 98.7°F
   4. 101°F

7. The nurse is aware that the following factors can affect a client's blood pressure. (Select all that apply)
   1. Obesity
   2. Gender
   3. Diurnal variations
   4. Medications
   5. Physical activity

8. When auscultating a blood pressure, the nurse identifies the Korotkoff sounds. When listening for these sounds, the nurse is able to determine the blood pressure by documenting:
   1. phase 1 as the systolic pressure and phase 5 as the diastolic pressure.
   2. phase 1 as the systolic pressure and the number just before phase 4 begins as the diastolic pressure.
   3. the number at the beginning of phase 2 as the systolic pressure and the end of phase 4 as the diastolic pressure.
   4. the number at the beginning of phase 2 as the systolic pressure and the end of phase 5 as the diastolic pressure.

9. A 19-year-old female presents to the clinic on a hot summer day for her annual exam. While she sits in the waiting area she is wearing dark sunglasses and a long-sleeve shirt. As her name is called she walks slowly into the examination room with her head down. When she sits down on the table you obtain a full set of vital signs and begin to ask her health history questions. The first piece of assessment data collected in this scenario would be:
   1. the vital signs.
   2. the health history.
   3. her physical appearance.
   4. the assessment has not begun yet.

10. A 65-year-old male client is recovering from a total knee replacement. Hospital policy requires a pain assessment be performed and documented every 4 hours and as needed. When using the numerical scale to determine intensity, the client states the pain is a 10 on a scale from 0 to 10. During the assessment he answers a phone call and begins to laugh and reposition himself in the bed with a smile on his face. Your response would be to:
    1. hold his pain medication because he obviously is not in that much pain.
    2. clarify the parameters of the numerical scale and, if the client does not understand the numerical scale, use the Wong-Baker Face Scale.
    3. administer the highest dose of pain medication ordered by the healthcare provider for the client's severe pain.
    4. wait until the next pain assessment is due in 4 hours and hope for more congruent data among the pain history and the observation of behaviors.

Pain Assessment 8

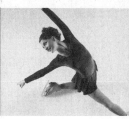

We cannot learn without pain.
—Aristotle

Pain is unique and has a different meaning to each individual. Each painful experience, combined with one's psychosocial background, brings a different response. The nurse must be able to perform an accurate pain assessment in order to develop an individualized plan of care for the client. This chapter will provide you with an understanding of various types of pain and assist in developing the skill of performing a pain assessment utilizing various tools.

OBJECTIVES

At the completion of these exercises you will be able to:

1. Define key terminology regarding pain.
2. Differentiate between acute and chronic pain.
3. Categorize various types of pain.
4. Explore pain assessment tools.
5. Identify factors that may influence a person's pain perception.
6. Perform a pain assessment.
7. Complete NCLEX®-style review questions related to the pain assessment.

RESOURCES

Pearson Nursing Student Resources

Find additional review materials at
nursing.pearsonhighered.com

Prepare for success with additional NCLEX®-style practice questions, interactive assignments and activities, Web links, animations and videos, and more!

Additional resources: *www.cancer.org*
www.pain-topics.org
www.jointcommission.org

CROSSWORD PUZZLE FOR KEY TERMS

Read each definition below and fill in the correct term on the puzzle grid. If the answer requires two words do not leave a blank space between the words. Use a pencil so you can erase easily.

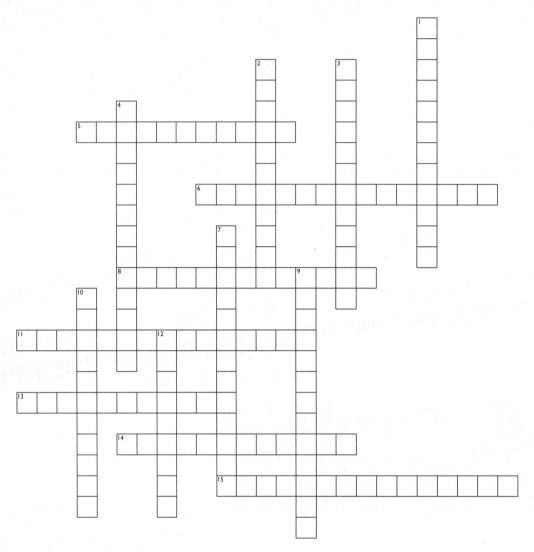

CLUES

Across

5. Painful sensation experienced in a missing body part or paralyzed area (**two words**)
6. Pain that is diffuse and arises from ligaments, tendons, bones, blood vessels, and nerves, which tends to last longer than cutaneous pain (**three words**)
8. Pain perceived at one location that then extends to nearby tissue (**two words**)
11. Pain that is highly resistant to relief (**two words**)
13. Receptors that transmit pain sensation
14. Excessive sensitivity to pain
15. Pain resulting from current or past damage to the peripheral or central nervous system rather than a particular stimulus (**two words**)

Down

1. Pain felt in a part of the body that is considerably removed or distant from the area actually causing the pain (**two words**)
2. Physiological processes related to pain perception
3. Pain that results from stimulation of pain receptors deep within the body such as the abdominal cavity, cranium, or thorax (**two words**)

4. Maximum amount and duration of pain that an individual is able to endure without relief **(two words)**
7. Pain that originates in the skin or subcutaneous tissue **(two words)**
9. Point at which the sensation of pain is perceived **(two words)**
10. Pain that is prolonged, usually recurring or persisting over 6 months **(two words)**
12. Pain that lasts only through the expected recovery period **(two words)**

ACUTE VERSUS CHRONIC PAIN

1. Review the characteristics of pain below. Place the letter that corresponds with each characteristic in the appropriate circle. Use each letter only once.

Characteristics

A. Prolonged over 6 months
B. Lasts only through recovery period
C. Client reports pain
D. Client often doesn't mention pain
E. Sympathetic nervous system response

F. Parasympathetic nervous system response
G. Restless and anxious client
H. Depressed and withdrawn client

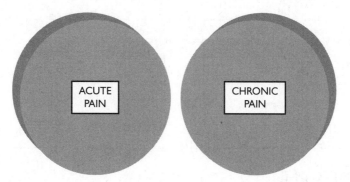

2. Identify the pain associated with each of the problems below as Acute or Chronic by writing an **A** for Acute or **C** for Chronic on the line provided.

_____ **1.** Ruptured appendix

_____ **2.** Pancreatic cancer

_____ **3.** Fibromyalgia

_____ **4.** Laceration to left third digit

_____ **5.** Childbirth

_____ **6.** Fractured hip

_____ **7.** Rheumatoid arthritis

_____ **8.** Myocardial infarction

_____ **9.** Inguinal hernia

_____ **10.** Degenerative disc disease

_____ **11.** Ischemic colon

_____ **12.** Renal calculi

From above, select one acute pain problem and one chronic pain problem and provide a rationale for your classification.

Acute Pain—

_____

_____

Chronic Pain—

_____

_____

CATEGORIES OF PAIN

Circle the most appropriate descriptor for each type of pain. Write the rationale for your answer on the line provided.

1. Torn anterior cruciate ligament

   Cutaneous Pain   **Deep Somatic Pain**   **Visceral Pain**

   Rationale: _____

2. Abrasions to the right arm

   Intractable Pain   **Neuropathic Pain**   **Cutaneous Pain**

   Rationale: _____

3. Osteosarcoma

   Radiating Pain   **Visceral Pain**   **Cutaneous Pain**

   Rationale: _____

4. Herpes Zoster

   Neuropathic Pain   **Intractable Pain**   **Referred Pain**

   Rationale: _____

5. A client reports pain in a leg that has been surgically amputated

   Intractable Pain   **Radiating Pain**   **Phantom Pain**

   Rationale: _____

6. Right shoulder pain from cholecystitis

   Intractable Pain   **Neuropathic Pain**   **Referred Pain**

   Rationale: _____

PAIN ASSESSMENT TOOLS

1. Draw an example of each scale in the space provided.

   1. The Numeric Rating Scale

   2. The Simple Verbal Descriptive Scale

   3. The Oucher Scale

2. Answer the following questions referring to the pain scales in Question 1.

   1. Which pain scale would be the most appropriate to use for a 5-year-old? Explain your answer.

   2. You are about to use the Simple Verbal Descriptive Scale to assess the pain intensity of your client. In the space provided below, describe how you would introduce this scale to your client in order to obtain accurate data.

3. Use a nursing database to research the FLACC scale.

   a. What database did you use?

   b. In the space below, write what each letter stands for.

      F—

      L—

      A—

      C—

      C—

   c. Explain how this scale is scored.

4. In the space below, design your own tool in order to assess a client's level of pain. Explain how the tool is to be used.

APPLICATION OF THE CRITICAL THINKING PROCESS

Mr. Pineapple (white Anglo-Saxon) and Mrs. Wong (Chinese) have had a total hip replacement. Mr. Pineapple has a client-controlled analgesic pump (PCA) and is receiving a small dose of morphine every 10 minutes. He scales his pain as an 8 on a numerical scale of 0 to 10. Mrs. Wong refused the morphine pump and prefers to use over-the-counter Motrin for the pain. She scales her pain as a 3 on a numerical scale of 0 to 10.

1. Which client is experiencing the greater amount of pain? Explain your answer.

2. Explain how two people who have had the same surgery can experience different levels of pain.

FACTORS INFLUENCING PAIN ASSESSMENT

Ms. Lemon is a 56-year-old female who was diagnosed with stomach cancer 18 months ago. She has undergone a partial gastrectomy (removal of the stomach) accompanied by radiation and chemotherapy for 6 months. She has recently been informed her cancer has metastasized to her liver. She has been experiencing pain for months. Her past history includes herniated discs from L_4–S_1, cholecystectomy, appendectomy, total knee replacement, and three caesarean sections.

1. Is Ms. Lemon experiencing acute pain or chronic pain? Provide a rationale for your decision.

Ms. Lemon comes to the outpatient infusion center for her chemotherapy. Prior to connecting Ms. Lemon to her chemotherapy infusion, you must complete a pain assessment. You ask her the following questions:

   Where is your pain located?

   Can you scale your pain on a scale of 0–10, 0 being no pain and 10 being the worst pain imaginable?

   Is the pain constant or intermittent?

2. List four additional questions that should be asked during this assessment.

   1.

   2.

   3.

   4.

Ms. Lemon states that her body constantly aches all over. A few times per day she gets a sharp pressure pain in her upper abdomen. She states her pain fluctuates from a 3 to an 8 on a scale of 0–10. She is using an opioid skin patch for pain that she changes every 3 days and is also taking OxyContin twice per day. She seems confused about the medications she is taking and fears that she will die from the medication and not the cancer.

3. You decide to develop a teaching plan for Ms. Lemon. In the space below, write one goal that would be important to achieve.

4. Write two objectives that would support your goal.

   1.

   2.

5. Explain how you would evaluate each objective listed above.

   1.

   2.

NCLEX®-STYLE REVIEW QUESTIONS

Read each question carefully. Choose the best answer for each question.

1. The nurse understands that pain is:
   1. subjective.
   2. objective.
   3. a similar experience for persons undergoing similar injuries, illnesses, and treatments.
   4. dependent on the nurse's perception of the client's experience.

2. The nurse understands that the receptors that transmit pain sensation are called:
   1. modulators.
   2. gait controllers.
   3. nociceptors.
   4. impulse regulators.

3. When performing a pain assessment, the nurse must consider which of the following factors? (Select all that apply)
   1. Psychological factors
   2. Sociocultural factors
   3. Behavioral factors
   4. Environmental factors
   5. Developmental factors

4. The nurse identifies an example of a mechanical stimulus that can excite pain receptors as:
1. frostbite.
2. renal calculi (kidney stones).
3. muscle spasm.
4. angina.

5. A client is experiencing acute pain. The nurse knows that the sympathetic nervous system will initially respond by:
1. decreasing the heart rate and blood pressure.
2. constricting pupils.
3. causing diaphoresis.
4. decreasing the respiratory rate.

6. An adult male is brought to an emergency department via ambulance because he was an unrestrained passenger in a motor vehicle accident. He states that he has a high tolerance for pain. The nurse interprets this statement as:
1. the client has a low pain threshold.
2. the client has a high pain threshold.
3. he has a limited pain reaction.
4. pain threshold is not the same as pain tolerance.

7. A middle-aged Chinese American female arrives at a women's health clinic complaining of a burning sensation when she voids bloody urine. After an examination, the nurse practitioner (NP) explains to the client that she has a very bad urinary tract infection. The NP writes her a prescription for an antibiotic, but the client refuses any pain medication. The nurse is aware that this may be due to:
1. the client's fear of narcotic addiction.
2. the client's Chinese culture may lead her to be stoic.
3. the minimal pain that is typically experienced with a urinary tract infection doesn't really require pain medication.
4. the client's lack of trust in nurse practitioners.

8. A young child is seen with a fractured right radius after falling from a trampoline. The nurse caring for this client knows it is best to:
1. send the parents to the waiting area so they don't have to see their child in pain.
2. encourage the parents to hold the child to provide comfort.
3. avoid using distraction techniques because it is best to have the child aware of what is going on at all times.
4. use the Numeric Rating Scale to assess the child's pain.

9. An older adult who lives in a long-term care facility has become increasingly lethargic in the past 24 hours. The client is transferred from the long-term care facility to the emergency department, where it is determined the client has appendicitis. The nurse recognizes which of the following statements as correct when dealing with pain in the older adult? (Select all that apply)
1. Lethargy and fatigue may be an indicator of pain.
2. The older adult may misinterpret pain as part of the aging process.
3. The older adult may have decreased sensations of pain.
4. The prevalence of pain is lower in the older adult population.
5. The older adult requires more pain medication due to physiological changes associated with aging.

10. An adult client suffers from migraine headaches and is seen frequently by the healthcare provider (HCP) for pain management. Which question would be inappropriate for the nurse to ask the client during a focused interview regarding pain?
1. "How bad is the pain now?"
2. "How long does the pain last?"
3. "Why are you smiling at me if you're having pain?"
4. "What were you doing just before the pain started?"

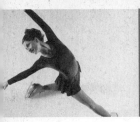

9 Nutritional Assessment

You only get out what you put in.
—Unknown

Nutritional health is a vital component of the overall health status of the individual. Some of the leading causes of death can be caused by poor dietary habits. This includes but is not limited to coronary artery disease and diabetes mellitus. Although nurses work collaboratively with members of other disciplines, such as dieticians and nutritionists, nurses must be capable of performing a nutritional assessment. The data collected will allow the nurse to incorporate dietary changes in the plan of care or make referrals to other disciplines in order to further assess a client's needs.

OBJECTIVES

At the completion of these exercises you will be able to:

1. Define key terminology regarding the Nutritional Assessment.
2. Complete a nutritional history.
3. Analyze anthropometric measurements.
4. Identify nutritional deficiencies that may lead to physical findings.
5. Examine the relationship between culture and nutrition.
6. Perform a Nutritional Assessment.
7. Evaluate Nutritional Assessment data.
8. Complete NCLEX®-style review questions related to nutrition.

RESOURCES

Pearson Nursing Student Resources

Find additional review materials at
nursing.pearsonhighered.com

Prepare for success with additional NCLEX®-style practice questions, interactive assignments and activities, Web links, animations and videos, and more!

Additional resources: *www.mypyramid.gov*

WORD SEARCH

Find and circle the correct term in the word search puzzle for each of the definitions listed below. The word may be horizontal, vertical, or diagonal.

```
R  T  B  A  H  Z  O  U  W  H  J  B  D  E  Z  Z  H  G  H  U  D  W  J  E  S
H  N  G  B  N  V  N  D  A  G  L  B  G  P  N  P  D  Z  T  N  G  G  D  Y  A
A  I  Z  R  M  H  G  K  A  I  B  E  Q  B  P  K  R  H  I  N  B  R  P  Q  D
N  X  C  Q  U  V  I  C  N  A  J  L  D  L  Y  U  T  E  M  N  A  A  X  Z  E
T  J  Y  D  Y  K  Q  D  G  Q  J  R  P  K  P  L  T  I  S  W  T  K  J  B  J
H  E  J  P  N  Z  M  F  U  V  N  C  V  D  A  O  E  O  W  R  R  N  W  Q  E
R  H  O  P  B  K  W  O  L  X  J  X  R  E  R  N  F  Q  L  P  O  F  G  E  T
O  H  D  N  U  F  W  I  A  F  Z  A  H  P  F  S  O  L  K  I  P  P  C  C  O
P  B  P  Q  L  O  D  G  R  Z  N  L  C  D  Z  N  A  F  T  S  H  K  H  U  Y
O  T  E  V  O  I  S  D  S  F  A  I  I  Z  X  C  G  I  Z  L  I  H  E  W  T
M  S  G  X  B  Q  I  U  T  N  T  X  K  L  E  H  R  V  V  W  C  W  I  K  E
E  T  A  L  P  T  C  D  O  A  A  S  E  R  K  T  K  R  V  I  P  S  L  V  A
T  X  A  N  O  C  U  I  M  L  I  M  T  R  U  A  T  G  E  H  A  D  O  M  I
R  G  O  Z  M  S  T  O  A  T  H  E  K  N  O  U  K  X  C  A  P  B  S  B  L
I  R  K  V  B  I  S  E  T  C  I  B  L  I  W  P  M  P  P  O  I  A  I  J  P
C  C  P  Z  R  G  U  I  I  D  E  A  T  J  N  B  H  Y  I  J  L  Q  S  B  P
F  U  Q  T  W  L  I  G  T  M  M  R  T  H  L  Y  X  T  C  E  L  R  M  F  U
Z  L  U  P  D  G  N  K  I  I  F  L  A  G  S  I  G  N  H  R  A  L  Q  R  F
J  N  B  S  I  F  T  V  S  Q  S  Y  E  N  A  L  T  Y  A  E  D  V  R  G
F  N  K  E  Z  C  Y  R  I  C  K  E  T  S  I  N  N  R  N  Q  L  L  S  O  N
T  E  U  K  C  X  A  P  T  T  O  W  K  Q  X  A  Y  F  T  G  L  M  Y  R  N
O  F  Q  K  O  I  L  O  N  Y  C  H  I  A  X  O  R  H  N  U  L  S  I  W  W
U  N  D  E  R  N  U  T  R  I  T  I  O  N  D  V  R  M  E  C  M  B  U  A  T
O  V  E  R  N  U  T  R  I  T  I  O  N  A  K  R  Q  Q  T  R  G  C  Y  K  K
I  Y  K  F  T  J  O  B  L  I  M  U  B  M  D  Q  A  A  J  A  S  C  N  P  A
```

CLUES

1. An imbalance, whether a deficit or excess, of the required nutrients of a balanced diet _____
2. A smooth tongue appearance caused by poor nutrition (**two words**) _____ _____
3. A clinical finding associated with poor nutritional health resulting in bowed legs _____
4. An abnormal condition of the lips characterized by scaling of the surface and by the formation of fissures in the corners of the mouth _____
5. A remembrance of all food, beverages, and nutritional supplements or products consumed in a set period of time such as a 24-hour period (**two words**) _____ _____
6. Dry mucosa as a result of poor nutrition _____
7. Dyspigmentation of the mouth or part of the mouth (**two words**) _____ _____
8. Inflammation or redness of the tongue _____
9. Spoon-shaped ridges in the cardia _____
10. Using vitamins, foods, nutrients, or herbs to achieve or maintain good health (**two words**) _____ _____
11. Any scientific measurement of the body _____
12. Excessive intake or storage of essential nutrients _____
13. Abnormal craving for or eating of nonfood items such as chalk or dirt _____
14. Another term for muscle mass or skeletal muscle (**two words**) _____ _____
15. Cracks at the corner of the mouth caused by poor nutrition (**two words**) _____ _____
16. Insufficient intake or storage of essential nutrients _____
17. Soft, yellow plaques on the lids at the inner canthus, which are sometimes associated with high cholesterolemia _____

THE NUTRITIONAL HISTORY

THE 24-HOUR DIET RECALL

Review the sample 24-hour Diet Recall. In the space provided below document all the food and beverages you consumed in the past 24 hours.

SAMPLE RECALL		MY PERSONAL RECALL	
TYPE OF FOOD	PORTION	TYPE OF FOOD	PORTION
Cheerios	1 cup		
Skim milk	1 cup		
Banana	1 small		
Orange juice	½ cup		
Almonds-dry roasted, unsalted	¼ cup		
Apple	1 small		
Water	16 oz		
Grilled cheese sandwich			
American cheese	2 slices		
Whole wheat bread	2 slices		
Tomato	1		
Deli pickle	1 cup		
Herbal tea	8 oz		
Water	16 oz		
Low-fat yogurt	¾ cup		
Fresh strawberries	¼ cup		
Water	16 oz		
Grilled chicken	8 oz		
Baked potato	1 small		
Steamed broccoli	1½ cups		
Chocolate pudding	1 cup		
Iced tea	32 oz		

BODY MASS INDEX

Use Table 9.4 in chapter 9 of the textbook to determine the body mass index for each client listed. Use the following key to interpret your findings and place the interpretation on the line.

U – Underweight   **H** – Healthy Weight   **OW** – Overweight   **OB** = Obese

_____ _____ **1.** 24-year-old female who is 5′ tall and weighs 143 lb

_____ _____ **2.** 62-year-old male who is 5′8″ tall and weighs 258 lb

_____ _____ **3.** 43-year-old female who is 5′3″ tall and weighs 120 lb

_____ _____ **4.** 37-year-old female who is 5′6″ tall and weighs 148 lb

_____ _____ **5.** 92-year-old female who is 5′2″ tall and weighs 95 lb

_____ _____ **6.** 68-year-old male who is 6′2″ tall and weighs 200 lb

_____ _____ **7.** 45-year-old male who is 6′ tall and weighs 175 lb

_____ _____ **8.** 55-year-old female who is 5′4″ tall and weighs 220 lb

_____ _____ **9.** 18-year-old male who is 5′9″ tall and weighs 175 lb

_____ _____ **10.** 57-year-old female who is 4′10″ tall and weighs 85 lb

ASSESSMENT FINDINGS

Identify each piece of data as either "N" for Normal or "A" for Abnormal by circling the letter below each finding. Write the potential nutritional deficit on the line below each abnormal finding.

1. Bleeding Gums

   N   A _____

2. Goiter

   N   A _____

3. Pallor

   N   A _____

4. Tongue Midline

   N   A _____

5. Brittle Hair

   N   A _____

6. Nail Bed Curvature of 160°

   N   A _____

7. Pitting Edema

   N   A _____

8. Bowed Legs

   N   A _____

9. Freckles

   N   A _____

10. Smooth Tongue

    N   A _____

CULTURAL CASE STUDIES

Read each scenario and complete the following questions.

> Crystal is a 27-year-old Chinese female who presents to the clinic with coughing, runny nose, and a headache. She is diagnosed with a rhinovirus (a cold). Crystal explains this is considered a "cold" illness in her culture.

1. What types of food and beverages would be appropriate for Crystal to have? Why?

> Rachel is a 36-year-old Jewish female who is hospitalized for a venous thromboembolism (VTE) in her right leg. She is very concerned about being in the hospital because Passover starts in 2 days.

2. What dietary restrictions may be expected?

3. What foods should be available for Rachel to eat during Passover?

> Jessie is a 56-year-old African American male who is hospitalized with uncontrolled hypertension. When performing a nutritional assessment, Jessie states "I love my wife's southern cooking." His favorite foods are chicken fried steak, greens with smoked ham hocks, candied yams, and fried peach pie.

4. Explain the relationship between Jessie's diagnosis and his diet.

5. Develop a goal and objectives for a teaching plan for Jessie.

   Goal—

   Objectives—

MY FOOD PYRAMID

Log on to the www.mypyramid.gov website. Use the Interactive Tools to develop your own food pyramid.

1. How many calories are suggested per day?

2. List the amount of each food in each group that is suggested.

Grains

Vegetables

Fruits

Milk

Meat and Beans

Oils

3. Compare the suggested food selections and portions with your personal 24-hour Diet Recall from the section The Nutritional History.

    1. Which food groups are you meeting appropriately?

    2. Which food groups demonstrate a deficiency?

    3. Which food groups demonstrate an abundance?

    4. Is the 24-hour Diet Recall the appropriate assessment tool to use for this exercise? If not, which assessment tool would be more appropriate?

5. Develop a 2-day menu that meets the recommended daily amounts of each food group according to your personal pyramid.

Example

Breakfast	Calories 210
Cheerios 1 cup	
Skim milk 1 cup	**Food Groups**
	Grains
	Milk

DAY 1		DAY 2	
Breakfast	Calories	Breakfast	Calories
	Food Groups		Food Groups
Snack	Calories	Snack	Calories
	Food Groups		Food Groups
Lunch	Calories	Lunch	Calories
	Food Groups		Food Groups
Snack	Calories	Snack	Calories
	Food Groups		Food Groups
Dinner	Calories	Dinner	Calories
	Food Groups		Food Groups

LAB ASSIGNMENT

Complete the Mini Nutritional Assessment (MNA) on another student in your clinical laboratory.

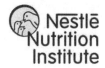 Nestlé
Nutrition
Institute

Mini Nutritional Assessment
MNA®

Last name:			First name:		
Sex:	Age:	Weight, kg:		Height, cm:	Date:

Complete the screen by filling in the boxes with the appropriate numbers. Add the numbers for the screen. If score is 11 or less, continue with the assessment to gain a Malnutrition Indicator Score.

Screening

A   Has food intake declined over the past 3 months due to loss of appetite, digestive problems, chewing or swallowing difficulties?
0 = severe decrease in food intake
1 = moderate decrease in food intake
2 = no decrease in food intake ☐

B   Weight loss during the last 3 months
0 = weight loss greater than 3kg (6.6lbs)
1 = does not know
2 = weight loss between 1 and 3kg (2.2 and 6.6 lbs)
3 = no weight loss ☐

C   Mobility
0 = bed or chair bound
1 = able to get out of bed / chair but does not go out
2 = goes out ☐

D   Has suffered psychological stress or acute disease in the past 3 months?
0 = yes   2 = no ☐

E   Neuropsychological problems
0 = severe dementia or depression
1 = mild dementia
2 = no psychological problems ☐

F   Body Mass Index (BMI) (weight in kg) / (height in m²)
0 = BMI less than 19
1 = BMI 19 to less than 21
2 = BMI 21 to less than 23
3 = BMI 23 or greater ☐

Screening score
(subtotal max. 14 points) ☐☐

12-14 points: Normal nutritional status
8-11 points: At risk of malnutrition
0-7 points: Malnourished

For a more in-depth assessment, continue with questions G-R

Assessment

G   Lives independently (not in nursing home or hospital)
1 = yes   0 = no ☐

H   Takes more than 3 prescription drugs per day
0 = yes   1 = no ☐

I   Pressure sores or skin ulcers
0 = yes   1 = no ☐

J   How many full meals does the patient eat daily?
0 = 1 meal
1 = 2 meals
2 = 3 meals ☐

K   Selected consumption markers for protein intake
• At least one serving of dairy products
  (milk, cheese, yoghurt) per day   yes ☐   no ☐
• Two or more servings of legumes
  or eggs per week   yes ☐   no ☐
• Meat, fish or poultry every day   yes ☐   no ☐
0.0   = if 0 or 1 yes
0.5   = if 2 yes
1.0   = if 3 yes ☐.☐

L   Consumes two or more servings of fruit or vegetables per day?
0 = no   1 = yes ☐

M   How much fluid (water, juice, coffee, tea, milk...) is consumed per day?
0.0 = less than 3 cups
0.5 = 3 to 5 cups
1.0 = more than 5 cups ☐.☐

N   Mode of feeding
0 = unable to eat without assistance
1 = self-fed with some difficulty
2 = self-fed without any problem ☐

O   Self view of nutritional status
0 = views self as being malnourished
1 = is uncertain of nutritional state
2 = views self as having no nutritional problem ☐

P   In comparison with other people of the same age, how does the patient consider his / her health status?
0.0 = not as good
0.5 = does not know
1.0 = as good
2.0 = better ☐.☐

Q   Mid-arm circumference (MAC) in cm
0.0 = MAC less than 21
0.5 = MAC 21 to 22
1.0 = MAC 22 or greater ☐.☐

R   Calf circumference (CC) in cm
0 = CC less than 31
1 = CC 31 or greater ☐

Assessment (max. 16 points) ☐☐.☐

Screening score ☐☐.☐

Total Assessment (max. 30 points) ☐☐.☐

Ref.   Vellas B, Villars H, Abellan G, et al. *Overview of MNA® - Its History and Challenges.* J Nut Health Aging 2006; 10: 456-465.
Rubenstein LZ, Harker JO, Salva A, Guigoz Y, Vellas B. Screening for Undernutrition in Geriatric Practice: *Developing the Short-Form Mini Nutritional Assessment (MNA-SF).* J. Geront 2001; 56A: M366-377.
Guigoz Y. The Mini-Nutritional Assessment (MNA®) *Review of the Literature – What does it tell us?* J Nutr Health Aging 2006; 10: 466-487.
® Société des Produits Nestlé, S.A., Vevey, Switzerland, Trademark Owners
© Nestlé, 1994, Revision 2009. N67200 12/99 10M
For more information: www.mna-elderly.com

Malnutrition Indicator Score

24 to 30 points   ☐   normal nutritional status

17 to 23.5 points   ☐   at risk of malnutrition

Less than 17 points   ☐   malnourished

NCLEX®-STYLE REVIEW QUESTIONS

Read each question carefully. Choose the best answer for each question.

1. The nurse is aware that undernutrition may lead to:
    1. muscle loss.
    2. a compromised immune system.
    3. poor wound healing.
    4. All of the above

2. When using a Food Diary/Record as part of a nutritional assessment, it is best for the nurse to:
    1. encourage the client to record his intake for one full week.
    2. encourage the client to record his intake for two sequential weekdays and a weekend day.
    3. encourage the client to record his intake for five weekdays and two full weekends.
    4. encourage the client to record his intake for 30 days.

3. The nurse understands that anthropometric measurements refer to:
    1. height, weight, body mass index, and abdominal circumference.
    2. the overall increase in the average size of humans through time.
    3. tracking the measurements of an individual from infancy through late adulthood.
    4. the use of the metric system when measuring height and weight ratios.

4. A 62-year-old male reports to the clinic for his annual physical assessment. His present weight is 174 lb, and his last recorded weight was 198 lb 4 months ago. He claims he has had a very poor appetite the last few months, and he denies doing any exercise. The nurse interprets this finding as a weight loss:
    1. of 2% and of no clinical significance.
    2. of 8% and of clinical significance.
    3. greater than 11% and of clinical significance.
    4. greater than 15% and of no clinical significance.

5. The equipment needed for the nurse to obtain skinfold thickness measurements includes:
    1. calipers.
    2. calipers and a flexible measuring tape.
    3. flexible measuring tape and 5-lb dumbbell.
    4. calipers, flexible measuring tape, and a 5-lb dumbbell.

6. An older adult Roman Catholic is hospitalized for a total knee replacement (TKR) on a Friday during Lent. Which menu item would you anticipate the client will order for dinner?
    1. Roasted chicken with brown rice
    2. Strip steak with baked potato
    3. Honey-glazed ham with carrots
    4. Veggie-topped personal pizza

7. A young adult is admitted through the emergency department for alcohol intoxication. The client has a long history of alcohol abuse. In order to complete a comprehensive initial assessment, the nurse anticipates which lab tests to be ordered in order to evaluate visceral protein status?
    1. Nitrogen, cholesterol, and transferrin
    2. Albumin, prealbumin, and transferrin
    3. Nitrogen, albumin, and cholesterol
    4. Cholesterol, triglycerides, and total iron binding

8. The nurse is aware that the culture of a client may influence the: (Select all that apply)
    1. method of food preparation.
    2. number of meals eaten in a day.
    3. types of herbs used.
    4. food selection for special occasions.
    5. food beliefs.

9. An 81-year-old male was brought to the emergency department due to a syncopal episode (fainting). A 12-lead EKG has revealed that Freddie has an arrhythmia called *Torsades de pointes*. This arrhythmia is commonly caused by:
   1. a magnesium deficiency.
   2. a sodium deficiency.
   3. an iron deficiency.
   4. a calcium deficiency.

10. When performing a nutritional assessment, it is important for the nurse to collect data regarding a client's functional capacity because the client may not be capable of: (Select all that apply)
    1. food shopping.
    2. feeding himself.
    3. preparing a meal.
    4. reading a food label.
    5. opening containers in preparing a meal.

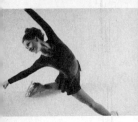

10 The Health History

We must know what knowledge is available, how we can obtain it, and why it is true.

—Socrates

The ability to conduct a comprehensive health history is an important aspect of nursing. Utilizing effective communication skills, the nurse will be able to collect data regarding a client's health status. This chapter will provide you the opportunity to develop communication skills while learning the components of the health history.

OBJECTIVES

At the completion of these exercises you will be able to:

1. Define key terminology regarding the health history.
2. Utilize communication skills.
3. Identify barriers to the communication process.
4. Develop interview questions for each component of the health history.
5. Interpret a genogram.
6. Create a personal genogram.
7. Apply the critical thinking process to case studies.
8. Obtain and document a health history.
9. Complete NCLEX®-style review questions to the health history.

RESOURCES

Pearson Nursing Student Resources
Find additional review materials at
nursing.pearsonhighered.com

Prepare for success with additional NCLEX®-style practice questions, interactive assignments and activities, Web links, animations and videos, and more!

CROSSWORD PUZZLE FOR KEY TERMS

Read each definition below and fill in the correct term on the puzzle grid. If the answer requires two words do not leave a blank space between the words. Use a pencil so you can erase easily.

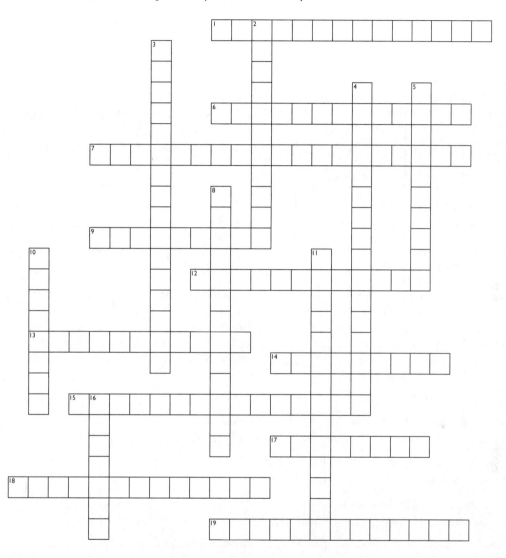

CLUES

Across

1. The ability to appreciate and respect another person's worth and dignity with a nonjudgmental attitude **(two words)**
6. A set of related traits, habits, or acts that affect a client's health **(two words)**
7. Actions that are used during the encoding/decoding process to obtain and disseminate information, develop relationships, and promote understanding of self and others **(two words)**
9. Paying undivided attention to what the client says and does
12. Restating the client's basic message to test whether it was understood
13. The ability to present oneself honestly and spontaneously
14. Giving full-time attention to verbal and nonverbal messages
15. A record or person other than the client that provides additional information about the client **(two words)**
17. The process of formulating a message for transmission to another person
18. Information about the client's health in his or her own words and based on the client's own perceptions **(two words)**
19. Exchange of information, feelings, thoughts, and ideas

Down

2. Tying together the various messages that the client has communicated throughout the interview
3. An interview that enables the nurse to clarify points to obtain missing information and to follow up on verbal and nonverbal cues identified in the health history **(two words)**
4. The client is assured of a positive outcome with no basis for believing it **(two words)**
5. A communication technique used in letting the client know that the nurse empathizes with the thoughts, feelings, or experiences expressed
8. The client is the best source because the client can describe personal symptoms, experiences, and factors leading to the current concerns **(two words)**
10. A pictorial representation of family relationships and medical history
11. The period before first meeting with the client in which the nurse reviews information and prepares for the initial interview
16. Understanding, being aware, being sensitive to the feelings, thoughts, and/or experiences of another

USING COMMUNICATION SKILLS

DO YOU SAY WHAT YOU MEAN TO SAY?

Requires: 2 students

1 piece of plain paper for each student

Markers or colored pencils

One student will draw a simple picture on a sheet of paper without having the other student see what has been drawn. An example would be a house, a flower, or a school bus. The objective is to have the second student replicate the exact picture by following only the verbal instructions provided by the student who drew the picture. The second student is not permitted to ask any questions at this time. The verbal instructions cannot include any words that would reveal what the picture should be. After the verbal instructions are complete and the picture has been drawn, compare the pictures and ask the following questions:

Student Providing Verbal Instructions

How difficult was it to describe your picture to your classmate?

How accurate was your classmate's drawing when compared to your original drawing?

Was it frustrating trying to provide instructions? Explain.

Would you have changed your verbal instructions in any way? Explain.

Student Receiving Verbal Instructions

How clear were the instructions that were provided to you?

How accurate was your drawing when compared to your classmate's original drawing?

Was it frustrating trying to interpret the verbal instructions that were provided to you? Explain.

Would you have changed the verbal instructions you received in any way? Explain.

Example

Drawing

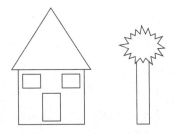

Examples of Verbal Instructions

The following statements can be used:

Draw a square on the bottom center of the paper.

Draw a triangle on the top of the square with the point facing upward.

Do not use statements similar to the following:

Draw a house.

Draw a tree next to the house.

IT'S ALL IN THE DETAILS

Requires: 3 students

Have student A tell a story about his/her childhood to student B without student C listening. The story can be about a special achievement, a fond memory, a special person, and so on. Student B may ask questions in order to obtain as many details about the story as possible to avoid misinterpretation. Student B may take notes. Student B must then repeat the story to Student C without any input from Student A. Student C may ask any questions of Student B in order to clarify any misinterpretation and to obtain as much detail as possible. When this communication process has been completed, discuss the following questions:

Student A

Do you feel student B was actively listening to you tell your story? Explain.

Did student B ask relevant questions about your story?

Did student B interrupt your story in order to obtain more detail that you would have mentioned if the listener had been more patient?

Do you feel student B understood the highlights of your story? Explain.

Describe how this exercise can be related to a nurse communicating information to the healthcare provider about a client.

Student B

Do you feel that student A provided you with enough information in the story to repeat it to student C?

Do you feel that student C was actively listening to you repeat the story? Explain.

Did student C ask relevant questions about the story?

Did student C interrupt your story in order to obtain more detail that you would have mentioned if the listener had been more patient?

Do you feel that you were able to obtain enough details about the story to accurately repeat the story to student C so that it was understood as Student A intended? Explain.

Describe how this exercise can be related to a nurse communicating information to another nurse about a client.

Student C

Do you feel student B provided you with enough information about the story to understand the story?

Did student B speak clearly and with organized thought? Explain.

Do you feel that you would have understood the story better if you heard it from student A instead of student B? Explain.

Describe how this exercise can be related to a nurse communicating information to a client or a client's family.

Students A, B, and C

Write the definition of each interactional skill on the line provided. Provide an example of how each interactional skill was used during this communication exercise. If the skill was not used, provide an example of how it could have been used.

1. **Attending:** _____

   Example _____

   _____

2. **Paraphrasing:** _____

   Example _____

   _____

3. **Direct Leading:** _____

   Example _____

   _____

4. **Focusing:** _____

 Example _____

 _____

5. **Questioning:** _____

 Example _____

 _____

6. **Reflecting:** _____

 Example _____

 _____

7. **Summarizing:** _____

 Example _____

 _____

BARRIERS TO COMMUNICATION

Read each dialogue and decide whether the nurse was therapeutic or nontherapeutic in his/her response by circling your answer. If the response was nontherapeutic, state the barrier and provide an alternate therapeutic response on the line provided.

1. *Client:* "I am so worried about my upcoming surgery tomorrow morning. I keep thinking something bad is going to happen."

 Nurse: "Don't waste another minute worrying about it. You will be just fine."

 Therapeutic　　　　　　　　**Nontherapeutic**

 Barrier: _____

 Alternate Response: _____

 _____

2. *Client:* "I've had pain in my leg for the past few days."

 Nurse: "Do you have any history of peripheral vascular disease (PVD) or venous thromboembolism (VTE)?"

 Therapeutic　　　　　　　　**Nontherapeutic**

 Barrier: _____

 Alternate Response: _____

 _____

3. *Client:* "Yesterday my healthcare provider spoke to me so fast when explaining the procedure planned for me tomorrow. I'm a bit concerned."

 Nurse: "It sounds like you may have some questions. Let me see if I can help clarify things for you."

 Therapeutic　　　　　　　　**Nontherapeutic**

 Barrier: _____

 Alternate Response: _____

 _____

4. *Client:* "When I started having pain in my chest at 2 a.m., I figured it was just indigestion from the fried food I ate for dinner last night."

   Nurse: "So you also figured you were a doctor last night, too."

   Therapeutic   **Nontherapeutic**

   Barrier: _____

   Alternate Response: _____

   _____

5. *Client:* "I cried all night last night thinking about how my cancer has spread. I'm just not ready to die. I feel like I haven't even truly lived."

   Nurse: "Oh, you should have watched the show I was watching last night on the comedy channel. My husband and I couldn't stop laughing."

   Therapeutic   **Nontherapeutic**

   Barrier: _____

   Alternate Response: _____

   _____

6. *Client:* "My husband was so angry with me last night and totally lost control."

   Nurse: "Let's discuss what you mean by *lost control.*"

   Therapeutic   **Nontherapeutic**

   Barrier: _____

   Alternate Response: _____

   _____

7. *Client:* "I think I had sex with someone who has a sexually transmitted disease."

   Nurse: "What makes you think that? Did you use any form of protection? How many partners have you had? Do you have a history of sexually transmitted disease?"

   Therapeutic   **Nontherapeutic**

   Barrier: _____

   Alternate Response: _____

   _____

8. *Client:* "It seems that diabetes is really much more serious than I thought. I'm going to have to rethink a lot of things I do each day."

   Nurse: "It sounds like you have some concerns about your diabetes. Would you like to discuss some of those concerns now?"

   Therapeutic   **Nontherapeutic**

   Barrier: _____

   Alternate Response: _____

   _____

COMPONENTS OF THE HEALTH HISTORY

Write two questions that may be asked for each component of the health history in the space provided.

1. **Biographical Data**

   A. _____

   B. _____

2. **Present Health or Illness**

   A. _____

   B. _____

3. **Past History**

   A. _____

   B. _____

4. **Family History**

   A. _____

   B. _____

5. **Psychosocial History**

   A. _____

   B. _____

6. **Review of Body Systems**

   Skin

   A. _____

   B. _____

   Hair

   A. _____

   B. _____

   Nails

   A. _____

   B. _____

   Head

   A. _____

   B. _____

   Neck

   A. _____

   B. _____

   Lymphatics

   A. _____

   B. _____

   Eyes

   A. _____

   B. _____

Ears

A. _____

B. _____

Nose

A. _____

B. _____

Mouth and Throat

A. _____

B. _____

Respiratory

A. _____

B. _____

Breasts and Axillae

A. _____

B. _____

Cardiovascular

A. _____

B. _____

Peripheral Vascular

A. _____

B. _____

Abdomen

A. _____

B. _____

Urinary

A. _____

B. _____

Male Reproductive

A. _____

B. _____

Female Reproductive

A. _____

B. _____

Musculoskeletal

A. _____

B. _____

Neurologic

A. _____

B. _____

GENOGRAMS

1. Review the genogram below and answer the following questions. Use the genogram symbols listed in chapter 10 of your textbook.

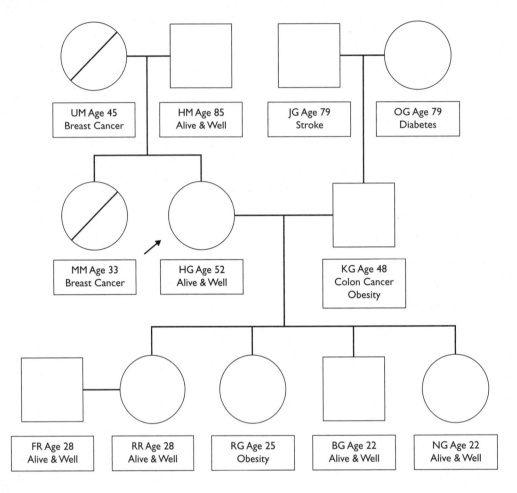

1. What are the initials of the client being interviewed?

2. How many women are in this family?

3. How many generations are represented in this genogram?

4. How many people are deceased in this family?

5. How many siblings does the client have?

6. What disease or illness is this client at risk for?

7. How can this genogram be used to improve the health of this client?

2. Create a personal genogram representing three generations of your family in the space provided. Make sure to develop a key in order to interpret the information you provide. Be sure to include gender, age, initials, relationships, and health status.

HEALTH HISTORY: TRUE OR FALSE

Read each statement and decide whether it is true or false. Circle your answer. If the answer is false, rewrite the statement to make it true.

1. Over-the-counter (OTC) medication should not be included in the medication history.

   True   **False**

   Correction _____

2. The client is the most reliable source of information.

   True   **False**

   Correction _____

3. Healthcare professionals may be considered secondary sources of information.

   True   **False**

   Correction _____

4. Collecting information about a client's health insurance is not part of the health history.

   True   **False**

   Correction _____

5. Birthplace is part of the psychosocial history.

   True   **False**

   Correction _____

6. Asking about a client's financial status is inappropriate and unnecessary in health care.

   True   **False**

   Correction _____

7. Pain may affect the client's ability to participate in the interview.

   True   **False**

   Correction _____

8. It is better to obtain a sexual history early on in the interview to get a potentially embarrassing portion completed first.

   True   **False**

   Correction _____

9. If a client reports identifying with American culture, further questioning is necessary.

True   **False**

Correction _____

10. The client's own words should never be used when documenting any portion of the health history.

True   **False**

Correction _____

APPLICATION OF THE CRITICAL THINKING PROCESS

Read the following scenario and answer the questions.

Scott Petrowski is a 38-year-old male who has cerebral palsy. He is being admitted to a long-term care facility by his mother, Magda Petrowski, who states she is getting too old to care for him by herself at home. The nurse is preparing to obtain a comprehensive health history as part of the admission process. The nurse is aware that this can be a very stressful time for both mother and son.

1. List three ways the nurse can help reduce the fears and anxiety of the client and family during this time.

    1.

    2.

    3.

2. What sources of data may be used to conduct this interview?

Mrs. Petrowski states multiple times in the interview that she is very upset having Scott leave her home. She holds his hand throughout much of the interview, and the nurse notes that at times her eyes become very teary.

3. Identify two ways the nurse can show empathy during this interview.

    1.

    2.

The nurse asks questions regarding the client's cultural beliefs, traits, and traditions. Mrs. Petrowski explains they are from a strong Polish family but is confused as to why this is so important for them to know.

4. The nurse responds by stating:

After one hour of continuous questioning, it is evident that Scott is becoming very restless. Mrs. Petrowski explains that he usually has his lunch at this time and does not like to stay in his wheelchair for long periods of time. The nurse is aware that the process is only about three-fourths complete.

5. The nurse's best action in this situation would be to:

OBTAINING DATA

Read the dialogue and answer the following questions.

The following dialogue is between a nurse and a client being admitted to a medical-surgical floor for cellulitis of the left leg.

Nurse: "Mr. Johnson, do you take any medications on a regular basis?"

Client: "I do take a blood pressure pill when I need it."

Nurse: "How do you know when you need your blood pressure pill?"

Client: "I can tell I need it when I start to get a headache and feel very stressed."

Nurse: "How many times per week do you take the pill?"

Client: "Maybe two or three times per week."

Nurse: "What are the instructions on the medication bottle?"

Client: "My doctor thinks I should take it every single day, but I don't think that is necessary."

Nurse: "How often do you have your blood pressure checked?"

Client: "About once per month and it's about 150 over 80."

Nurse: "Can you tell me the name and dosage of the medication you take?"

Client: "It's a little green pill. I don't remember the name, but my doctor said it is a low dose."

1. The above information falls under which category of health history data?

2. Explain why it was necessary for the nurse to ask so many questions in this scenario.

3. Complete the following grid using the data collected from the above dialogue:

Medication	Dose	Frequency	Duration	Purpose	Effect

4. List any questions the nurse should ask to complete the data collection.

HEALTH HISTORY DOCUMENTATION

Select a classmate or family member who is willing to participate in a health history interview. Arrange for a suitable time and location for your interview. Be sure to explain that all the data collected will be kept confidential—no name will be used (initials only). Document the information on the form provided.

Nurses' Health History Sheet from:

HEALTH HISTORY EXERCISE

A. Interview your laboratory partner and complete the following selected portions of the health history.

I. BIOGRAPHICAL DATA

Name: _____

Address: _____

_____

_____

DOB: _____ Age: _____ Sex: _____

Marital Status: _____

Birth Place: _____

Race: _____ Ethnic Origin: _____

Occupation: _____

_____

____

Religion: _____

Health Insurance: _____

_____

_____

Source of Information: _____

_____

_____

II. PRESENT HEALTH-ILLNESS

Identification of Health Concerns: _____

_____

_____

_____

_____

Current Medications: (Name, Dose, Purpose,
    Duration, Effect, Frequency)

RX: _____

_____

_____

_____

OTC: _____

_____

_____

_____

III. PAST HISTORY

Medical History: (Date, Treatment, Outcome) _____

_____

_____

Surgery: (Date, Procedure, Outcome) _____

_____

_____

IV. FAMILY HISTORY

Nuclear Family: (Initials, Age(s), Relationship,
    Health Status, Diagnosis)

_____

_____

_____

_____

_____

_____

_____

V. PSYCHOSOCIAL HISTORY (Summary of Perceptions)

Educational History: (Highest Level, Date) _____

_____

_____

Occupational History: (Title, Date, Descending
    Order from Most Recent)

_____

_____

_____

_____

_____

Significant Other: (Initials and Title) _____

_____

Support Systems: (Initials and Titles) _____

_____

_____

_____

_____

_____

VI. REVIEW OF SYSTEMS

Nutrition

Height: _____ Weight: _____

Changes: (Date, Reason) _____

_____

Appetite: _____

Menu: Sample for 24 Hours _____

_____

_____

_____

Fluids Not Included in Menu: (Type and Amount) ___

_____

Likes: _____

_____

Dislikes: _____

_____

Snacks: _____

_____

Religious Restrictions: _____

_____

Vitamins/Food/Dietary Supplements: _____

_____

The Abdomen _____

Bowel Elimination: _____

_____

Pattern: _____

_____

Change in Pattern: _____

_____

Characteristics: _____

   Color: _____

   Consistency: _____

   Change: _____

Hemorrhoids/Bleeding: _____

Laxatives/Enemas: _____

Appliances: _____

Other: _____

_____

_____

Urinary System

Pattern: _____

Change in Pattern: _____

_____

Color: _____   Appliances/Devices: _____

_____   _____

Stream: _____   Other: _____

_____   _____

Continence: _____   _____

_____

Nocturia: _____

Barbarito, C. & D'Amico, D. (2000). *Comprehensive Health Assessment:* A Student Workbook. Dubuque, IA: Kendall Hunt Publishing Co., 25–28.

NCLEX®-STYLE REVIEW QUESTIONS

Read each question carefully. Choose the best answer for each question.

1. A client is injured after falling from a bicycle. The best question for the nurse to include when attempting to gather more details about a client's injuries would be:
   1. "Did you fall on concrete?"
   2. "Do you think you broke any bones?"
   3. "Describe how you landed when you fell off the bike?"
   4. "Are you having any pain now?"

2. The nurse understands the term used to select words, body language, and signs to develop a message is called:
   1. encoding.
   2. transmitting.
   3. decoding.
   4. interactional skills.

3. A new graduate nurse has just started working in a woman's health clinic where many of the clients speak very little English. The nurse often uses a translator in order to conduct her interviews. When using a translator it is important for the nurse to:
   1. look at the translator while speaking clearly to them.
   2. pause frequently.
   3. speak loudly with more hand gestures than normal.
   4. ask the translator to use any slang or idiomatic language.

4. A young adult is carried into the emergency department by two friends. The client is barely conscious. The nurse suspects some form of substance abuse. The nurse attempts to obtain information from the client's friends, who are very hesitant to share any information. This is most likely because they:
   1. are a secondary source of information and may not be reliable.
   2. have had bad past experiences in the emergency department.
   3. fear legal implications.
   4. are embarrassed for their friend.

5. The nurse identifies which of the following situations as one where a client health history may be impossible to obtain?
   1. A 90-year-old male admitted through the emergency department from a nursing home with no family present
   2. A 6-month-old infant who was left in a safe haven crib at a church
   3. A 36-year-old female who arrives at the hospital in active labor
   4. A 76-year-old female who is in a rehabilitation facility for a stroke she had 3 months ago that has left her with expressive aphasia

6. The nurse uses a pictorial display of a client's family relationships and health issues. This is called a:
   1. family tree.
   2. pictogram.
   3. genealogy.
   4. genogram.

7. When obtaining information about a client's medication history, it is important for the nurse to ask the client:
   1. name, purpose, dosage, and the client's understanding of the medication.
   2. name, dosage, frequency, and manufacturer of the medication.
   3. name, dosage, frequency, and expiration date of the medication.
   4. name, purpose, dosage, frequency, duration, and client's understanding of the medication.

8. During an interview, a client denies having any medical history. Later, the client states, "I've been taking blood pressure medication for 10 years." The nurse's response should be:
   1. "Tell me the reason your healthcare provider has prescribed blood pressure medication for you."
   2. "What you are saying to me does not make any sense."
   3. "Why are you taking blood pressure medication?"
   4. "You realize that if you are taking blood pressure medication you have a history of high blood pressure, right?"

9. A woman calls the health center stating that there is something wrong with her son's penis. She uses slang terminology during the phone call. The nurse's most professional response would be:
   1. "Ma'am, I will not continue this conversation with you unless you use the proper terminology."
   2. "I would just like to clarify that you are referring to your son's penis."
   3. hang up the phone; it is most likely a prank call.
   4. use the same terminology that the client is comfortable with.

10. The nurse includes which of the following in the review of systems? (Select all that apply)
    1. Breast and axillae
    2. Emotional history
    3. Reproductive history
    4. Eye history
    5. Smoking history

Skin, Hair, and Nails 11

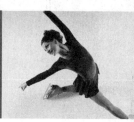

All the world is a laboratory to the inquiring mind.
—Martin H. Fischer

The integumentary system includes the skin, hair, and nails. It can reveal vital information about multiple systems when thoroughly and accurately assessed. This chapter will focus on gathering both subjective and objective data, as well as analysis of the data collected.

OBJECTIVES

At the completion of these exercises you will be able to:

1. Define key terminology associated with the integumentary system.
2. Review the anatomy and physiology of the integumentary system.
3. Select the equipment necessary to complete the assessment of the integumentary system.
4. Identify the correct techniques for assessment of the integumentary system.
5. Analyze data related to assessment of the integumentary system.
6. Recognize factors that can influence assessment findings.
7. Document an assessment of the integumentary system.
8. Apply critical thinking in analysis of a case study.
9. Relate *Healthy People 2020* objectives to the integumentary system.
10. Complete NCLEX®-style review questions related to the integumentary system.

RESOURCES

Pearson Nursing Student Resources

Find additional review materials at
nursing.pearsonhighered.com

Prepare for success with additional NCLEX®-style practice questions, interactive assignments and activities, Web links, animations and videos, and more!

Additional resources: *www.skincancer.org*

CROSSWORD PUZZLE FOR KEY TERMS

Read each definition below and fill in the correct term on the puzzle grid. If the answer requires two words do not leave a blank space between the words. Use a pencil so you can erase easily.

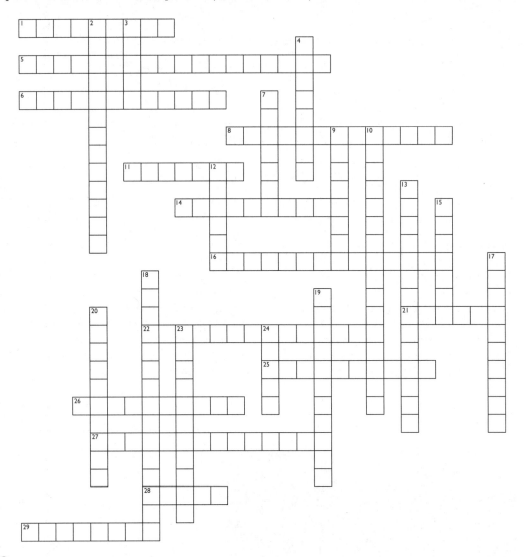

CLUES

Across

1. The outermost layer of skin on the body
5. Small parasitic insects that live on the scalp and neck **(two words)**
6. Dark, coarse, long hair that appears on eyebrows, the scalp, and the pubic region **(two words)**
8. A cheesy-white substance that coats the skin surfaces at birth **(two words)**
11. A fold of epidermal skin along the base of the nail that protects the root and sides of each nail
14. A dark line running from the umbilicus to the pubic area of pregnant women **(two words)**
16. Sudden patchy or complete loss of body hair for unknown cause **(two words)**
21. A fine, downy hair in newborns that is most prominent on the upper chest, shoulders, and back
22. Glands in the axillary and anogenital regions that are dormant until the onset of puberty **(two words)**
25. Bruising resulting from the escape of blood from a ruptured blood vessel into the tissues
26. Pale, fine, short hair that appears over the entire body except for the lips, nipples, palms of hands, soles of feet, and parts of external genitals **(two words)**
27. Gray, blue, or purple spots in the sacral and buttocks areas of newborns that fade during the first year of life **(two words)**
28. Thin plates of keratinized epidermal cells that shield the distal ends of the fingers and toes
29. Itching

Down

2. Glands that produce a clear perspiration mostly made of water and salt **(two words)**
3. Areas of tiny white facial papules
4. Patchy, depigmented skin
7. A fibrous protein that gives the epidermis its tough, protective qualities
9. The mask of pregnancy
10. Skin conditions or changes to the skin that occur following a primary lesion **(two words)**
12. A moon-shaped crescent which appears on the nail body over the thickened nail matrix
13. The initial lesions of a disease **(two words)**
15. Skin pigment produced in the melanocytes in the stratum basale
17. An inflammation of the cuticle
18. Oil glands that secrete sebum **(two words)**
19. Profuse perspiration or sweating
20. A cellular layer of subcutaneous tissue consisting of loose connective tissue
23. Separation of the nail plate from the nail bed
24. An increased accumulation of fluid in a dependent part that is caused by an accumulation of fluid in the intercellular spaces

ANATOMY & PHYSIOLOGY REVIEW

For each diagram below label the structures as indicated by the lines.

1.

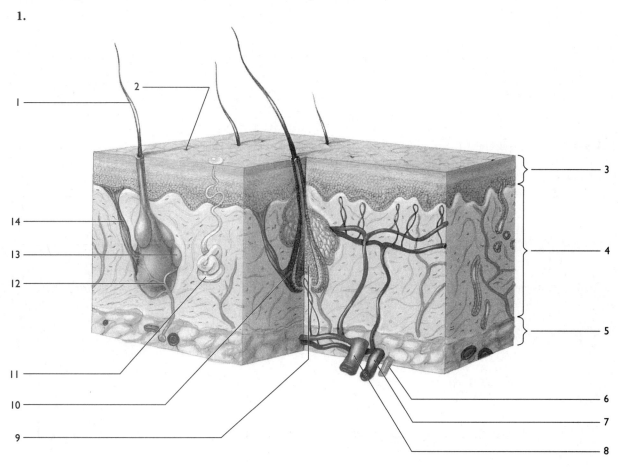

2.

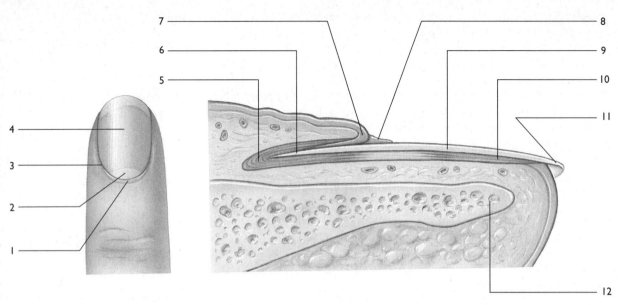

3. Read each statement. On the line provided indicate if the data is a function of the skin, subcutaneous gland, or neither.

1. Perceives pain _____

2. Creates perspiration _____

3. Synthesizes vitamin D _____

4. Protects against environmental toxins _____

5. Creates mucus _____

6. Protects against bacterial growth _____

7. Excretes vitamin D _____

8. Lubricates _____

9. Perceives touch _____

10. Converts vitamin C into uric acid _____

EQUIPMENT SELECTION

Prior to beginning the physical assessment of a client's skin, hair, and nails, it is important to gather the appropriate assessment equipment. Place a check mark next to each piece of equipment that you would need to perform this assessment.

EQUIPMENT		
Cotton balls	Lubricant	Stethoscope
Cotton-tipped applicator	Magnifying glass	Tape measure
Drape sheet	Otoscope	Test tubes
Examination gown	Penlight	Thermometer
Flashlight	Ruler (cm or in.)	Tongue blade
Gauze	Skinfold calipers	Vision chart
Gloves	Skin-marking pen	Watch with second hand
Goggles	Slides	Wood's lamp

ASSESSMENT TECHNIQUES

Review each assessment technique. If the technique is correct, circle the number. If the technique is incorrect, write the correct assessment technique on the line provided.

1. When examining a client's skin, it is best to have the client fully disrobed and in a supine position on an examination table.

2. Explain that you will be touching the client in various areas with different parts of your hand.

3. It is best to determine a client's skin temperature using the ulnar surface of the hand.

4. When palpating for skin texture, it is best to use the palmar surface of fingers and finger pads.

5. Skin turgor can be assessed on the adult by using the forefinger and thumb to grasp the skin superior to the clavicle or on the lateral aspect of the wrist.

6. The assessment technique used to grade edema on a 4-point scale is inspection.

7. When assessing a client's scalp and hair, it is best to divide the hair at 1-inch intervals.

8. When assessing for hair texture, it is appropriate to roll a few strands of hair between your thumb and forefinger.

_____

_____

9. Capillary refill can be assessed by depressing the cuticle briefly to blanch and then quickly releasing.

_____

_____

10. The spooning technique can be performed to assess clubbing.

_____

_____

ASSESSMENT FINDINGS

Read each assessment finding. Determine if the finding is normal or abnormal. Write an A for abnormal and an N for normal on each line provided.

_____ 1. Pallor	_____ 11. +2 edema
_____ 2. Warm and dry	_____ 12. Ecchymoses
_____ 3. Jaundice	_____ 13. Tinea capitis
_____ 4. Free from odor	_____ 14. Thick hair
_____ 5. Freckles	_____ 15. Brittle hair
_____ 6. Fine network of thin veins on the eyelids	_____ 16. Bluish tint to nail beds
_____ 7. Fine sheen of perspiration	_____ 17. Gray scaly patches on scalp
_____ 8. Smooth and firm	_____ 18. 160° nail curvature
_____ 9. Pruritus	_____ 19. Spoon nails
_____ 10. Decreased skin turgor	_____ 20. Senile lentigines

FACTORS THAT INFLUENCE PHYSICAL ASSESSMENT FINDINGS

Fill in the blank to complete each statement about expected findings in assessment of the integumentary system.

1. Melasma occurs more frequently in _____ women.

2. Sparse body hair is common in the _____ culture.

3. When assessing dark skinned clients for skin color changes, it is best to inspect the _____, _____, _____, and _____.

4. The fine, downy hair on a newborn is replaced with _____ hair within a few months.

5. The older adult has a (an) _____ in sweat gland activity.

6. Many _____ females develop striae gravidarum.

7. Adolescents are prone to _____ because of the increased production of sebum.

8. Infants have inefficient _____ regulation.

9. Indian and Arabic females may decorate their skin with _____.

10. Compulsive behaviors related to stress may be demonstrated by _____ or _____.

ABNORMAL FINDINGS

Write the name of each lesion on the first line next to each illustration. On the second line write two associated characteristics. Finally, on the third line provide an example of that type of lesion.

Example

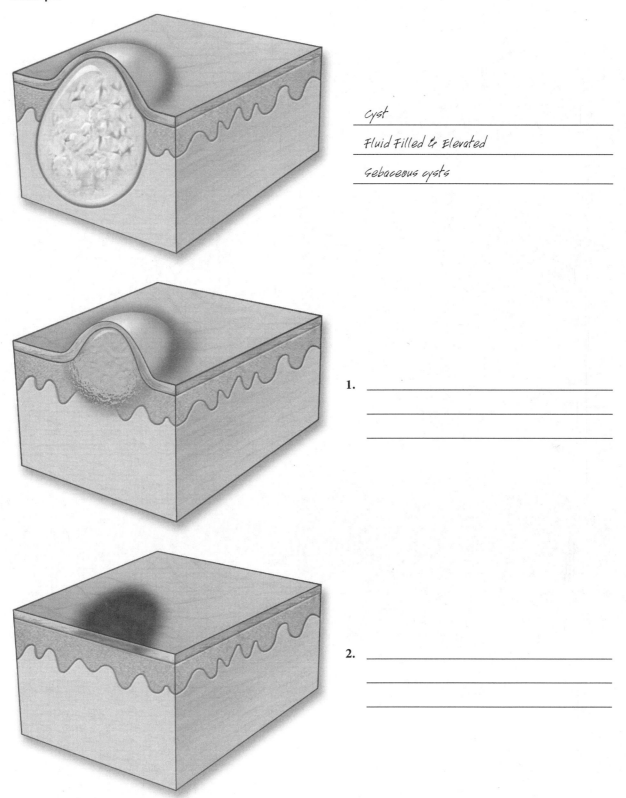

Cyst

Fluid Filled & Elevated

Sebaceous cysts

1. _____

_____

_____

2. _____

_____

_____

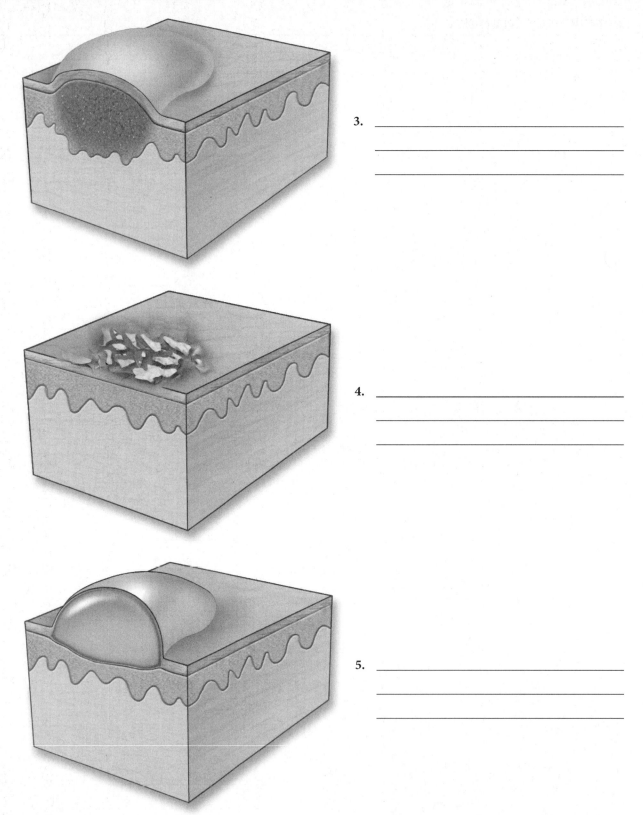

3. _____

_____

_____

4. _____

_____

_____

5. _____

_____

_____

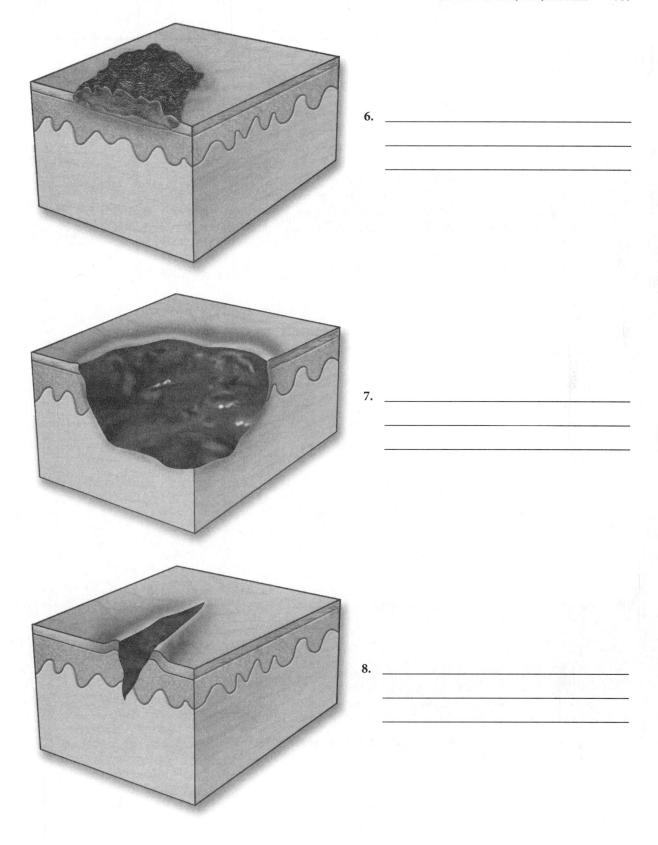

6. _____

_____

_____

7. _____

_____

_____

8. _____

_____

_____

APPLICATION OF THE CRITICAL THINKING PROCESS

Read the following scenarios and answer the questions.

SCENARIO A

Mr. Young is a 22-year-old male who presents to a clinic with symptoms of a common cold. After gathering data for a health history, you learn that he has worked for his father's landscape company since he was 16 years old. When assessing his posterior thorax for breath sounds, you notice a 5 mm × 2 mm lesion on the posterior neck. When you question Mr. Young about this lesion, he states "I could feel something there but I thought it was a patch of dry skin." He also states that it has been there for at least 6 months. You learn that Mr. Young does not apply sunscreen to his body when he is landscaping and often removes his shirt when he feels too hot. As you continue to assess the lesion, you note it has rounded pearly edges with a central mild ulceration.

1. Identify two subjective behaviors presented by Mr. Young:

   A.

   B.

2. Identify two objective behaviors noted by the nurse:

   A.

   B.

3. Two risk factors identified by Mr. Young are:

   A.

   B.

4. What type of lesion do you suspect this to be?

During the remainder of the assessment, you learn that Mr. Young intermittently experiences a stinging sensation at the site of the lesion. He began experiencing this when he first noticed the lesion 6 months ago.

5. Place the data collected into the OLDCART & ICE assessment. If the assessment is incomplete, write questions that the nurse should ask to complete the assessment.

   O

   L

   D

C

A

R

T

I

C

E

6. Explain the ABCDE criteria for skin cancer screening.

   A

   B

   C

   D

   E

7. Read the following *Healthy People 2020* objective: "Reduce the rate of sunburn."

   Explain how a nurse could have used this objective to prevent skin cancer in Mr. Young.

SCENARIO B

Julia is a 6-year-old girl who was sent to the school nurse's office for an itch on her scalp. She states it started the night before and is becoming very annoying. After putting on a pair of clean gloves, you begin to inspect her long, light blonde hair and note tiny white nits along multiple hair shafts. You also note her scalp in the occipital region is reddened and excoriated. You determine that Julia has pediculosis capitis. (Additional resources may be necessary to complete this scenario.)

1. List the subjective and objective data gathered that lead you to this conclusion.

   Subjective Data:

   Objective Data:

2. Can Julia be sent back to class? Explain.

3. What teaching must be done and with whom in this situation?

4. State your learning goal for the client and (or) parent.

5. Write two objectives to support your above learning goal.

   A.

   B.

6. Explain how you will evaluate the goal stated above in question 4.

ASSESSMENT AND DOCUMENTATION

Perform an integumentary assessment on your lab partner and document your findings on the provided documentation form. You can download the form from the Pearson Student Resources site.

NCLEX®-STYLE REVIEW QUESTIONS

Read each question carefully. Choose the best answer for each question.

1. The nurse knows that which of the following are major functions of the skin? (Select all that apply)
   1. Perception of pain and pressure
   2. Regulation of body temperature
   3. Vitamin E synthesis
   4. Protection of fluid and electrolyte loss
   5. Protection against bacterial invasion

2. The nurse knows that which of the following are considered vascular lesions? (Select all that apply)
   1. Port wine stain
   2. Hematoma
   3. Petechia
   4. Keloid
   5. Pustule

3. During a skin assessment, the nurse notices a lesion that is coiled and twisted in shape. The nurse will document this as:
   1. linear.
   2. annular.
   3. gyrate.
   4. confluent.

4. A client is asking a nurse questions about skin cancer. The nurse explains to the client that the least common but most serious type of skin cancer is:
   1. basal cell carcinoma.
   2. squamous cell carcinoma.
   3. malignant melanoma.
   4. Kaposi's sarcoma.

5. A nurse is assessing the nails of a newly admitted client to a long-term care facility. She notes redness, swelling, and tenderness to the cuticle of the third and fourth left digits. This is also known as:
   1. hirsutism.
   2. paronychia.
   3. onycholysis.
   4. folliculitis.

6. When assessing a client's nails, the nurse notices horizontal white bands in multiple fingers. This could indicate:
   1. arteriosclerosis.
   2. hepatic or renal disease.
   3. hypoxia.
   4. vitamin deficiencies.

7. Skin turgor assesses the elasticity and mobility of the skin. The nurse knows that which of the following is true about skin turgor? Skin turgor is: (Select all that apply)
   1. decreased in dehydrated clients.
   2. decreased in clients with scleroderma.
   3. decreased in clients who have lost large amounts of weight.
   4. increased in clients with connective tissue disorders that harden the skin.
   5. increased turgor results in tenting of the skin.

8. Which of the following lesions would the nurse consider abnormal when assessing the skin of an older adult client?
   1. Cherry angiomas
   2. Cutaneous tags
   3. Senile lentigines
   4. Chloasma

9. A nurse working in the emergency department is assessing a rectal temperature on an Asian newborn. The nurse notices a bluish-purple discoloration to the sacral area. The nurse's next step should be to:
   1. notify the Division of Youth and Family Services for suspected abuse.
   2. bring the child to the attention of the healthcare provider immediately because of suspected trauma.
   3. continue with her assessment and disregard the finding.
   4. seek clarification with the parents that the discoloration is a Mongolian spot.

10. Spoon nails are commonly associated with:
    1. iron deficiency.
    2. vitamin B_1 deficiency.
    3. vitamin D deficiency.
    4. deficiency of fat-soluble vitamins.

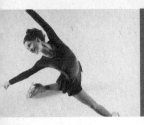

12 Head, Neck, and Related Lymphatics

The will to win is important, but the will to prepare is vital.
—Joe Paterno

The head and neck may appear to be a small region in relation to the rest of the body; however, a thorough assessment of this region can lead to vital information in other body systems. This chapter will focus on gathering both subjective and objective data, as well as analysis of the data collected.

OBJECTIVES

At the completion of these exercises you will be able to:

1. Define key terminology associated with the head, neck, and related lymphatics.
2. Review the anatomy and physiology of the head, neck, and related lymphatics.
3. Select the equipment necessary to complete the assessment of the head, neck, and related lymphatics.
4. Identify the correct techniques for assessment of the head, neck, and related lymphatics.
5. Analyze data related to assessment of the head, neck, and related lymphatics.
6. Recognize factors that can influence assessment findings.
7. Assess the head, neck, and related lymphatics on a laboratory partner.
8. Document an assessment of the head, neck, and related lymphatics.
9. Apply critical thinking in analysis of a case study.
10. Relate *Healthy People 2020* objectives to the head, neck, and related lymphatics.
11. Complete NCLEX®-style review questions related to assessment of the head, neck, and related lymphatics.

RESOURCES

Pearson Nursing Student Resources

Find additional review materials at
nursing.pearsonhighered.com

Prepare for success with additional NCLEX®-style practice questions, interactive assignments and activities, Web links, animations and videos, and more!

Additional resources: *www.CDC.gov*

WORD SEARCH

Find and circle the correct term in the word search puzzle for each of the definitions listed below. The word may be horizontal, vertical, or diagonal.

```
C  H  O  V  T  G  S  B  T  H  Y  O  I  D  K  B  H  V  P  U  C  S  H
L  Y  M  P  H  A  D  E  N  O  P  A  T  H  Y  A  L  I  H  A  K  T  V
Z  P  A  V  Y  Y  Y  L  G  O  I  T  E  R  E  C  Q  L  J  Q  C  T  N
E  O  N  L  R  K  K  L  C  L  O  P  L  S  Q  R  V  D  A  G  M  V  Q
V  T  T  V  O  X  R  S  R  R  H  E  N  L  Z  O  E  R  Y  R  X  K  S
D  H  E  N  I  C  A  P  A  Y  V  T  M  Q  A  M  B  Q  C  V  T  I  E
Z  Y  R  R  D  R  C  A  N  G  F  F  O  Z  L  E  A  X  V  W  L  L  M
W  R  I  J  G  E  N  L  I  V  L  Y  Z  F  M  G  V  H  J  L  G  P  A
D  O  O  N  L  L  K  S  O  Z  M  A  Z  O  C  A  D  V  O  N  S  O  H
O  I  R  O  A  G  Z  Y  S  S  D  G  R  K  O  L  F  C  A  Z  U  I  A
W  D  T  R  N  U  W  W  Y  Y  J  D  D  B  D  Y  I  I  E  T  T  Z  T
N  I  R  G  D  T  V  A  N  U  N  E  D  O  Z  T  R  B  D  C  U  G  L
S  S  I  K  N  J  R  N  O  Y  Y  A  K  E  R  T  D  F  X  G  R  Z  A
Y  M  A  Y  T  R  T  I  S  X  X  R  O  O  R  C  C  R  C  F  E  K  S
N  E  N  Q  Q  S  D  S  T  U  X  C  T  O  W  M  F  M  U  K  S  L  H
D  B  G  L  A  L  G  W  O  K  Q  Q  I  G  O  O  L  Z  M  D  Y  E  D
R  W  L  K  D  N  T  Z  S  P  V  R  L  F  H  G  N  R  L  A  F  Q  U
O  T  E  K  I  L  M  G  I  X  E  M  E  W  K  P  X  Z  L  H  X  Q  B
M  L  V  H  W  F  K  V  S  T  A  A  F  S  T  O  P  N  C  P  N  I  E
E  A  S  F  V  G  Q  Z  S  R  O  B  J  K  X  P  S  U  K  J  F  T  S
D  U  W  X  Z  O  C  O  E  N  C  W  K  F  D  T  C  U  J  E  F  Z  U
C  K  T  V  H  Y  P  E  R  T  H  Y  R  O  I  D  I  S  M  T  P  R  X
P  B  Z  W  I  L  C  E  H  Y  D  R  O  C  E  P  H  A  L  U  S  V  K
```

CLUES

1. A disorder caused by overproduction of growth hormone by the pituitary gland _____
2. A landmark area of the anterior neck bordered by the mandible, the midline of the neck, and the anterior aspect of the sternocleidomastoid (**two words**) _____ _____
3. The first cervical vertebra, which carries the skull _____
4. The second cervical vertebra, which supports the movement of the head _____
5. A temporary disorder affecting cranial nerve VII and producing unilateral facial paralysis (**two words**) _____ _____
6. A condition that results in cranial deformity due to premature fusion of the cranial bones _____
7. Abnormality in which increased adrenal hormone production leads to a rounded "moon" face, ruddy cheeks, prominent jowls, and excess facial hair (**two words**) _____ _____
8. A chromosomal defect that causes varying degrees of mental retardation (**two words**) _____ _____
9. Enlargement of the thyroid gland that is commonly visible as swelling of the anterior neck _____
10. The enlargement of the head caused by inadequate drainage of the cerebrospinal fluid, resulting in abnormal growth of the skull _____
11. A bone that is suspended in the neck approximately 2 cm above the larynx _____

12. The excessive production of thyroid hormones, resulting in enlargement of the gland, exophthalmos, fine hair, weight loss, and other alterations _____

13. Metabolic disorder causing enlarged thyroid due to iodine deficiency _____

14. The enlargement of lymph nodes, which is often caused by infection, allergies, or a tumor _____

15. A landmark area of the posterior neck bordered by the trapezius muscle, the sternocleidomastoid muscle, and the clavicle (**two words**) _____ _____

16. Nonmovable joints that connect two bones _____

17. The largest gland of the endocrine system, which is butterfly shaped and is located in the anterior portion of the neck (**two words**) _____ _____

18. A spasm of the sternocleidomastoid muscle on one side of the body _____

ANATOMY & PHYSIOLOGY REVIEW

1. For each diagram below, label the structures as indicated by the lines.

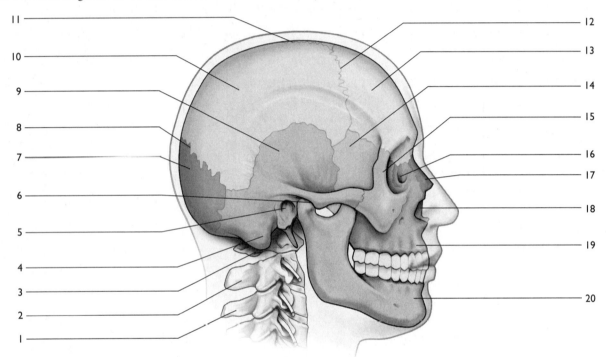

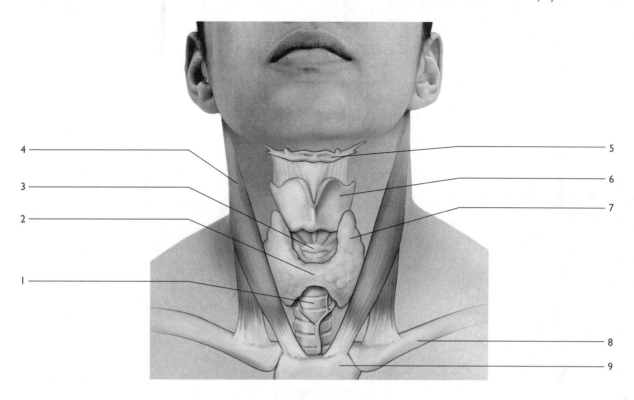

4
3
2
1

5
6
7
8
9

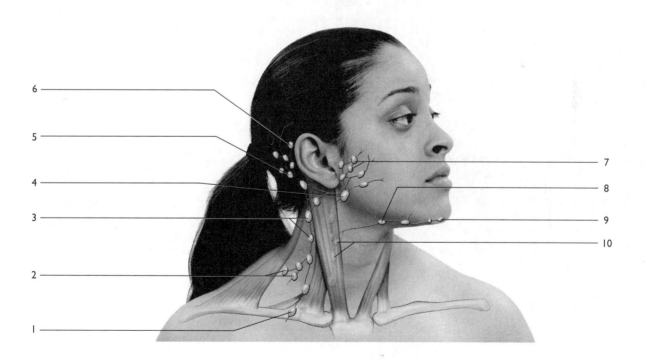

6
5
4
3
2
1

7
8
9
10

2. List the anatomical landmarks used for the anterior triangle of the neck:

    1.

    2.

    3.

3. List the anatomical landmarks used for the posterior triangle of the neck:

    1.

    2.

    3.

4. Use a pencil to shade in the anterior and posterior triangles of the neck.

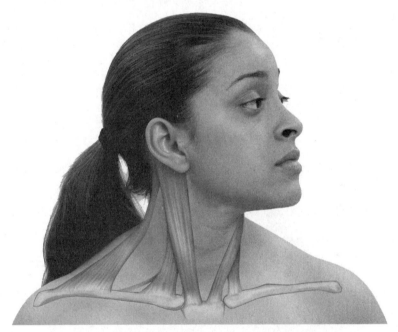

EQUIPMENT SELECTION

Prior to beginning the physical assessment of a client's head, neck, and lymphatics, it is important to gather the appropriate equipment. Place a check mark next to each piece of equipment that you would need to perform this assessment.

EQUIPMENT		
Cotton balls	Lubricant	Sphygmomanometer
Cotton-tipped applicator	Nasal speculum	Stethoscope
Culture media	Ophthalmoscope	Tape measure
Dental mirror	Otoscope	Test tubes
Doppler ultrasonic stethoscope	Penlight	Thermometer
Drape sheet	Reflex hammer	Tongue blade
Examination gown	Ruler	Transilluminator
Flashlight	Skinfold calipers	Tuning fork
Gauze	Skin-marking pen	Vaginal speculum
Gloves	Slides	Vision chart
Goggles	Small towel	Watch with second hand
Goniometer	Specimen containers	Water in cup

ASSESSMENT TECHNIQUES

Review each assessment technique. If the technique is correct, circle the number. If the technique is incorrect, write the correct assessment technique on the line provided.

1. When examining a client's head and neck, it is best to have the client fully disrobed and in a supine position on an examination table.

    _____

    _____

2. Explain that you will be touching the client in various areas with different parts of your hand.

    _____

    _____

3. Explain to the client the need to remove items that would interfere with the assessment, such as hair clips, hats, scarves, or veils.

    _____

    _____

4. Palpate for the temporal artery between the trachea and sternocleidomastoid using the finger pads.

    _____

    _____

5. When palpating the thyroid gland by standing behind the client, the examiner's left hand will push the trachea to the right. The thyroid would be palpated with the examiner's right hand.

    _____

    _____

6. The thyroid cannot be auscultated for bruits.

    _____

    _____

7. Lymph nodes are palpated by exerting moderate pressure in a vertical motion.

   _____

   _____

8. The best order to examine the lymph nodes of the head and neck is from the cervical chains to the jaw followed by the supraclavicular region.

   _____

   _____

9. The trachea should be palpated using the thumb and the index finger.

   _____

   _____

10. Percussion of the trachea is best done with a bimanual method.

    _____

    _____

ASSESSMENT FINDINGS

Read each assessment finding. Identify the finding as normal or abnormal by writing an A for abnormal and an N for normal on each line provided.

_____ 1. Nasolabial folds equal

_____ 2. Facial movements smooth

_____ 3. TMJ crepitation

_____ 4. Nuchal rigidity

_____ 5. Smooth trachea

_____ 6. Non-palpable thyroid

_____ 7. Lymphadenopathy

_____ 8. Tenderness to the temporal artery

_____ 9. Jugular vein distention

_____ 10. Movement of the trachea when client swallows

_____ 11. Scaliness of the scalp

_____ 12. Normocephalic

_____ 13. Unilateral facial paralysis

_____ 14. Slight tremors of the lips

_____ 15. Torticollis

_____ 16. Hyperextension of the neck

_____ 17. Goiter

_____ 18. Thyroid bruit

_____ 19. Non-palpable occipital node

_____ 20. Tenderness to scalp

FACTORS THAT INFLUENCE PHYSICAL ASSESSMENT FINDINGS

Fill in the blank to complete each statement.

1. Thyroid disorders are common in areas where _____ is limited.

2. The ability for an infant to control his/her head occurs at about _____ months.

3. The older female adult may develop coarse hair on the _____.

4. A disorder that may be seen in infants whose mothers ingest significant amounts of alcohol during pregnancy is called _____ _____ _____.

5. The posterior fontanel is a _____ shape.

6. The _____ adult loses subcutaneous fat in the face.

7. Psychological stress may lead to physical pain, most commonly in the _____ or _____.

8. The thyroid may _____ in size during pregnancy.

9. In the Muslim culture it is common for the females to cover their _____ and _____.

10. The range of motion (ROM) of the cervical spine may be limited because of _____ of the vertebrae.

APPLICATION OF THE CRITICAL THINKING PROCESS

Read the scenario and answer the following questions.

Ronnie is a 22-year-old African American male who works for the environmental services department at a small community hospital. He cleans client rooms upon discharge and maintains the cleanliness of the hallways. Everyone at the hospital knows Ronnie because he is always friendly and always smiling. Over the past 2 months, Ronnie hasn't been his usual cheerful self and has appeared very sweaty and anxious at times while performing his typical duties. When asked if anything is wrong, he simply states "I haven't been sleeping well at night." He also apprehensively reveals that his stomach "hasn't been right" and that he has been having "frequent episodes of diarrhea." His face appears thinner, and he admits to losing 12 lb in the past month or so.

1. List five pieces of subjective data in the above scenario:

   1.

   2.

   3.

   4.

   5.

Ronnie is seen in the emergency department the next day, when he complains of heart palpitations and a slight uncontrollable tremor in his left hand.

2. List five questions the nurse should ask Ronnie upon his arrival to the emergency department.

   1.

   2.

   3.

   4.

   5.

During the health history, the nurse notices that Ronnie has exophthalmus. When further investigating this finding, Ronnie states he seldom looks at himself in a mirror and has not noticed the bulging of his eyes. He states that he thinks he may need a stronger eyeglass prescription because his vision has been more blurry than usual.

3. Define exophthalmus.

4. What may be responsible for Ronnie's variety of signs and symptoms?

5. Write three focused interview questions that would assist in gathering further data for Ronnie.

   1.

   2.

   3.

6. Use OLDCART & ICE to identify data related to pain.

7. List the questions the nurse should ask to complete the pain assessment.

HEALTHY PEOPLE 2020

A *Healthy People 2020* objective is:

Increase the proportion of motorcyclists using helmets.

1. What are the laws in your city or town related to helmet use for cyclists? Is this a local or state ordinance?

2. Discuss how a nurse can use this objective to promote and maintain the health and optimal function of the structures of the head and neck.

ASSESSMENT AND DOCUMENTATION

Perform a head, neck, and lymphatic assessment on your lab partner and document your findings on the provided documentation form. You can download the form from the Pearson Student Resources site.

NCLEX®-STYLE REVIEW QUESTIONS

Read each question carefully. Choose the best answer for each question.

1. The nurse knows that mobility in the cervical spine is greatest at the level of:
   1. C_1, C_2, and C_3.
   2. C_3, C_4, and C_5.
   3. C_4, C_5, and C_6.
   4. C_5, C_6, and C_7.

2. The nurse understands that the anterior fontanelle is formed by the:
   1. coronal suture, the frontal suture, and the sagittal suture.
   2. sagittal suture, the lambdoidal suture, and the coronal suture.
   3. coronal suture, the frontal suture, and the lambdoidal suture.
   4. sagittal suture, the frontal suture, and the lambdoidal suture.

3. Which of the following questions would be inappropriate for the nurse to ask when conducting a focused interview with a client who has suffered an acute head injury?
    1. "Did anyone witness your injury?"
    2. "Have you experienced nausea or vomiting since your injury?"
    3. "Where on your head are you experiencing pain?"
    4. "How often do you wash your hair?"

4. The nurse knows that enlarged palpable lymph nodes may be indicative of:
    1. malignancy or infection.
    2. infection or thrombosis.
    3. vascular occlusion or malignancy.
    4. thrombosis or vascular occlusion.

5. An infant is diagnosed with fetal alcohol syndrome. The nurse performs an assessment and knows that which of the following assessment findings support this diagnosis?
    1. deformed upper lip
    2. widened palpebral fissures
    3. deep nasolabial folds
    4. "moon" face

6. The nurse understands an increased production of growth hormone can lead to:
    1. hydrocephalus.
    2. craniosynostosis.
    3. Cushing's syndrome.
    4. acromegaly.

7. A client presents to a busy urban emergency department complaining of pain that radiates from the base of the cervical spine to the right frontal region of the head. The client describes the pain as a dull, steady ache that began in the morning and has gradually increased in intensity throughout the day. The nurse identifies these symptoms most likely indicate a:
    1. cluster headache.
    2. tension headache.
    3. spinal headache.
    4. classic migraine.

8. The nurse is examining a client's neck. Which of the following movements of the neck will the nurse assess when testing range of motion (ROM)? (Select all that apply)
    1. Lateral flexion
    2. Rotation
    3. Hyperextension
    4. Abduction
    5. Forward flexion

9. An adult client presents to the outpatient clinic with a 2-day history of shortness of breath. While at the clinic, the client's respiratory rate increases rapidly, and the client appears cyanotic. The nurse notes the client's trachea is deviated from the midline. The nurse identifies that this client is most likely experiencing:
    1. pneumothorax.
    2. lung cancer.
    3. myocardial infarction.
    4. pulmonary embolism.

10. The nurse is assessing a client's ear. The top of the ear should be equal to the:
    1. pinna.
    2. nasolabial folds.
    3. brow.
    4. lateral canthus.

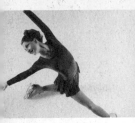

13 Eye

It is better to trust the eyes than the ears.
—German Proverb

The eye is a sensory organ that is responsible for vision. A thorough assessment of the eye will include structural, visual, and neuromuscular testing. This chapter will focus on gathering both subjective and objective data, as well as analysis of the data collected.

OBJECTIVES

At the completion of these exercises you will be able to:

1. Define key terminology associated with the eye.
2. Review the anatomy and physiology of the eye.
3. Select the equipment necessary to complete an assessment of the eye.
4. Identify the correct techniques for assessment of the eye.
5. Analyze objective and subjective data related to assessment of the eye.
6. Recognize factors that can influence assessment findings.
7. Perform an assessment of the eye on your laboratory partner.
8. Document an assessment of the eye.
9. Apply critical thinking in analysis of a case study.
10. Relate *Healthy People 2020* objectives to the eye.
11. Complete NCLEX®-style review questions related to the assessment of the eye.

RESOURCES

Pearson Nursing Student Resources

Find additional review materials at
nursing.pearsonhighered.com

Prepare for success with additional NCLEX®-style practice questions, interactive assignments and activities, Web links, animations and videos, and more!

Additional resources: *www.CDC.gov*

CROSSWORD PUZZLE FOR KEY TERMS

Read each definition below and fill in the correct term on the puzzle grid. If the answer requires two words do not leave a blank space between the words. Use a pencil so you can erase easily.

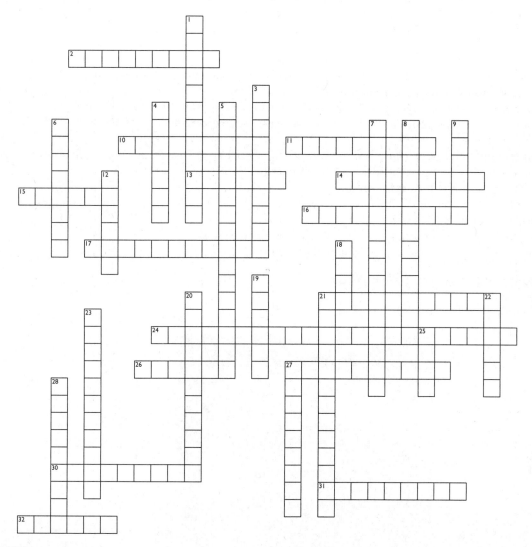

CLUES

Across

2. Rapid fluttering or constant involuntary movement of the eye
10. Outward turning of the eye
11. Prolonged dilation of the pupil of the eye
13. Nearsightedness
14. Farsightedness
15. The window of the eye
16. Decreased ability of the eye lens to change shape to accommodate for near vision
17. Inflammation of the eyelid
21. A condition in which the refraction of light is spread over a wide area rather than on a distinct point on the retina
24. The simultaneous response of one pupil to the stimuli applied to the other (**two words**)
26. The outermost layer of the eye
27. The normal refractive condition of the eye
30. The eyelids
31. The creamy yellow area on the retina of the eye where the optic nerve leaves the eye (**two words**)
32. The inner back surface of the internal eye

Down

1. A clear, fluidlike substance found in the anterior segment of the eye that helps maintain ocular pressure **(two words)**
3. A condition in which the axes of the eyes cannot be directed at the same object
4. The vascular pigmented mid-layer of the eye
5. Swelling of the soft tissue in the periorbital area **(two words)**
6. A condition that causes the lens to thicken and yellow
7. The opening between the upper and lower eyelids **(two words)**
8. A clear gel in the posterior eye that is refractory and maintains intraocular pressure **(two words)**
9. The third and innermost membrane, the sensory portion of the eye
12. A hyperpigmented spot on the temporal aspect of the retina responsible for central vision
18. A biconvex, situated directly behind the pupil that is flexible and transparent
19. One eyelid drooping
20. Movement of the two eyes so that the coordination of an image falls at corresponding points of the two retinas
21. The ability of the eye to automatically adjust clear vision from far to near or a variety of distances
22. Prolonged constriction of the pupil of the eye
23. The total area of vision in which objects can be seen while the eye remains focused on a central point **(two words)**
25. The circular, colored muscular aspect of the eye's middle layer
27. The inversion of the lid and lashes caused by muscle spasm of the eyelid
28. The eversion of the lower eyelid caused by muscle weakness

ANATOMY & PHYSIOLOGY REVIEW

1. For each diagram below, write the name of the structure indicated by each line.

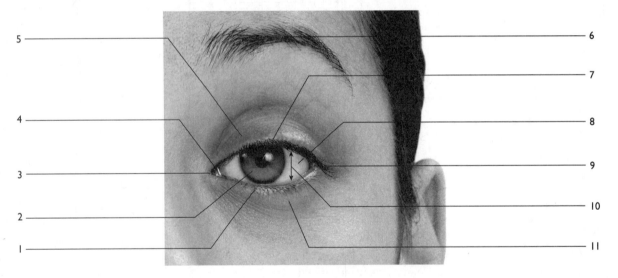

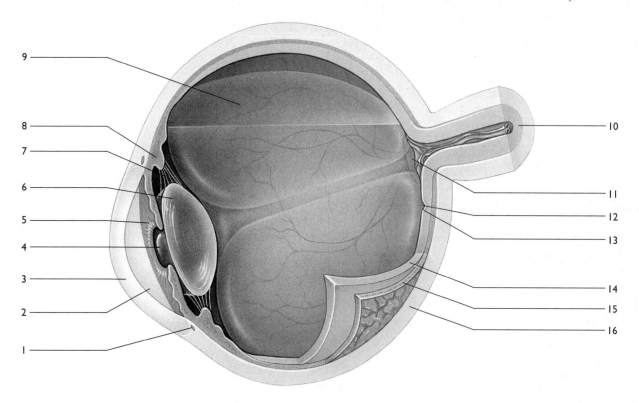

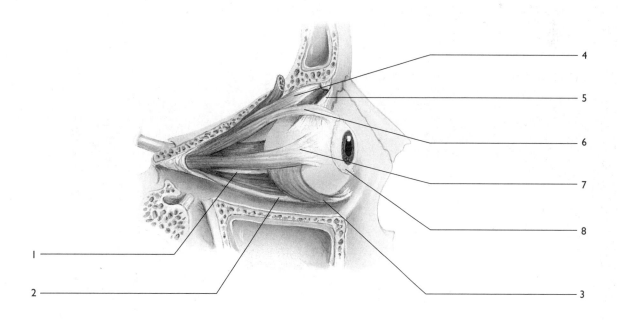

2. Read each statement carefully. Identify each as True or False by circling the word True or False. If the statement is False, rewrite the statement correctly in the space provided.

1. Light rays travel in a straight line and must refract in order for vision to occur.

   True   **False**

   Correction: _____

2. The crystalline lens is solely responsible for the refraction of light rays.

   True   **False**

   Correction: _____

3. When refraction occurs, the rays are reflected to the cornea for the most accurate vision.

   True   **False**

   Correction: _____

4. Aqueous humor is a refractory medium.

   True   **False**

   Correction: _____

5. The anterior and posterior segments of the eye are separated by the retina.

   True   **False**

   Correction: _____

6. A retinal image is conducted to the occipital nerve.

   True   **False**

   Correction: _____

7. The optic chiasm is the site for crossover of the nerve fingers.

   True   **False**

   Correction: _____

8. Impulses from the eye are transmitted to the temporal lobe of the brain for interpretation.

   True   **False**

   Correction: _____

3. Label each picture with the cranial nerves responsible for the eye movement.

1 _____

2 _____

3 _____

4 ——————————————————————————

5 ——————————————————————————

6 ——————————————————————————

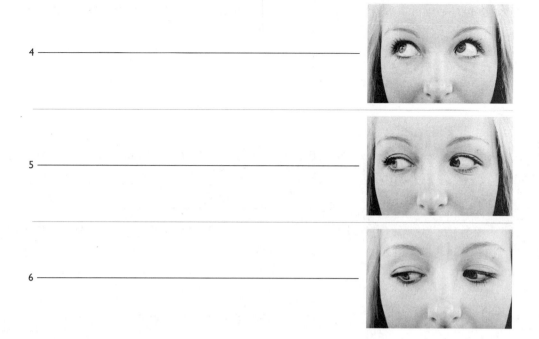

EQUIPMENT SELECTION

Prior to beginning the physical assessment of a client's skin, hair, and nails, it is important to gather the appropriate assessment equipment. Place a check mark next to each piece of equipment that you would need to perform this assessment.

EQUIPMENT					
	Acuity chart		Lubricant		Sphygmomanometer
	Cotton-tipped applicator		Nasal speculum		Stethoscope
	Culture media		Ophthalmoscope		Tape measure
	Dental mirror		Otoscope		Test tubes
	Doppler ultrasonic stethoscope		Penlight		Thermometer
	Drape sheet		Reflex hammer		Tongue blade
	Eye cover		Ruler		Transilluminator
	Flashlight		Skinfold calipers		Tuning fork
	Gauze		Skin-marking pen		Vaginal speculum
	Gloves		Slides		Vision chart
	Goggles		Small towel		Watch with second hand
	Goniometer		Specimen containers		Wood's lamp

ASSESSMENT TECHNIQUES

Review each assessment technique. If the technique is correct, circle the number. If the technique is incorrect, write the correct assessment technique on the line provided.

1. Position the client approximately 40 inches away from the Rosenbaum Chart to assess near vision.

   _____

   _____

2. When assessing distant vision with the Snellen Chart, ask the client to remove eyeglasses first and then repeat with eyeglasses on.

   _____

   _____

3. When positioning a client to test the six cardinal fields of gaze, the nurse should be at eye level with the client.

_____

_____

4. In order to assess the corneal light reflex, the nurse should instruct the client to stare directly into the penlight.

_____

_____

5. When testing visual fields by confrontation, the client should be sitting about 1 foot from the nurse.

_____

_____

6. When testing visual fields by confrontation, the client should cover one eye with a card while the nurse covers his/her own opposite eye.

_____

_____

7. The corneal reflex is stimulated by gently wisping a piece of cotton on the cornea.

_____

_____

8. In order to evaluate pupillary response, the nurse should dim the lighting in the room.

_____

_____

9. To examine the client's right eye, the nurse should hold the ophthalmoscope in his left hand.

_____

_____

10. If a client's vision is hyperopic, the diopter wheel should be rotated into the plus numbers.

_____

_____

ASSESSMENT FINDINGS

Read each assessment finding. Identify the finding as normal or abnormal by writing an A for abnormal and an N for normal on each line provided.

_____ 1. 20/200 vision

_____ 2. Nystagmus

_____ 3. PERRLA

_____ 4. Bilateral blinking when one cornea is touched

_____ 5. Equal distance between palpebral fissures

_____ 6. Fine network of thin veins on the external eyelids

_____ 7. Red reflex of the pupil

_____ 8. Pink conjunctiva

_____ 9. Ptosis of the lids

_____ 10. Symmetrical reflection of light on the cornea

_____ 11. Dark spots on the retina

_____ 12. Emmetropia

_____ 13. Lack of convergence

_____ 14. Opaque lens

_____ 15. Irregular shape to the optic disc

_____ 16. Small white spot in the center of the macula

_____ 17. Firm eyeballs

_____ 18. Convergence

_____ 19. Presbyopia

_____ 20. Round and equal pupils

FACTORS THAT INFLUENCE PHYSICAL ASSESSMENT FINDINGS

Fill in the blank to complete each statement.

1. In the assessment of a 3-week-old baby girl with both parents of Irish descent, you expect the irises of her eyes to be _____ in color.

2. A female, 7 months pregnant, has been wearing her eyeglasses instead of her contacts for the past 2 weeks. This is most likely because pregnant women are prone to _____ _____.

3. A 5-year-old visits the eye doctor for the first time. He learns that his eyes will be adult size when he is _____ years old.

4. A 52-year-old female, visiting a plastic surgeon, is complaining about a drooping appearance of her eyes. The surgeon explains to the client the drooping is caused by a loss of _____.

5. A 3-year-old from an underdeveloped area of Africa is experiencing blindness due to a deficiency of vitamin _____.

6. A 38-year-old female visits the tanning parlor three times per week. She also enjoys sunbathing as frequently as she can. She does not like to wear sunglasses or eye shields because she does not like the "tan lines." These practices will increase her risk for _____.

7. A general contractor who is responsible for building a science lab at the local junior college has learned it is important to wear _____ _____ when he goes to work.

8. A 25-year-old female is being told by her ophthalmologist that she needs eyeglasses. He explains that her Hispanic culture has the _____ rates of visual impairments compared to other cultures.

9. An African American female has been diagnosed with diabetes. She is concerned because she has learned that uncontrolled diabetes can lead to diabetic retinopathy. This complication may lead to _____.

10. When the nurse is assessing the eyes of an Asian client, prominent _____ _____ are noted.

APPLICATION OF THE CRITICAL THINKING PROCESS

Read the scenario and answer the following questions.

Jordan is a 5-year-old girl in kindergarten. After recess she complains to her teacher that her right eye is bothering her. The teacher sends her to the school nurse who looks at Jordan and believes she has pink eye (conjunctivitis).

1. What physical assessment findings would support the school nurse's assumption?

2. How will the nurse test Jordan's visual acuity? Explain your answer.

The school nurse continues to assess Jordan. The nurse plans to assess Jordan's pain level.

3. List two pain scales that would be appropriate for the nurse to use.

4. After Jordan is sent home with her mother, the school nurse visits the kindergarten class to review good hand hygiene practices with the students. Why would the nurse select this as a topic at this time?

HEALTHY PEOPLE 2020

A *Healthy People 2020* objective is:

Reduce the number of occupational eye injuries.

1. Name three occupations where eye safety should be a priority.

   1.

   2.

   3.

2. Discuss how an occupational health nurse can use this objective to promote and maintain health and function of the structures of the eye.

ASSESSMENT AND DOCUMENTATION

Perform an eye assessment on your lab partner and document your findings on the provided documentation form. You can download the form from the Pearson Student Resources site.

NCLEX®-STYLE REVIEW QUESTIONS

Read each question carefully. Choose the best answer for each question.

1. In which environment is mydriasis most likely to occur?
   1. A movie theatre
   2. A park
   3. An examination room
   4. A swimming pool

2. The nurse knows that which of the following is (are) true about the conjunctiva? (Select all that apply)
   1. Lines the interior of the eyelids
   2. Produces a lubricating fluid
   3. Protects the eye
   4. Is normally red in color
   5. Is not responsive to pain

3. The nurse is aware that there are _____ extraocular muscles for each eye.
   1. 4
   2. 5
   3. 6
   4. 8

4. Which of the following questions would be necessary when conducting a focused interview related to the eye? (Select all that apply)
   1. Have you ever been diagnosed with diabetes?
   2. Have you ever been diagnosed with hypertension?
   3. Have you ever been diagnosed with multiple myeloma?
   4. Have you ever been diagnosed with glaucoma?
   5. Have you ever been diagnosed with urticaria?

5. A 1-year-old appears to have "cross eyes." The nurse explains this problem to the mother by stating it can be caused by:
    1. trauma at birth.
    2. antiseizure medication she was taking during pregnancy.
    3. an eye infection when the baby was born.
    4. weakness of the eye muscle.

6. During the ophthalmoscope exam on a client with hyperopic vision, the nurse should rotate the diopter wheel to:
    1. minus numbers.
    2. plus numbers.
    3. There are no numbers on the diopter wheel.
    4. Plus and minus numbers are irrelevant to hyperopic vision.

7. When using the ophthalmoscope to inspect a client's ocular fundus, the nurse understands that it is best to:
    1. begin with the diopter on –10.
    2. rotate the wheel to the plus numbers if the client's vision is myopic.
    3. approach the client from a 15-degree angle toward the client's nose.
    4. rotate the wheel to the minus numbers if the client's vision is hyperopic.

8. The nurse is aware that the condition in which the refraction of light is spread over a wide area rather than on a distinct point on the retina is called:
    1. strabismus.
    2. astigmatism.
    3. retinal detachment.
    4. glaucoma.

9. A first grader is brought to the school nurse because he was hit in the eye with a ball during recess. After assessing the client, the nurse documents periorbital edema of the right eye. Periorbital edema refers to:
    1. swelling of the soft tissue surrounding the eye.
    2. inversion of the lid and lashes.
    3. redness around the cornea.
    4. a papular appearance of the lower lid.

10. The nurse is aware that the leading cause of blindness in the United States is:
    1. glaucoma.
    2. congenital birth defects.
    3. diabetic retinopathy.
    4. chronic eye infections.

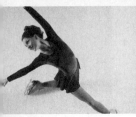

14 Ears, Nose, Mouth, and Throat

Knowing is not enough; we must apply. Willing is not enough; we must do.
—Bruce Lee

The ears, nose, mouth, and throat are important structures of the head and neck. Assessment of these structures provides valuable information about the health of the respiratory and neurologic systems and the abdomen with which they are related. This chapter focuses on methods and techniques to gather subjective data, objective data, and analysis of the data related to the ears, nose, mouth, and throat.

OBJECTIVES

At the completion of these exercises you will be able to:

1. Define key terminology associated with the ears, nose, mouth, and throat.
2. Review the anatomy and physiology of the ears, nose, mouth, and throat.
3. Select the equipment necessary to complete an assessment of the ears, nose, mouth, and throat.
4. Identify the correct techniques for assessment of the ears, nose, mouth, and throat.
5. Analyze subjective and objective data related to the assessment of the ears, nose, mouth, and throat.
6. Recognize factors that can influence assessment findings.
7. Assess the ears, nose, mouth, and throat on a laboratory partner.
8. Document an assessment of the ears, nose, mouth, and throat.
9. Apply critical thinking in analysis of a case study.
10. Relate objectives in *Healthy People 2020* to the assessment of the ears, nose, mouth, and throat.
11. Complete NCLEX®-style review questions related to assessment of the ears, nose, mouth, and throat.

RESOURCES

Pearson Nursing Student Resources
Find additional review materials at
nursing.pearsonhighered.com

Prepare for success with additional NCLEX®-style practice questions, interactive assignments and activities, Web links, animations and videos, and more!

Additional resources: *www.CDC.gov*

WORD SEARCH

Find and circle the correct term in the word search puzzle for each of the definitions listed below. The word may be horizontal, vertical, or diagonal.

```
C G K C F M Y Y D H R O M B N K H F A N F D X
I G K M E D W Q H P U N T G A G R Y K K V G E
Q Y D P A R A N A S A L S I N U S E S L E O E
W R V T S O U H X J N D Z H B O T Q N B R L S
C Y Y T X P V M E M P R T G F T N L U G C O V
R L N R Q J O K E L Z C M R S O J T E I V N D
K A Y K L V W L T N I A M T I R N T R Y I G O
L W B P H I B Q O V S X Z T W A A U S L V S T
H M N K T T C B I B N C C T I L A N N P R S I
P I M R F N O W N X U U Q H A N U Q C E A C T
G P A D L C L N Z V D L C P O M A H T G K Z I
H Z S S S L D N G N P A E I W C S S Q B H P S
L I T H V D S Y O M T H T D T I I E A S Y Y E
Y J O R T T O C R S R C K R S L C O E B E K X
V N I M D L R V U V U L A U B A O L P L B L T
W F D K R I E E R D T A C R F F C U I Y L V E
S M I M A Q S R N I X Y E G V I H M N X V J R
O V T L Y E P O C G B V N W S X L W N O E C N
I S I V L W C T K S E N L S Y T E E A H M J A
L L S S A E J E E F A O R H P A W A C H M Q
I B L L N U J R Y N T R N A S A L P O L Y P S
M I H O F D P O X N O E L T R A G U S X E Y M
U V B T Y M P A N I C M E M B R A N E U J V N
```

CLUES

1. The transmission of sound through the tympanic membrane to the cochlea and auditory nerve **(two words)**
   _____ _____
2. The external portion of the ear _____
3. The transmission of sound through the bones of the skull to the cochlea and auditory nerve **(two words)**
   _____ _____
4. Yellow-brown wax secreted by glands in the external auditory canal _____
5. A spiraling chamber in the inner ear that contains the receptors for hearing _____
6. Occurs on the lip or corner of the mouth caused by a herpes simplex virus **(two words)** _____ _____
7. The bony and cartilaginous auditory tube that connects the middle ear with the nasopharynx **(two words)**
   _____ _____
8. Lesions or blisters on the lips may be caused by the herpes simplex virus **(two words)** _____
   _____
9. The external large rim of the auricle of the ear _____
10. A small flap of flesh at the inferior end of the auricle of the ear _____
11. Inflammation of the mastoid that may be the result of a middle ear or a throat infection _____
12. Smooth, pale, benign growths found along the turbinates of the nose **(two words)** _____ _____
13. Bones of the middle ear _____
14. Swimmer's ear **(two words)** _____ _____
15. The anterior portion of the roof of the mouth formed by bones _____

16. Mucous-lined, air-filled cavities that surround the nasal cavity (**two words**) _____ _____
17. The external portion of the ear _____
18. High frequency hearing loss that occurs over time _____
19. A small projection of the external ear that is positioned in front of the external auditory canal _____
20. The eardrum (**two words**) _____ _____
21. A fleshy pendulum that hangs from the edge of the soft palate in the back of the mouth _____

ANATOMY & PHYSIOLOGY REVIEW

1. For each diagram below write the name of the structure each line is leading to.

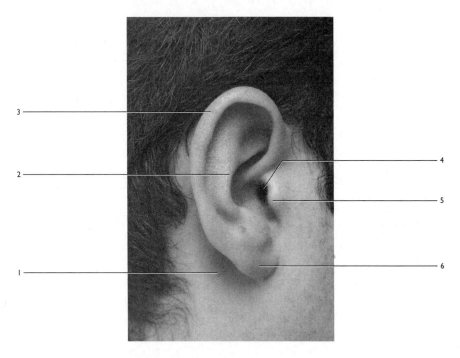

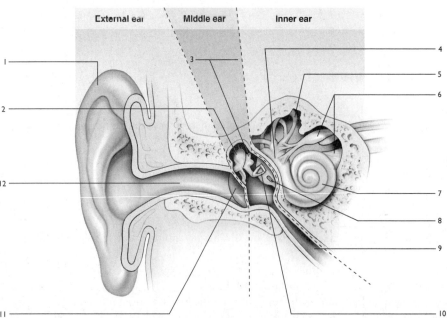

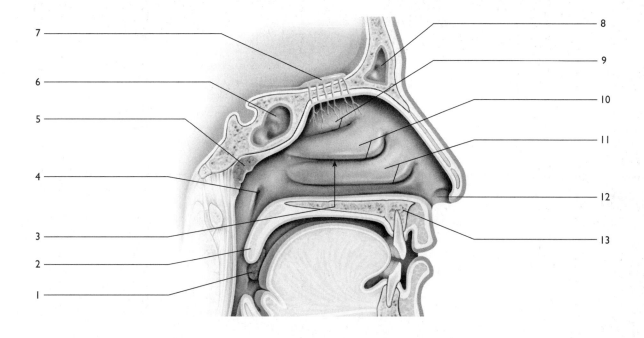

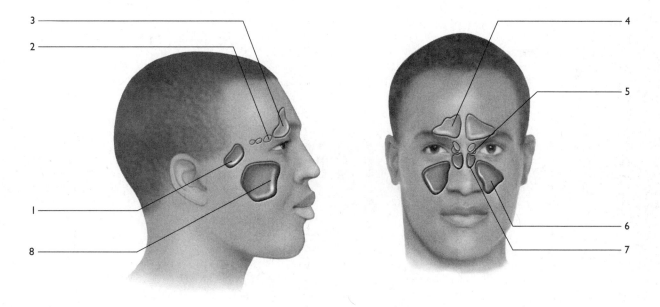

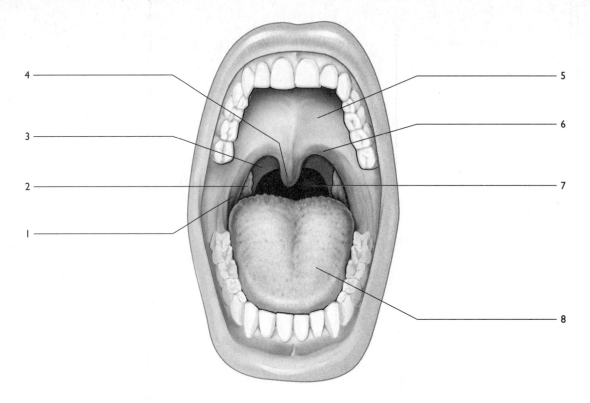

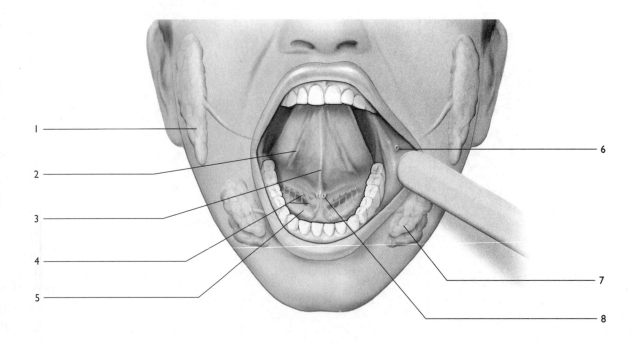

2. Using numbers 1–10, identify the pathway of sound waves through the structures below, as sound travels from the external ear to the brain. Next, circle all the structures that are included in the middle ear.

_____ Malleus   _____ Cranial Nerve VIII

_____ Cochlea   _____ Auditory Canal

_____ Auditory Cortex   _____ Incus

_____ Pinna   _____ Oval Window

_____ Stapes   _____ Tympanic Membrane

EQUIPMENT SELECTION

Prior to beginning the physical assessment of a client's ears, nose, mouth, and throat, it is important to gather the appropriate assessment equipment. Place a check mark next to each piece of equipment that you would need to perform this assessment.

EQUIPMENT		
Cotton balls	Lubricant	Speculum covers
Cotton-tipped applicator	Nasal speculum	Stethoscope
Culture media	Ophthalmoscope	Tape measure
Dental mirror	Otoscope	Test tubes
Doppler ultrasonic stethoscope	Penlight	Thermometer
Examination gown	Reflex hammer	Tongue blade
Eye cover	Ruler	Transilluminator
Flashlight	Skinfold calipers	Tuning fork
Gauze	Skin-marking pen	Vaginal speculum
Gloves	Slides	Vision chart
Goggles	Specimen containers	Watch with second hand
Goniometer	Sphygmomanometer	Wood's lamp

ASSESSMENT TECHNIQUES

Review each assessment technique. If the technique is correct, circle the number. If the technique is incorrect, write the correct assessment technique on the line provided.

1. After palpating the auricle, the nurse should push on the tragus.

   _____

   _____

2. In order to perform an otoscopic examination, the nurse should use the largest speculum that fits most comfortably in the auditory canal.

   _____

   _____

3. When inspecting the auditory canal of an adult client with the otoscope, the nurse should pull the pinna up, back, and out.

   _____

   _____

4. The nurse uses only one monosyllable word when performing the whisper test.

   _____

   _____

5. The nurse is assessing a client's hearing and places the tuning fork on the angle of the mandible in order to assess bone conduction during the Rinne test.

_____

_____

6. The nurse places the tuning fork at the midline of the posterior portion of the frontal bone during the Weber test.

_____

_____

7. During the Romberg test, the nurse asks the client to stand with feet together and eyes closed.

_____

_____

8. When using a nasal speculum, the nurse should stabilize the client's head with his/her dominant hand.

_____

_____

9. The nurse palpates the maxillary sinuses by pressing his/her thumbs below the client's superior orbital ridge.

_____

_____

10. When inspecting a client's salivary glands, the nurse should look for the Stensen's ducts near the frenulum.

_____

_____

11. To assess a client's throat, the nurse asks the client to say "aah" and then uses the tongue blade to swipe the posterior wall of the pharynx.

_____

_____

ASSESSMENT FINDINGS

Read each assessment finding. Identify the finding as normal or abnormal by writing an A for abnormal and an N for normal on each line provided.

_____ 1. Bone conduction longer than tympanic air conduction during the Rinne test

_____ 2. Moist cerumen

_____ 3. Negative Romberg test

_____ 4. Dark pink nasal mucosa

_____ 5. Erythema to tympanic membrane

_____ 6. Smooth vascular ventral surface of tongue

_____ 7. Symmetrical lips

_____ 8. Sweet fruity breath

_____ 9. Midline nasal septum

_____ 10. Patent external auditory meatus of ear

_____ 11. White patches on membrane

_____ 12. Lateralized sound during the Weber test

_____ 13. Equal-sized nares

_____ 14. Maxillary sinus tenderness

_____ 15. Movable tragus

_____ 16. Absence of red glow from transillumination of the sinuses

_____ 17. Hard palate intact

_____ 18. Exudate in posterior pharynx

_____ 19. Patent nares

_____ 20. Gingival hyperplasia

FACTORS THAT INFLUENCE PHYSICAL ASSESSMENT FINDINGS

Fill in the blank to complete each statement.

1. The auditory canal in infants has a (an) _____ curve.

2. Hyperemia of the sinuses in the pregnant female may lead to _____ and _____.

3. Gradual hearing loss in the older adult is called _____.

4. Salivation begins at _____ months of age.

5. The hair at the opening of the auditory meatus becomes more _____ with age.

6. Cerumen in the Asian and Native American cultures may appear _____ in consistency and _____ in color.

7. Clients who participate in activities that increase exposure to loud sounds or music are at increased risk for _____ _____.

8. Cleft lip and palate occur with greatest frequency in the _____ culture.

9. Tics, jaw clenching, and lip biting are all common behaviors that may be assessed in a client who has been experiencing _____.

10. Tooth decay is _____ common among Caucasians.

APPLICATION OF THE CRITICAL THINKING PROCESS

Read the scenario and answer the following questions.

Kenny is a 2-year-old boy who stuck cotton-tipped swabs in both his ears and ran around the house. Unfortunately, he tripped over the dog and hit his head on the stairs. His mother rushed to him as he began to scream. She became extremely alarmed when she pulled the cotton-tipped swab out of his left ear and noted blood. She immediately brought him to his healthcare provider's office.

1. List five focused interview questions the nurse should ask.

   1.

   2.

   3.

   4.

   5.

During the pain assessment, Kenny will not look at or speak to the nurse. He hides his head in his mother's lap and cries. He kicks his left leg on the floor and squirms. His mother attempts to console him by stroking his hair and reassuring him that the nurse is there to help. This seems to help a bit.

2. State why using a FLACC scale for a pain assessment would be appropriate in this situation.

3. What score would Kenny receive using the FLACC scale? _____

4. With the potential of a perforated tympanic membrane, should the nurse proceed to perform the otoscope examination? Explain.

5. Is it necessary to assess Kenny's hearing? Explain.

ASSESSMENT AND DOCUMENTATION

Perform an ears, nose, mouth, and throat assessment on your lab partner and document your findings on the provided documentation form. You can download the form from the Pearson Student Resources site.

NCLEX®-STYLE REVIEW QUESTIONS

Read each question carefully. Choose the best answer for each question.

1. The nurse knows that the eustachian tube connects the middle ear with the:
   1. cochlea.
   2. vestibule.
   3. nasopharynx.
   4. sphenoid sinus.

2. The nurse encourages parents to begin dental checkups for children beginning at what age?
   1. As soon as the first tooth erupts
   2. 3–4 years
   3. 6–7 years
   4. Once the child loses the first deciduous tooth

3. The nurse knows that taste buds are innervated by the:
   1. trigeminal and facial nerves.
   2. facial and glossopharyngeal nerves.
   3. olfactory and vagus nerves.
   4. glossopharyngeal and hypoglossal nerves.

4. A certified nurse midwife is caring for a client who is 28 weeks pregnant and complaining of sinus pressure and a runny nose. The nurse recognizes that these are common complaints during pregnancy due to:
   1. elevated estrogen levels causing hyperemia to the sinuses.
   2. elevated progesterone levels causing hyperemia to the sinuses.
   3. a decreased immune response.
   4. These are not common complaints during pregnancy.

5. An older adult presents to a community health center with "ringing in her ears." Which of the following questions would be appropriate for the nurse to ask during the focused interview? (Select all that apply)
   1. "What medications have you been taking?"
   2. "Are you exposed to loud noises?"
   3. "Have you felt dizzy or nauseated?"
   4. "Do you have any pets at home?"
   5. "Do you have dentures?"

6. An adult client presents to the community health center complaining of nasal congestion, sore throat, and fever. The nurse takes the client's history and performs a physical assessment. Which of the following findings should the nurse record in the subjective section of the client's chart? (Select all that apply)
   1. Oral temperature 101.5°F
   2. Difficulty swallowing
   3. Pharynx with erythema
   4. Throat pain 5 (scale 0–10)
   5. Nighttime chills

7. If the nurse is unable to visualize the tympanic membrane during the otoscope examination, the next step would be to:
   1. reposition the auricle with the otoscope in place.
   2. remove the otoscope, reposition the auricle, and reinsert the otoscope.
   3. move on to the other ear and document "unable to identify" in the notes.
   4. seek out urgent care for the client because the tympanic membrane is most likely ruptured.

8. An adolescent is having his hearing checked by the school nurse. Interpret the following findings:
   Weber test– no lateralization
   Rinne test– AC 15 sec, BC 15 sec Right ear
   AC 30 sec, BC 15 sec Left ear
   1. Sensorineural hearing loss in the right ear
   2. Conductive hearing loss in the left ear
   3. Conductive hearing loss in the right ear
   4. All findings are within the expected range.

9. The nurse expects the nasal mucosa of a client suffering from seasonal allergies would be most likely to appear:
   1. swollen and red.
   2. swollen and pink.
   3. bleeding.
   4. pale and boggy.

10. A mother frantically carries her toddler into the emergency department stating he fell down a flight of stairs and hit his head multiple times. The child is lethargic and pale. Upon a thorough assessment, it is noted that the tympanic membrane has a bluish tinge to it. The nurse notes this as:
    1. a perforated tympanic membrane.
    2. epistaxis.
    3. hemotympanum.
    4. a normal finding.

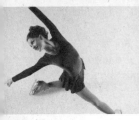

15 Respiratory System

Keep breathing.
—Sophie Tucker

The exchange of oxygen and carbon dioxide is essential for proper functioning of all body systems. The ability of the nurse to recognize subtle changes related to the respiratory status of the client through physical assessment can prevent acute, chronic, and life-threatening situations.

This chapter will focus on gathering both subjective and objective data related to the respiratory assessment, as well as analysis of the data collected.

OBJECTIVES

At the completion of these exercises you will be able to:

1. Define key terminology associated with the respiratory system.
2. Review the anatomy and physiology of the respiratory system.
3. Select the equipment necessary to complete the respiratory assessment.
4. Identify the correct techniques for assessment of the respiratory system.
5. Analyze data related to assessment of the respiratory system.
6. Recognize factors that can influence assessment findings.
7. Assess the respiratory system on a laboratory partner.
8. Document an assessment of the respiratory system.
9. Apply critical thinking in analysis of a case study.
10. Relate objectives in *Healthy People 2020* to the assessment of the respiratory system.
11. Complete NCLEX®-style review questions related to the assessment of the respiratory system.

RESOURCES

Pearson Nursing Student Resources
Find additional review materials at
nursing.pearsonhighered.com

Prepare for success with additional NCLEX®-style practice questions, interactive assignments and activities, Web links, animations and videos, and more!

Additional resources: *www.CDC.gov*
www.lungsusa.org

CROSSWORD PUZZLE FOR KEY TERMS

Read each definition below and fill in the correct term on the puzzle grid. If the answer requires two words do not leave a blank space between the words. Use a pencil so you can erase easily.

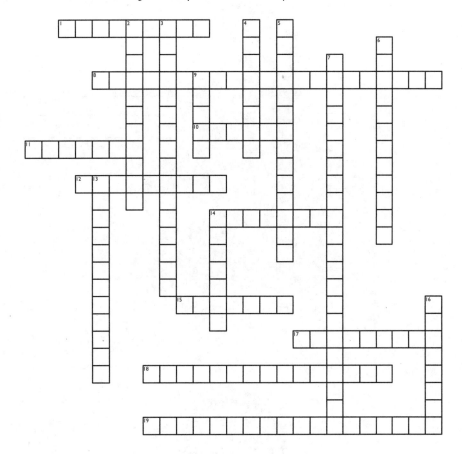

CLUES

Across

1. Thoracic reference points and specific anatomical structures used to help provide an exact location
8. Auscultation of voice sounds, client whispers word (**two words**)
10. The regular, even-depth, rhythmic pattern of inspiration and expiration
11. A range of whistling or snoring sounds
12. The superior or upper portion of the sternum
14. A flat percussion tone that is soft and of short duration
15. High-pitched squeaky or sibilant breath sounds
17. A long, low-pitched hollow sound elicited with percussion over the lungs
18. Loud, high-pitched sounds heard in the upper airways and region of the trachea (**two words**)
19. Added sounds heard during auscultation of the chest (**two words**)

Down

2. Part of the thorax that contains the heart, trachea, esophagus, and major blood vessels of the body
3. Consists of an inspiratory and expiratory phase of breathing (**two words**)
4. Auscultation of voice sounds, client says "E"
5. Harsh, high-pitched sound heard over the trachea when the client inhales and exhales (**two words**)
6. Auscultation of voice sounds, client says "ninety-nine"
7. Sounds that are medium in loudness and pitch, heard as auscultation moves from the large central airways toward the periphery of the lungs (**two words**)
9. Discontinuous sounds that are intermittent, nonmusical, and brief
13. The sternal angle (**three words**)
14. Shortness of breath
16. The palpable vibration on the chest wall when the client speaks

ANATOMY & PHYSIOLOGY REVIEW

1. For each diagram below write the name of the structure each line is leading to.

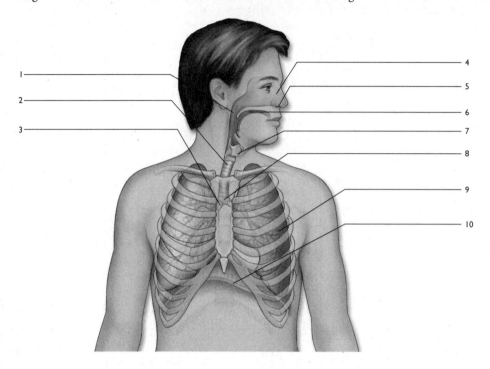

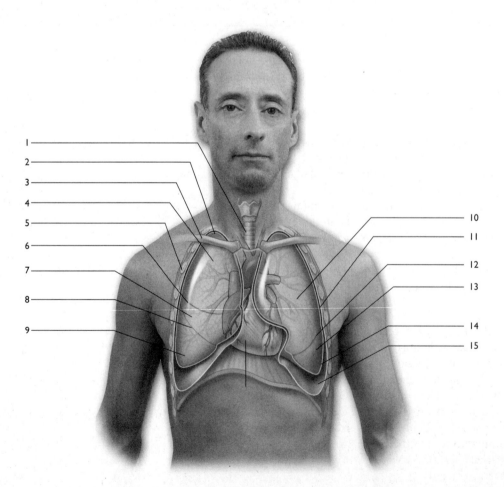

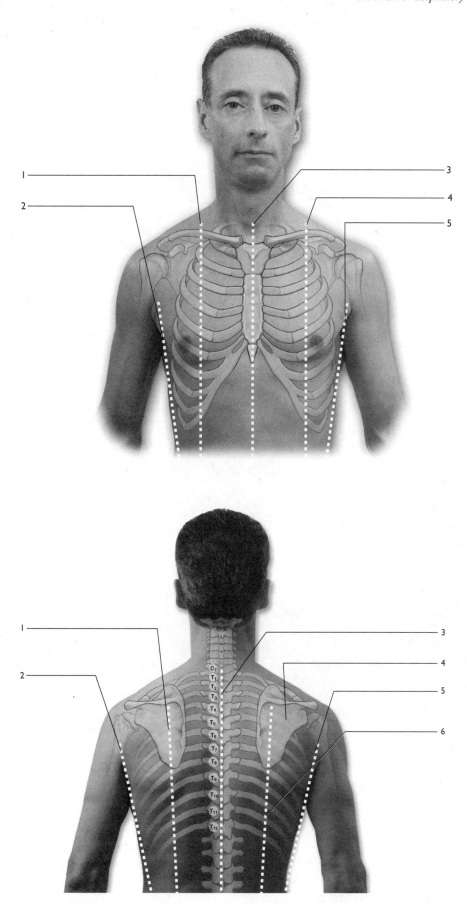

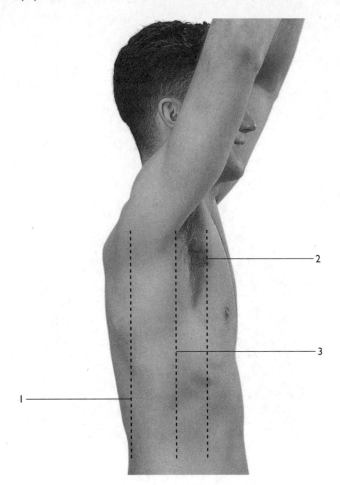

2. Read each statement. Write an I if the action occurs during inspiration and an E if it occurs during expiration on the line provided.

_____ 1. Diaphragm contracts

_____ 2. Recoil of the lungs

_____ 3. Contraction of the intercostal muscles

_____ 4. Diaphragm relaxes

_____ 5. Alveolar pressure decreases

_____ 6. Lung expansion

_____ 7. Increase in size of thoracic cavity

_____ 8. Passive phase of breathing

_____ 9. Relaxation of the intercostal muscles

_____ 10. Rise of the diaphragm

_____ 11. Decrease in size of thoracic cavity

_____ 12. Diaphragm lowers

EQUIPMENT SELECTION

Prior to beginning the physical assessment of a client's respiratory system, it is important to gather the appropriate assessment equipment. Place a check mark next to each piece of equipment that you would need to perform this assessment.

EQUIPMENT		
Cotton balls	Lubricant	Stethoscope
Cotton-tipped applicator	Nasal speculum	Tape measure
Culture media	Ophthalmoscope	Test tubes
Dental mirror	Otoscope	Thermometer
Doppler ultrasonic stethoscope	Penlight	Tissues
Examination gown	Reflex hammer	Transilluminator
Examination light	Ruler (metric)	Tuning fork
Face mask	Skinfold calipers	Vaginal speculum
Gauze	Skin-marking pen	Vision chart
Gloves	Slides	Watch with second hand
Goggles	Specimen containers	Water
Goniometer	Sphygmomanometer	Wood's lamp

ASSESSMENT TECHNIQUES

Review each assessment technique. If the technique is correct, circle the number. If the technique is incorrect, write the correct assessment technique on the line provided.

1. When counting a respiratory rate, it is important to inform the client that you are counting the rate.

2. When palpating and counting the ribs and intercostal spaces of the posterior thorax, the nurse should instruct the client to flex the neck, round the shoulders, and lean forward.

3. The nurse can palpate for respiratory expansion by placing the palmar surface of his hands on the posterior lower chest of the client.

4. The ulnar surface of the hand or the finger pads can be pressed against the chest wall to assess tactile fremitus.

5. During percussion of the thorax, the client should hold his breath.

6. During percussion of the thorax, the nurse should begin at the apices of the lungs.

7. To properly assess for diaphragmatic excursion, the nurse should begin to percuss at the level of T7 or T8 of the vertebral column.

   _____

   _____

8. When auscultating lung sounds, the nurse should move the stethoscope to the next area after listening through a full respiratory cycle.

   _____

   _____

9. When auscultating voice sounds using egophony, the nurse should ask the client to say "ninety-nine" each time the stethoscope is placed on the thorax.

   _____

   _____

10. Assessment of the anterior thorax is not performed with female clients who have large breast tissue because of interference in sound perception.

   _____

   _____

ASSESSMENT FINDINGS

Read each assessment finding. Identify if the finding is normal or abnormal. Write an A for abnormal and an N for normal on each line provided.

_____	1. Pallor of skin		_____	11. Midline sternum
_____	2. Symmetrical chest movement		_____	12. Even height of scapulae
_____	3. Firm muscle mass over thorax		_____	13. Posterior thorax non-tender
_____	4. Vibrations over chest wall while client speaks		_____	14. Vesicular sounds between the scapulae
_____	5. Respiratory rate 26 in an adult		_____	15. Pink undertones of skin for Caucasians
_____	6. Unilateral delay in chest expansion		_____	16. Resonance on percussion of lung fields
_____	7. Eupnea		_____	17. Intercostal muscle retraction
_____	8. Costal angle less than 90 degrees		_____	18. Stridor
_____	9. Atelectasis		_____	19. Bibasilar rales
_____	10. Anterior/posterior diameter equal to the transverse diameter		_____	20. Lateral deviation of thoracic spinous process

FACTORS THAT INFLUENCE PHYSICAL ASSESSMENT FINDINGS

Fill in the blank to complete each statement.

1. During fetal development gas exchange occurs at the _____.

2. The respiratory rate _____ from infancy into childhood.

3. During the third trimester of pregnancy, it is common for eupnea to change to _____.

4. There is less expansion of the _____ cavity in the older adult.

5. Oxygen consumption can increase by _____% throughout pregnancy.

6. The heating and cooling ducts in office buildings may carry airborne organisms that cause workers to have frequent respiratory _____.

7. Children in _____ socioeconomic groups have a higher incidence of asthma.

8. In the infancy period, the lateral and anterior-posterior diameters of the chest are _____.

9. Costal breathing is expected after _____ years of age.

10. The costal angle _____ during pregnancy.

11. As altitude increases, the partial pressure of oxygen _____.

12. Forced hot air heating systems can cause _____ to membranes of the body.

RESPIRATORY PATTERNS

Match the name of each wave pattern in Column A with its associated waveform in Column B by writing the waveform's letter on the line provided.

Column A

_____ 1. Cheyne Stokes

_____ 2. Hyperventilating

_____ 3. Bradypnea

_____ 4. Eupnea

_____ 5. Tachypnea

_____ 6. Eupnea with a sigh

_____ 7. Hypoventilating

_____ 8. Obstructive breathing with prolonged expiration

Column B (WAVEFORMS)

A.

B.

C.

D.

E.

F.

G.

H.

AUSCULTATION REVIEW

1. Using the diagram below place an X over each area that the nurse should place the stethoscope when auscultating breath sounds. Then number the Xs in the order in which you will proceed. Provide a rationale for your pattern.

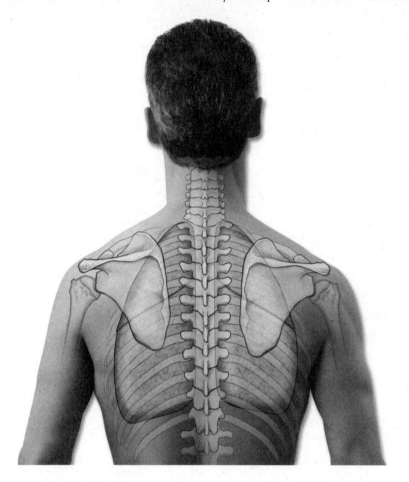

Auscultation Pattern Rationale: _____

_____

2. Match the auscultated sound in Column A with the description in Column B by writing the description's letter on the line provided.

Column A

_____ 1. Crackles

_____ 2. Stridor

_____ 3. Vesicular

_____ 4. Egophony

_____ 5. Bronchophony

_____ 6. Bronchial

_____ 7. Wheeze

_____ 8. Friction rub

_____ 9. Ronchi

_____ 10. Bronchovesicular

_____ 11. Tracheal

_____ 12. Whispered pectoriloquy

Column B

A. Inspiration louder than expiration

B. Moist bubbling sound

C. "EEEEEEEE" or "AAAAAA"

D. Grating, rubbing sound

E. Continuous snoring/rattling sound

F. Inspiration equal to expiration

G. Harsh high-pitched sound

H. "Ninety-nine"

I. High-pitched shrill sound

J. "One, Two, Three"

K. Loud crowing sound

L. Expiration greater than inspiration

APPLICATION OF THE CRITICAL THINKING PROCESS

Read the scenario and answer the following questions.

Keith is a 20-year-old male who plays guitar in a band. He is 6 feet tall and weighs 165 lb. His medical-surgical history indicates an appendectomy at age 14 and an allergy to citrus fruits. He has been smoking 1–2 packs of cigarettes per day for about 3 years and admits to occasionally smoking marijuana (about 2–3 times per month). During a concert performance with his band, he suddenly felt a pain under his left rib cage. He began to experience shortness of breath and thought for a second he was going to faint. He quickly ran off the stage and sat down in a back room. A friend ran to his side and noticed that Keith was having some difficulty breathing and called for medical assistance.

When presenting in the emergency department, Keith's vital signs were BP 142/90, HR 120, RR 36, and T 99.2°F (tympanic).

1. List three focused interview questions the nurse should ask Keith at this time:

   1.
   2.
   3.

During a pain assessment, the nurse collects the following data: The client experienced a sudden onset of pain under his left rib cage that he scaled as an 8 on the numeric pain scale; taking a deep breath makes the pain worse.

2. Using the OLDCART & ICE acronym, list any information that has not been collected regarding the pain assessment.

3. Upon physical assessment, it is noted that Keith's skin color is pale and his breathing is rapid and labored. His chest expansion is asymmetrical, and he has absent breath sounds in his left lower lobe. His oxygen saturation level is 91% on room air. Upon collecting this data, the nurse must determine if Keith should be seen by the doctor immediately or if he can wait in the waiting area. State what the nurse's decision should be and provide a rationale.

4. After careful assessment and diagnostic testing, it is determined that Keith has a spontaneous pneumothorax of his left lung.

   1. Define pneumothorax.

   2. List three assessment findings from the above data that support this medical diagnosis.

      1.
      2.
      3.

5. Write nursing diagnoses for Keith in this scenario using NANDA or the PES method.

   1. Nursing Diagnosis: _____

   2. Nursing Diagnosis: _____

6. Using your presented nursing diagnosis, write an anticipated outcome. How would you evaluate this outcome?

HEALTHY PEOPLE 2020

A *Healthy People 2020* objective is:

Reduce the number of workdays missed among persons with current asthma.

1. List four asthma triggers.

    1.

    2.

    3.

    4.

2. Discuss how an occupational health nurse can use this objective to promote and maintain health and function of the respiratory system among employees.

ASSESSMENT AND DOCUMENTATION

Perform an assessment of the respiratory system on your lab partner and document your findings on the provided documentation form. You can download the form from the Pearson Student Resources site.

NCLEX®-STYLE REVIEW QUESTIONS

Read each question carefully. Choose the best answer for each question.

1. The nurse identifies the structures of the lower respiratory tract as the:
    1. pharynx, the bronchi, and the lungs.
    2. trachea, the bronchi, and the lungs.
    3. sinuses, the larynx, and the bronchi.
    4. larynx, the bronchi, and the lungs.

2. The nurse understands the action associated with expiration is:
    1. respiratory muscles contract.
    2. chest expansion.
    3. alveolar pressure decreases.
    4. negative intrapleural pressure decreases.

3. The nurse identifies signs of respiratory distress to include: (Select all that apply)
    1. circumoral cyanosis.
    2. respiratory rate of 22.
    3. intercostal muscle retractions.
    4. nasal flaring.
    5. periorbital edema.

4. A 19-year-old female arrives at the university clinic complaining of asthma-like symptoms. The nurse would most likely hear which of the following sounds upon auscultation?
   1. Loud, moist, bubbling sounds
   2. Low-pitched, grating sounds
   3. High-pitched, continuous sounds
   4. Crackling sounds

5. When auscultating for bronchophony, the nurse should instruct the client to:
   1. repeat the letter "E."
   2. repeat the number "ninety-nine."
   3. repeat the words "one, two, three."
   4. take in a deep breath and hold it.

6. An adult male client has suffered from emphysema for approximately 5 years. When percussing his posterior lung fields, the nurse is most likely to hear:
   1. hyperresonance.
   2. dullness.
   3. flatness.
   4. resonance.

7. Which client would most likely have the largest measured diaphragmatic excursion?
   1. A 22-year-old runner
   2. A 68-year-old smoker
   3. A 3-year-old
   4. A 35-year-old female who is 32 weeks pregnant

8. When auscultating lung sounds, which of the following assessment findings would require further investigation by the nurse? Inspiration is:
   1. greater than expiration over the peripheral lung fields.
   2. less than expiration over the trachea.
   3. equal to expiration at the sternal border between the scapulae.
   4. greater than expiration over the trachea.

9. During a focused interview, the nurse asks the client if she sleeps using two or three pillows. This question is important because the client may: (Select all that apply)
   1. snore.
   2. experience orthopnea.
   3. be prone to respiratory infections if she is sleep deprived.
   4. be obese.
   5. have a history of deep vein thrombosis.

10. The nurse identifies the following muscles as accessory muscles for respiratory function. (Select all that apply)
   1. Trapezius
   2. Scalene
   3. Sternocleidomastoid
   4. Pectorals
   5. Gracilis

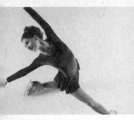

16 Breasts and Axillae

Patience and perseverance have a magical effect before which difficulties disappear and obstacles vanish.
—John Quincy Adams

Breasts are unique to the individual. They go through many changes throughout each month based on hormone fluctuations, weight fluctuations, and some medications. The ability of the nurse to recognize these changes through assessment and educate clients to perform their own assessments is crucial in early diagnosis of disease. This chapter will focus on gathering both subjective and objective data related to the breast and axillae assessment, as well as analysis of the data collected.

OBJECTIVES

At the completion of these exercises you will be able to:

1. Define key terminology associated with the breasts and axillae.
2. Review the anatomy and physiology of the breasts and axillae.
3. Select the equipment necessary to complete the breast and axillae assessment.
4. Identify the correct techniques for assessment of the breasts and axillae.
5. Analyze data related to assessment of the breasts and axillae.
6. Recognize factors that can influence assessment findings.
7. Assess the breasts and axillae on a laboratory partner.
8. Document an assessment of the breasts and axillae.
9. Apply critical thinking in analysis of a case study.
10. Relate objectives in *Healthy People 2020* to the breasts and axillae.
11. Complete NCLEX®-style review questions related to the assessment of the breasts and axillae.

RESOURCES

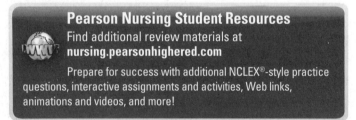

Pearson Nursing Student Resources

Find additional review materials at
nursing.pearsonhighered.com

Prepare for success with additional NCLEX®-style practice questions, interactive assignments and activities, Web links, animations and videos, and more!

Additional resources: *www.CDC.gov*

WORD SEARCH

Find and circle the correct term in the word search puzzle for each of the definitions listed below. The word may be horizontal, vertical, or diagonal.

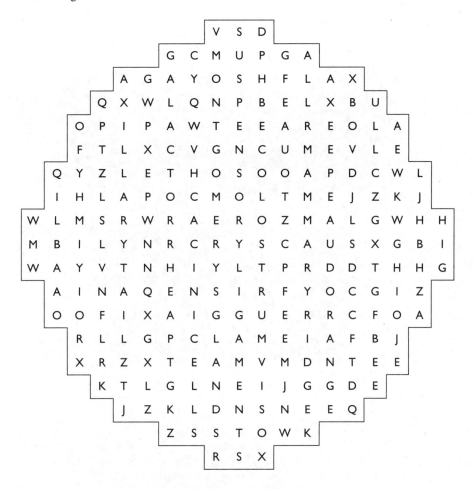

```
              V  S  D
           G  C  M  U  P  G  A
        A  G  A  Y  O  S  H  F  L  A  X
        Q  X  W  L  Q  N  P  B  E  L  X  B  U
     O  P  I  P  A  W  T  E  E  A  R  E  O  L  A
     F  T  L  X  C  V  G  N  C  U  M  E  V  L  E
     Q  Y  Z  L  E  T  H  O  S  O  O  A  P  D  C  W  L
     I  H  L  A  P  O  C  M  O  L  T  M  E  J  Z  K  J
  W  L  M  S  R  W  R  A  E  R  O  Z  M  A  L  G  W  H  H
  M  B  I  L  Y  N  R  C  R  Y  S  C  A  U  S  X  G  B  I
  W  A  Y  V  T  N  H  I  Y  L  T  P  R  D  D  T  H  H  G
     A  I  N  A  Q  E  N  S  I  R  F  Y  O  C  G  I  Z
     O  O  F  I  X  A  I  G  G  U  E  R  R  C  F  O  A
     R  L  L  G  P  C  L  A  M  E  I  A  F  B  J
     X  R  Z  X  T  E  A  M  V  M  D  N  T  E  E
        K  T  L  G  L  N  E  I  J  G  G  D  E
           J  Z  K  L  D  N  S  N  E  E  Q
              Z  S  S  T  O  W  K
                 R  S  X
```

CLUES

1. Glandular tissue in each breast that produces milk (**two words**)_____ _____
2. A circular pigmented field of wrinkled skin containing the nipple _____
3. Tail of Spence (**two words**) _____ _____
4. Thick yellow discharge that may leak from breasts in the month prior to birth in preparation for lactation _____
5. Lactation not associated with childbearing or breastfeeding _____
6. Benign temporary breast enlargement in one or both breasts in males _____
7. "Milk line," which extends from each axilla to the groin (**two words**)_____ _____
8. The sebaceous glands on the areola, which enlarge and produce a secretion that protects and lubricates the nipples (**two words**) _____ _____
9. "Orange peel" appearance caused by edema from blocked lymphatic drainage in advanced cancer (**two words**) _____ _____
10. Cooper's ligaments (**two words**) _____ _____

ANATOMY & PHYSIOLOGY REVIEW

1. For each diagram below write the name of the structure indicated by each line.

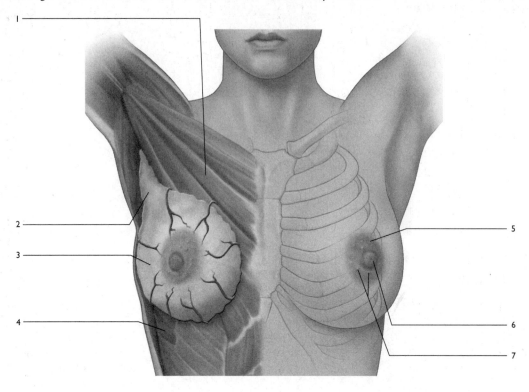

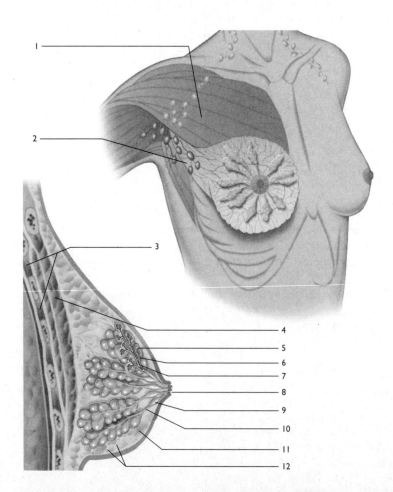

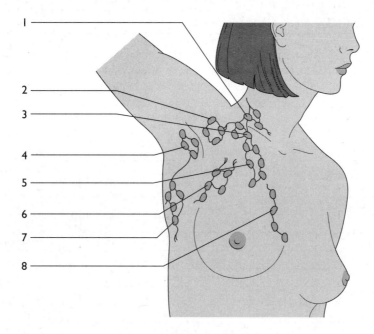

2. Place a check mark [✓] next to each statement that is **TRUE** about the physiology of the breast. If the statement is **FALSE** rewrite the statement correctly in the space provided.

_____ **1.** Breast tissue starts to change at the onset of puberty between the ages of 14 and 16.

Correction: _____

_____ **2.** Decreased levels of progesterone and increased levels of estrogen cause changes in fat deposits, ductile maturity, and pigmentation of the breasts.

Correction: _____

_____ **3.** Breast growth may be asymmetrical.

Correction: _____

_____ **4.** Each breast has 5 to 10 lobes of glandular tissue.

Correction: _____

_____ **5.** Acini cells produce milk that is emptied into the lactiferous ducts and carried to the nipple.

Correction: _____

_____ **6.** Each breast lobe is composed of 20 to 40 lobules.

Correction: _____

_____ **7.** Blood is supplied to the breasts by the Montgomery artery.

Correction: _____

_____ **8.** Spence glands are sebaceous glands that produce oils to lubricate and moisturize the areola and nipple.

Correction: _____

EQUIPMENT SELECTION

Prior to beginning the physical assessment of a client's breasts and axillae, it is important to gather the appropriate assessment equipment. Place a check mark next to each piece of equipment that you would need to perform this assessment.

EQUIPMENT					
	Cotton balls		Lubricant		Sphygmomanometer
	Cotton-tipped applicator		Nasal speculum		Stethoscope
	Culture media		Ophthalmoscope		Tape measure
	Dental mirror		Otoscope		Test tubes
	Doppler ultrasonic stethoscope		Penlight		Thermometer
	Drape sheet		Pillow (small)		Tongue blade
	Examination gown		Ruler		Transilluminator
	Flashlight		Skinfold calipers		Tuning fork
	Gauze		Skin-marking pen		Vaginal speculum
	Gloves		Slides		Vision chart
	Goggles		Small rolled towel		Watch with second hand
	Goniometer		Specimen containers		Wood's lamp

ASSESSMENT TECHNIQUES

Review each assessment technique. If the technique is correct, circle the number. If the technique is incorrect, write the correct assessment technique on the line provided.

1. The client should be in a supine position at the beginning of a breast assessment.

   _____

   _____

2. Explain to the female client that at least three positions will be used during the assessment of the breasts.

   _____

3. Inspection of the breasts can be done with the client's hands pressed together at the level of the waist.

   _____

4. Inspection of the breasts can be done with the client leaning back on the exam table.

   _____

5. When palpating one breast, the nurse should cover the breast that is not being examined.

   _____

6. The nurse should place a small pillow or rolled towel under the breast that is not being examined.

   _____

7. The finger pads of the first three fingers should be used in a slightly rotary motion during palpation of the breast.

   _____

   _____

8. The only pattern that covers the entire breast is the concentric circle pattern.

    _____

    _____

9. If a female client has pendulous breasts, the nurse should place one hand under the breast to support it while the other hand is palpating.

    _____

    _____

10. The nipple should be compressed between the second and third digit.

    _____

    _____

ASSESSMENT FINDINGS

Read each assessment finding. Identify the finding as normal or abnormal by writing an A for abnormal and an N for normal on each line provided.

_____ 1. Dimpling

_____ 2. Oval areolae

_____ 3. Nipple discharge

_____ 4. Presence of axillary hair

_____ 5. Non-palpable axillary lymph nodes

_____ 6. Unilateral areola tenderness

_____ 7. Inverted nipples for two weeks

_____ 8. Pendulous breasts

_____ 9. Bilateral venous patterns

_____ 10. Breasts fall freely and evenly when sitting or standing

_____ 11. Peau d'orange

_____ 12. Slight asymmetry of breasts

_____ 13. Smooth skin over the breast

_____ 14. Galactorrhea

_____ 15. Gynecomastia

_____ 16. Uninterrupted breast contour

_____ 17. Firm pectoral muscles

_____ 18. Thick breast skin

_____ 19. Red scaly areolae

_____ 20. Supernumerary nipple

FACTORS THAT INFLUENCE PHYSICAL ASSESSMENT FINDINGS

Fill in the blank to complete each statement.

1. Swollen breast tissue in a newborn may be caused by _____.

2. In the female, fatty tissue will replace _____ tissue at menopause.

3. Research has suggested that a high-fat diet may _____ a female's risk of developing breast cancer.

4. Infants may produce a thin discharge from the breasts known as _____ _____. This secretion will subside as the maternal _____ decreases.

5. Women with very small, very large, or asymmetrical breasts are at higher risk for _____ disturbance.

6. The nipples become _____ and _____ in the older adult.

7. Asian and Hispanic women have the _____ rates of breast cancer.

8. During pregnancy, the nipples and areolae become _____ in color and _____ in size.

9. Many women avoid doing _____ because their culture has prohibited looking at or touching oneself.

10. Adolescent male "breast buds" usually disappear within _____ of onset.

THE BREAST SELF-EXAM (BSE)

Fill in the blanks to complete each sentence. Next, number the steps of the breast self-exam in the order that the nurse would teach a female client (1 being the first step and 10 being the last).

_____ Compare breasts for _____, _____, _____, and _____.

_____ Observe breast in front of a _____.

_____ Many women palpate their breasts while they _____.

_____ Examine the nipples for _____ and recent _____.

_____ Palpation of the breast should be done with the _____ _____.

_____ Observe breasts in _____ positions.

_____ Instruct the client to palpate from the periphery of the breasts to the _____.

_____ Compress the nipple with the _____ and _____.

_____ A technique for palpation of the breasts is _____ _____.

_____ Instruct the client not to forget the _____ _____.

APPLICATION OF THE CRITICAL THINKING PROCESS

Read the scenario and answer the following questions.

Jill is a 34-year-old female Gravida 3 Para 2. She delivered a healthy baby 5 weeks ago and is breastfeeding with support from a lactation nurse at the hospital. Last night, Jill began feeling extremely fatigued, but attributed this to lack of sleep as her newborn is up several times at night to breastfeed. She also noticed a slight burning sensation when the baby fed from her left breast last night, and today she notes that the breast is slightly swollen and tender. She is concerned that something might be wrong and calls the lactation nurse at the hospital.

1. What three focused interview questions could the lactation nurse ask this client?

   1. _____
   2. _____
   3. _____

The lactation nurse asks Jill to come to the hospital for an assessment. Inspection reveals the breasts are asymmetrical, with the left being larger than the right with slightly reddened skin. The left breast is warm, firm, and tender to the touch. The areola appears cracked and tender. The nurse assesses Jill's vital signs, which reveal BP 104/68, HR 102, RR 18, and Temp 100.8°F (orally).

2. Identify three assessment findings found during inspection.

   1. _____
   2. _____
   3. _____

3. Identify three assessment findings found during palpation.

   1. _____
   2. _____
   3. _____

The nurse begins to assess Jill's pain by asking about the exact location of the pain, when the pain began, and for the client to rate the pain on a numeric scale. Jill states the discomfort started the previous evening and rated her pain as a 6 on a numerical scale of 0–10.

4. Document the pain-related data collected using the OLDCART & ICE pain assessment.

5. What questions should be asked to complete the pain assessment?

The lactation nurse suspects that Jill has developed mastitis of the left breast from a clogged milk duct. The nurse places a call to the healthcare provider for prescriptive treatment. Jill expresses concern that she could have prevented this from happening. The lactation nurse determines that Jill could benefit from education about measures to prevent mastitis.

6. Write one teaching goal and three objectives for this scenario.

   Goal:

   Objectives:
   1.
   2.
   3.

HEALTHY PEOPLE 2020

Please read the *Healthy People 2020* objective and answer the following questions.

A *Healthy People 2020* objective is:

**Increase the proportion of women aged 40 years and older who have received
a breast cancer screening based on the most recent guidelines.**

1. What is included in a breast cancer screening?

2. Discuss how a women's health nurse can use this *Healthy People 2020* objective to promote and maintain health and function of the client's breasts.

ASSESSMENT AND DOCUMENTATION

Perform a breast and axillae assessment on your lab partner and document your findings on the provided documentation form. You can download the form from the Pearson Student Resources site.

NCLEX®-STYLE REVIEW QUESTIONS

Read each question carefully. Choose the best answer for each question.

1. The nurse notes the areola is speckled with _____ glands.
   1. sebaceous
   2. serous
   3. apocrine
   4. mucus

2. Which of the following lymph nodes does not drain the breast and axillae?
   1. Brachial nodes
   2. Internal mammary nodes
   3. Interpectoral nodes
   4. Superficial cervical chain

3. A school nurse is teaching a group of young girls about puberty. The nurse explains that breast tissue will begin to enlarge during puberty between the ages of:
   1. 7 and 10.
   2. 9 and 13.
   3. 12 and 16.
   4. 14 and 18.

4. A female client visits a nurse midwife for a 2-month postpartum visit. The client is breastfeeding and states she has not performed a breast self-exam (BSE) since before the baby was born. The nurse midwife instructs the client that BSEs:
   1. are not advised while breastfeeding.
   2. should be performed after a completed breastfeeding.
   3. should be performed prior to the first feed of the day.
   4. can be done anytime while breastfeeding because menstruation is ceased.

5. Which statement by the nurse best explains changes in breast tissue during menopause? The breast tissue experiences:
   1. an increase in glandular tissue.
   2. a decrease in fatty tissue.
   3. relaxation of the suspensory ligaments.
   4. an increase in erectile sensitivity to the nipple.

6. A 14-year-old girl is having an annual physical. She appears quite embarrassed during the examination and shyly asks the nurse if it is normal for one of her breasts to be larger than the other. The nurse's response should be:
   1. "Breast development may not be the same on both sides; this is quite normal."
   2. "We will schedule you for a breast ultrasound."
   3. "Let's find out if your mother's breasts are the same way."
   4. "Do you have a history of breast cancer in the family?"

7. A nurse is working in a health and wellness center on a university campus. She was asked by a sorority to give a presentation during Breast Cancer Awareness month. In the presentation, the nurse decides to include which of the following guidelines from the American Cancer Society?
   1. Women in their 20s have an option to perform a monthly breast self-exam (BSE).
   2. A breast exam should be performed by a healthcare provider every 5 years after the age 25.
   3. All females should have a baseline mammography at age 50.
   4. All females over age 40 should perform a BSE once per week.

8. A 19-year-old female college student just finished reading an article in a fashion magazine on breast cancer. It really upset her, because her aunt died of breast cancer 2 years ago. The student decides that it is time for her to start thinking about performing breast self-examination (BSE). Unsure of what to do, she consults the nurse at the college health service. The nurse includes which of the following statements regarding BSE?
   1. "It is best to perform BSE about 5 days prior to your menstrual period."
   2. "It is best to perform BSE about 5 days after your menstrual period."
   3. It is best to perform BSE during your menstrual period."
   4. "We don't have to worry about BSE at our age."

9. The nurse knows that the incidence of breast cancer in the female is highest in the:
   1. axillary tail.
   2. upper inner quadrant.
   3. lower outer quadrant.
   4. lower inner quadrant.

10. Which of the following would the nurse document as an abnormal assessment finding during the menstrual cycle?
    1. Breast tenderness
    2. Breast pain
    3. Breast swelling
    4. Nipple discharge

Cardiovascular System 17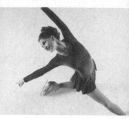

There is no instinct like that of the heart.
—Lord Byron

The cardiovascular system is responsible for the continuous circulation of blood throughout the body.

The physiology of the cardiac cycle consists of blood flow and electrical conduction. Understanding this cycle is an important aspect in performing a complete cardiovascular assessment. This chapter will focus on gathering both subjective and objective data related to the cardiovascular system, as well as analysis of the data collected.

OBJECTIVES

At the completion of these exercises you will be able to:

1. Define key terminology associated with the cardiovascular system.
2. Review the anatomy and physiology of the cardiovascular system.
3. Select the equipment necessary to complete the cardiovascular assessment.
4. Identify the correct techniques for assessment of the cardiovascular system.
5. Analyze data related to assessment of the cardiovascular system.
6. Recognize factors that can influence assessment findings.
7. Assess the cardiovascular system on a laboratory partner.
8. Document an assessment of the cardiovascular system.
9. Apply critical thinking in analysis of a case study.
10. Relate objectives in *Healthy People 2020* to the cardiovascular system.
11. Complete NCLEX®-style review questions related to the assessment of the cardiovascular system.

RESOURCES

Pearson Nursing Student Resources
Find additional review materials at
nursing.pearsonhighered.com

Prepare for success with additional NCLEX®-style practice questions, interactive assignments and activities, Web links, animations and videos, and more!

Additional resources: *www.americanheart.org*
www.CDC.gov

CROSSWORD PUZZLE FOR KEY TERMS

Read each definition below and fill in the correct term on the puzzle grid. If the answer requires two words do not leave a blank space between the words. Use a pencil so you can erase easily.

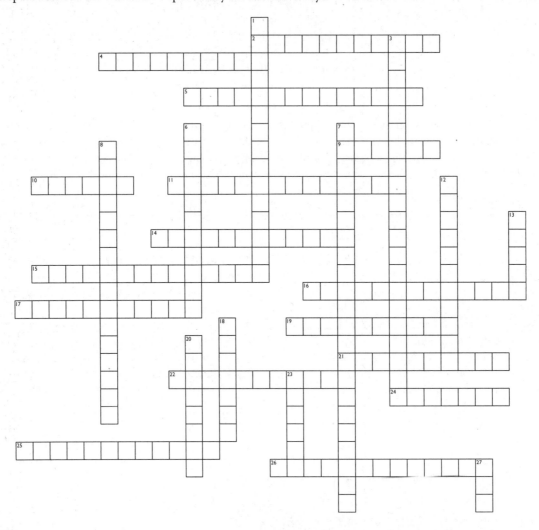

CLUES

Across

2. The innermost layer of the heart
4. The outer layer of the heart wall
5. Expressways of conducting fibers that spread the electrical current through the ventricular myocardial tissue **(two words)**
9. Soft vibratory sensations assessed by palpation with either the fingertips or palm flattened to the chest
10. Initiates the electrical impulse **(two words)**
11. The chamber that pushes unoxygenated blood out to the pulmonary vessels **(two words)**
14. The amount of blood that is ejected with every heartbeat **(two words)**
15. Fibers that fan out and penetrate into the myocardial tissue to spread the current into the tissues themselves **(two words)**
16. The amount of blood ejected from the left ventricle in one minute **(two words)**
17. The chamber that receives unoxygenated blood from the periphery of the body **(two words)**
19. The second, thick, muscular layer of the heart
21. The chamber that receives oxygenated blood from the pulmonary system **(two words)**
22. Soft, yellow plaques on the lids at the inner canthus, which are sometimes associated with high cholesterolemia
24. The flat, narrow center bone of the upper anterior chest
25. The event of one complete heartbeat, the contraction and relaxation of the atria and ventricles **(two words)**
26. The most powerful of all heart chambers **(two words)**

Down

1. Valves that separate the ventricles from the vascular system (**two words**)
3. A condition caused by bacterial infiltration of the lining of the heart's chambers (**two words**)
6. A thin sac composed of a fibroserous material that surrounds the heart
7. Valves that separate the atria from the ventricles within the heart (**two words**)
8. The area where the heart sits obliquely within the thoracic cavity between the lungs and above the diaphragm (**two words**)
12. Atypical sounds of the heart often indicating a functional or structural abnormality (**two words**)
13. A group of heart sounds that elicit a loud blowing sound
18. The phase in which the ventricles contract
20. The phase of ventricular relaxation in which the ventricles relax and are filled as the atria contract
23. Node, located in the wall of the right atrium, capable of initiating electrical impulses in the event of SA node failure (**two words**)
27. Electrical representations of the cardiac cycle are documented by deflections on recording paper

ANATOMY & PHYSIOLOGY REVIEW

1. For each diagram below write the name of the structure indicated by each line.

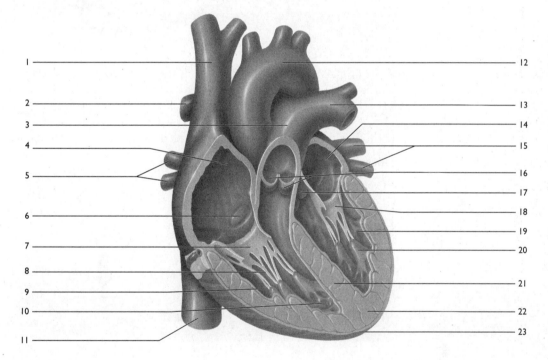

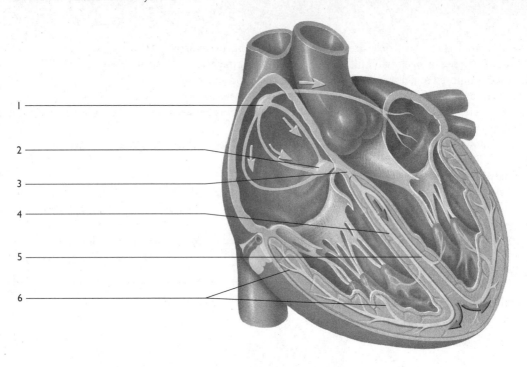

1
2
3
4
5
6

2. Starting with the vena cava, follow a drop of blood through the heart. Place the structure in the boxes provided. Be sure to use proper sequential order.

Aorta	Aortic Valve	Left Atrium	Left Ventricle
Lungs	Mitral Valve	Pulmonary Artery	Pulmonary Vein
Pulmonic Valve	Right Atrium	Right Ventricle	
Tricuspid Valve	Vena Cava		

3. Circle the term that is associated with each cardiac event.

   1. Ventricular contraction

   Systole   Diastole

   2. Filling of the ventricles

   Systole   Diastole

   3. Relaxation of the ventricles

   Systole   Diastole

   4. Blood is expelled into the pulmonary artery

   Systole   Diastole

   5. Closure of the tricuspid valve

   Beginning of Systole   Beginning of Diastole

   6. Closure of the pulmonic valve

   Beginning of Systole   Beginning of Diastole

   7. Closure of the mitral valve

   Beginning of Diastole   End of Diastole

   8. Closure of the aortic valve

   Beginning of Systole   End of Systole

4. Label each part of the ECG.

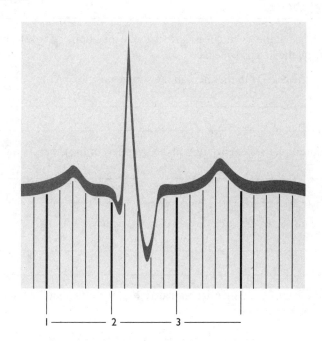

Answer the following questions related to the ECG pattern.

1. The P wave represents: _____.

2. The P wave lasts _____ seconds.

3. The QRS interval represents: _____.

4. The QRS interval lasts _____ seconds.

5. The QT interval represents: _____.

6. The QT interval lasts _____ seconds.

7. The PR interval represents: _____.

8. The PR interval lasts _____ seconds.

EQUIPMENT SELECTION

Prior to beginning the physical assessment of a client's cardiovascular system, it is important to gather the appropriate assessment equipment. Place a check mark next to each piece of equipment that you would need to perform this assessment.

EQUIPMENT					
	Cotton balls		Lubricant		Sphygmomanometer
	Cotton-tipped applicator		Nasal speculum		Stethoscope
	Culture media		Ophthalmoscope		Tape measure
	Dental mirror		Otoscope		Test tubes
	Doppler ultrasonic stethoscope		Penlight		Thermometer
	Drape sheet		Reflex hammer		Tongue blade
	Examination gown		Ruler		Transilluminator
	Flashlight		Skinfold calipers		Tuning fork
	Gauze		Skin-marking pen		Vaginal speculum
	Gloves		Slides		Vision chart
	Goggles		Small towel		Watch with second hand
	Goniometer		Specimen containers		Wood's lamp

ASSESSMENT TECHNIQUES

Review each assessment technique. If the technique is correct, circle the number. If the technique is incorrect, write the correct assessment technique on the line provided.

1. Begin the assessment of the heart with the client in the supine position.

   _____

   _____

2. Inspection of the cardiovascular system begins with an overview of the general skin color.

   _____

   _____

3. The nail beds should be inspected in the cardiovascular assessment.

   _____

   _____

4. During inspection of the external and internal jugular veins, the nurse should be sure the client's head is turned slightly toward the side being examined.

   _____

   _____

5. When assessing for jugular vein distention, the client should be in a supine position with the head of the examination table elevated to a 45-degree angle.

   _____

   _____

6. When inspecting the chest for pulsations, the client should be in a high Fowler's position and then a low Fowler's position.

_____

_____

7. Palpate each carotid artery separately.

_____

_____

8. When beginning to auscultate heart sounds, the client should breathe normally.

_____

_____

9. Initially when auscultating for cardiac murmurs, use the diaphragm of the stethoscope.

_____

_____

10. In order to determine a pulse deficit, the nurse will auscultate the apical pulse while simultaneously palpating a carotid pulse.

_____

_____

ASSESSMENT FINDINGS

Read each assessment finding. Identify the finding as normal or abnormal. Write an A for abnormal and an N for normal on each line provided.

_____ 1. Uniform skin color
_____ 2. Bradycardia
_____ 3. Xanthelasma
_____ 4. Apical heart rate 110 in the adult
_____ 5. Blue nail beds
_____ 6. Precordial heaves
_____ 7. Tetralogy of Fallot in the infant
_____ 8. Patchy hair distribution on legs of adults
_____ 9. QRS interval 0.08
_____ 10. S1 louder than S2 at the left SB, second ICS

_____ 11. +1 edema in the feet of an adult
_____ 12. Ruddy skin tone
_____ 13. Periorbital edema
_____ 14. Rhythmic head bobbing
_____ 15. Visible carotid pulsations
_____ 16. S3 and S4 in the adult
_____ 17. PR interval 0.12
_____ 18. Bounding pulse at rest for the adult
_____ 19. Ventricular gallop
_____ 20. S2 louder than S1 at the left MCL fifth ICS

FACTORS THAT INFLUENCE PHYSICAL ASSESSMENT FINDINGS

Fill in the blank to complete each statement.

1. The _____ _____, a passageway between the atria in the fetus, closes shortly after birth.
2. The blood pressure of a full-term infant is _____ than that of a preterm newborn.
3. Alcoholism may cause ventricular ectopy, which can lead to _____ cardiac output.
4. Cocaine causes a (an) _____ in the oxygen demands on the heart.
5. Blood volume may increase as high as _____ percent during pregnancy.
6. The most common type of murmur that reveals itself during pregnancy is a _____ murmur.
7. Hypertension is most common in the _____ and _____ cultures.

8. Caucasians have _____ serum cholesterol levels than African Americans.

9. The heart walls of an older adult may _____.

10. Ventricular compliance in the older adult may _____.

APPLICATION OF THE CRITICAL THINKING PROCESS

SCENARIO 1

Heena is a 62-year-old Indian female who was brought to the emergency department with dizziness and lightheadedness. She states she continues to get a strange sensation in her chest that she cannot describe. Her vital signs are BP 106/52, HR 112, RR 20, and T 98.7 (oral). Heena denies any medical or surgical history. She denies alcohol or tobacco use. She takes an antacid only when she experiences some heartburn, but denies any other medication use.

The nurse immediately places Heena on a cardiac monitor that reveals this rhythm:

MCL$_6$

1. Identify the above rhythm: _____

   _____

2. Identify two characteristics of this rhythm.

   1. _____

   2. _____

3. Describe any relationship between the identified rhythm and the client's complaint of dizziness and lightheadedness.

4. The nurse continues to assess Heena. The nurse asks Heena if she is experiencing any pain at this time; Heena stated no. The nurse's next question should be:

5. Heena's heart rate decreases to 89 beats per minute and she indicates she is starting to feel a little better. The cardiologist asks the nurse to monitor the client. List three factors that should be "monitored" during this time.

   1. _____

   2. _____

   3. _____

SCENARIO 2

Earl is an 81-year-old male who was diagnosed with congestive heart failure (CHF) 2 years ago. His condition has been managed by medication and careful monitoring. During his visit to the CHF clinic, the nurse discovers that Earl has gained 4 lb in the past 3 days.

1. Discuss if this is a normal or abnormal finding.

2. List three signs or symptoms that may be associated with congestive heart failure.

    1.

    2.

    3.

Vicki, a student nurse, is spending the day at the CHF clinic. Her preceptor has asked her to check Earl's heart rate. Vicki checks a radial pulse for 30 seconds and multiplies it by 2 and reports her findings to her preceptor. The preceptor appeared to be upset with Vicki's method of collecting this data.

3. What assessment technique would have been appropriate in collecting this data? Provide a rationale.

HEALTHY PEOPLE 2020

A *Healthy People 2020* objective is:

Reduce coronary heart disease deaths.

1. Define coronary heart disease.

2. List two risk factors for coronary heart disease that cannot be changed.

    1.

    2.

3. List two risk factors for coronary heart disease that can be changed.

    1.

    2.

4. Discuss how a nurse educator can use this objective to promote and maintain health and function of the cardio-vascular system.

ASSESSMENT AND DOCUMENTATION

Perform a cardiovascular assessment on your lab partner and document your findings on the provided documentation form. You can download the form from the Pearson Student Resources site.

NCLEX®-STYLE REVIEW QUESTIONS

Read each question carefully. Circle the letter that best answers each question.

1. Which of the following statements is true about the blood flow through the heart?
    1. Blood will travel through the pulmonary vein before it travels through the tricuspid valve.
    2. Oxygenated blood will travel through the pulmonary artery prior to being ejected from the left ventricle.
    3. Deoxygenated blood will travel through the pulmonic valve into the pulmonary artery.
    4. Blood passes through the mitral valve before it passes through the tricuspid valve.

2. The cardiac output equation is:
    1. cardiac output = stroke volume × heart rate for one minute.
    2. cardiac output = stroke volume × body surface area.
    3. cardiac output = cardiac index × heart rate for one minute.
    4. cardiac output = cardiac index × stroke volume.

3. A cardiac cycle is completed in:
    1. 0.12 second.
    2. 0.2 second.
    3. 0.8 second.
    4. 1.2 seconds.

4. A 34-week-pregnant African American female visits the Women's Health Clinic for a routine exam. Her blood pressure reading in the supine position is 162/88. The nurse's next step would be to:
    1. further assess and monitor the client for preeclampsia.
    2. further assess and monitor the client for a systolic murmur.
    3. provide the client with fluids for obvious dehydration.
    4. continue with the routine assessment and obtain her weight.

5. A 4-day-old newborn develops cyanosis of the skin and lips. After extensive diagnostic testing, a diagnosis of Tetralogy of Fallot is made. The nurse caring for this newborn discovers that the parents have little understanding of what this actually means. The nurse is aware that this condition includes which combination of cardiac defects?
    1. Atrial septal defect, coarctation of the aorta, right ventricular hypertrophy, and pulmonary stenosis
    2. Dextroposition of the aorta, pulmonary stenosis, atrial flutter, and mitral valve prolapse
    3. Atrial septal defect, left ventricular hypertrophy, pulmonary stenosis, and ventricular septal defect
    4. Dextroposition of the aorta, pulmonary stenosis, right ventricular hypertrophy, and ventricular septal defect

6. The nurse would associate which assessment finding as a pulse deficit?
    1. An absent pulse in more than one extremity
    2. An apical pulse of 88 and a carotid pulse of 78
    3. An apical pulse of 88 and a carotid pulse of 88
    4. An apical pulse of 88 and a carotid pulse of 98

7. When assessing for signs of increased central venous pressure, the nurse decides to inspect the jugular veins. With the client lying at a 45-degree angle, it is noted that the jugular veins distend 4.1 cm above the sternal angle. The nurse interprets this as:
    1. a normal finding.
    2. an abnormal finding but not indicative of increased central venous pressure.
    3. an abnormal finding and indicative of increased central venous pressure.
    4. inaccurate data due to the fact that the client should have been sitting at a 90-degree angle.

8. A middle-aged client with high cholesterol asks the nurse about starting an exercise regimen for a healthy heart. The nurse should be sure to mention that:
    1. only aerobic exercise is beneficial to the heart.
    2. only nonaerobic exercise is beneficial to the heart.
    3. a combination of aerobic and nonaerobic exercise is beneficial.
    4. people who have high cholesterol should not exercise.

9. A 36-year-old male is having a comprehensive history and physical performed. Which of the following pieces of data revealed in his medical history are relevant to the cardiac component of this exam?
    1. Splenectomy
    2. Rheumatic fever as a child
    3. Lactose intolerance
    4. Fractured left scapula

10. A nurse on the telemetry unit at a community hospital has been assigned a 45-year-old female with the diagnosis of "atypical chest pain." She is informed in report that the client has mitral valve regurgitation. The nurse understands that upon auscultation of the cardiac sounds of the client, a:
    1. high-pitched, harsh, blowing sound may be revealed.
    2. low, rumbling sound may be revealed.
    3. soft, blowing sound may be revealed.
    4. medium, coarse, clicking sound may be revealed.

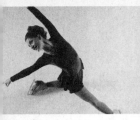

18 Peripheral Vascular System

I look to the future because that's where I'm going to spend the rest of my life.
—George Burns

The peripheral vascular system consists of vessels that carry blood throughout the body. High pressures in this system result in hypertension, known as "the silent killer."

This chapter will focus on gathering both subjective and objective data related to the peripheral vascular system, as well as analysis of the data collected.

OBJECTIVES

At the completion of these exercises you will be able to:

1. Define key terminology associated with the peripheral vascular system.
2. Review the anatomy and physiology of the peripheral vascular system.
3. Select the equipment necessary to complete the peripheral vascular assessment.
4. Identify the correct techniques for assessment of the peripheral vascular system.
5. Analyze data related to assessment of the peripheral vascular system.
6. Recognize factors that can influence assessment findings.

7. Assess the peripheral vascular system on a laboratory partner.
8. Document an assessment of the peripheral vascular system.
9. Apply critical thinking in analysis of a case study.
10. Relate objectives in *Healthy People 2020* to the peripheral vascular system.
11. Complete NCLEX®-style review questions related to the assessment of the peripheral vascular system.

RESOURCES

Pearson Nursing Student Resources
Find additional review materials at
nursing.pearsonhighered.com

Prepare for success with additional NCLEX®-style practice questions, interactive assignments and activities, Web links, animations and videos, and more!

Additional resources: *www.strokecenter.org*
www.CDC.gov
www.americanheart.org

WORD SEARCH

Find and circle the correct term in the word search puzzle for each of the definitions listed below. The word may be horizontal, vertical, or diagonal.

```
H W P W E Q A X P U L S E T C A P I L L A R I E S
H P E R I P H E R A L V A S C U L A R S Y S T E M
A O U Y M Z M E L Y M P H A T I C V E S S E L S A
R V M A Q J V S I S S D N I Q D W Q T E L J G E N
T E O A L I V C P P J R U S A D K N D W K T P V U
E N P Z N N F M V Y O R L N Q B O S A A S W Q U A
R O Z Q N S F Z L H B Q F E D E M A W E V Z A T L
I U B U U P S H M B X J W U W E S V T B I U Y G C
A S H N E J P I Y M L G M C S N V S T L D M D J O
L I U G A U E T G V F A S E O E N Q M B Q U W S M
I N T J R L V Q N N V R I P D E J K R J U Q F B P
N S C A T S E X E M W T K O L Q U J A O Z F T Y R
S U A A E F G Y V P I E N L B V O B Y B Q S P Z E
U F F J R V T N W S V R A O S T K F N M H Y S J S
F F B G I X C D O S A I Z R R W W V A A M O M G S
F I L C E O Q C E E P A R Z O H C E U D G F C M I
I C A O S F I D L G Q L X J I C O I D T N G C J O
C I X O J R O H N R B A D M M Q A N S S D E M S N
I E C H A N C I R H Z N L L N H I S D T R B L G T
E N E V H O B L H B E E J M L I U H I K D A A A E
N C A P R B Y V C H S U W S B Y Y L S S U H J W S
C Y M T U U U K U P X R H I K G I R E X J U G M T
Y Y I L H P B L V Q Y Y R A P I E J A S F G V J S
L P C E Z O P S A T C S Z Q I A K N S H A N X H Q
E G G H X S T T X S H M X T M Q D M E J B L A K Y
```

CLUES

1. Test used to determine patency of the radial and ulnar arteries **(two words)** _____ _____
2. A bulging caused by a weakness in the wall of an artery **(two words)** _____ _____
3. Inadequate arterial circulation, usually due to the buildup of fatty plaque or calcification of the arterial wall **(two words)** _____ _____
4. Tubular elastic-walled vessels that carry oxygenated blood throughout the body _____
5. A loud blowing sound most often associated with a narrowing of an artery _____
6. The smallest vessels of the circulatory system that exchange gases and nutrients between the arterial and venous system _____
7. Flattening of the angle of the nail and enlargement of the tips of the fingers is a sign of oxygen deprivation in the extremities _____
8. An increased accumulation of fluid in the intracellular spaces in a dependent part of the body _____
9. Node located on the medial surface of the arm above the elbow that drains the ulnar surface of the forearm and the third, fourth, and fifth digits **(two words)** _____ _____
10. Diagnostic maneuver in which pain in the lower leg may increase with sharp dorsiflexion of the foot **(two words)**
_____ _____

11. Vessels that extend from the capillaries that collect lymph in organs and tissues **(two words)** _____
    _____

12. Rounded lymphoid tissues that are surrounded by connective tissue **(two words)** _____ _____

13. A maneuver to determine the length of varicose veins **(three words)** _____ _____
    _____

14. Blood vessels of the body that together with the heart and the lymphatic vessels make up the body's circulatory
    system **(three words)** _____ _____ _____

15. Wave of pressure felt at various points in the body due to the force of the blood against the walls of the arteries
    _____

16. A condition in which the arterioles in the fingers develop spasms, causing intermittent skin pallor or cyanosis and
    then rubor **(two words)** _____ _____

17. Distended and dilated veins that have a diminished blood flow and an increased intravenous pressure
    _____

18. Tubular-walled vessels that carry deoxygenated blood from the body periphery back to the heart _____

19. Inadequate circulation in the venous system usually due to incompetent valves in deep veins or a blood clot in the
    veins **words)** _____ _____

ANATOMY & PHYSIOLOGY REVIEW

1. For each diagram below write the name of the structure indicated by each line.

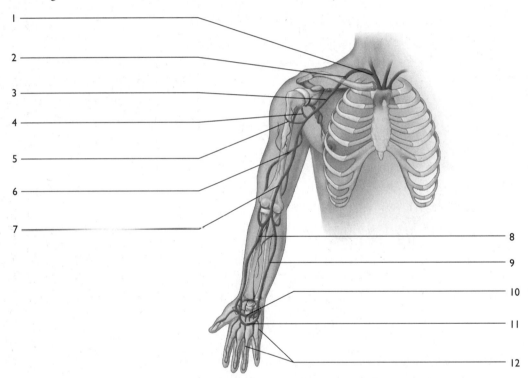

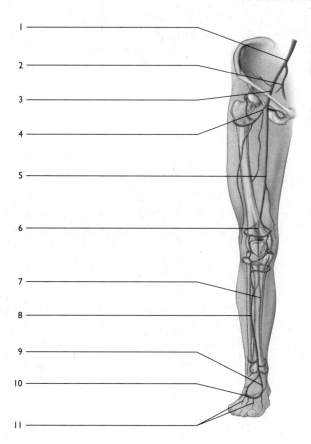

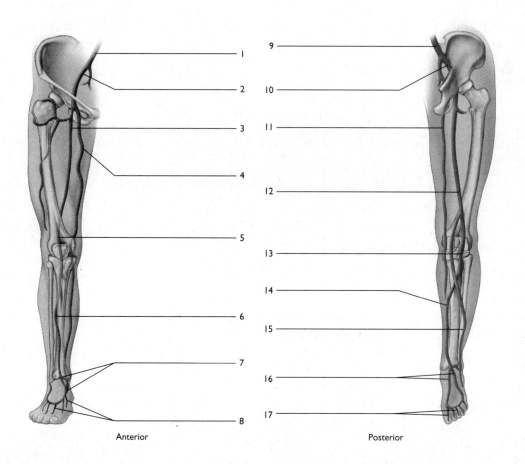

Anterior   Posterior

2. Label each vessel characteristic with a V for veins or an A for arteries.

_____ 1. Carry oxygenated blood   _____ 6. Receive blood from capillaries

_____ 2. Contain valves   _____ 7. Have thick walls

_____ 3. Have thin walls   _____ 8. Have higher pressure

_____ 4. Carry blood to the heart   _____ 9. Carry blood away from the heart

_____ 5. Carry deoxygenated blood   _____ 10. Are more elastic

EQUIPMENT SELECTION

Prior to beginning the physical assessment of a client's peripheral vascular system, it is important to gather the appropriate assessment equipment. Place a check mark next to each piece of equipment that you would need to perform this assessment.

EQUIPMENT		
Cotton balls	Lubricant	Sphygmomanometer
Cotton-tipped applicator	Nasal speculum	Stethoscope
Culture media	Ophthalmoscope	Tape measure
Dental mirror	Otoscope	Test tubes
Doppler ultrasonic stethoscope	Penlight	Thermometer
Drape sheet	Reflex hammer	Tongue blade
Examination gown	Ruler	Tourniquet
Flashlight	Skinfold calipers	Transilluminator
Gauze	Skin-marking pen	Tuning fork
Gloves	Slides	Vaginal speculum
Goggles	Small towel	Watch with second hand
Goniometer	Specimen containers	Wood's lamp

ASSESSMENT TECHNIQUES

Review each assessment technique. If the technique is correct, circle the number. If the technique is incorrect, write the correct assessment technique on the line provided.

1. In the adult, a blood pressure may be obtained on all extremities when performing a complete peripheral vascular assessment.

_____

_____

2. In order to palpate the carotid artery, the examiner must place the first two or three finger pads between the trachea and the sternocleidomastoid muscle and press firmly.

_____

_____

3. In order to assess for capillary refill, the examiner must apply pressure to one of the client's fingernails for 1 second and then quickly release the pressure.

_____

_____

4. In order to assess the brachial artery, the examiner must palpate lateral to the biceps tendon.

_____

_____

5. When performing the Allen's test, the client should sit with arms over the head.

_____

_____

6. The epitrochlear lymph node should be easily palpable behind the elbow to the groove between the biceps and triceps muscles.

_____

_____

7. The manual compression test should be performed with the client standing.

_____

_____

8. During a Trendelenburg's test, the tourniquet should be applied around the upper thigh while the client is standing.

_____

_____

9. The client's knee should be flexed 90 degrees while assessing the Homan's sign.

_____

_____

10. If the examiner has difficulty palpating the popliteal artery while the client is supine, the client can rotate to a prone position and flex the knee.

_____

_____

ASSESSMENT FINDINGS

Read each assessment finding. Identify the finding as normal or abnormal by writing an A for abnormal and an N for normal on each line provided.

_____ 1. Radial pulse 62 bpm in an adult
_____ 2. BP 138/94 in an adult
_____ 3. +2 peripheral pulses in the older adult
_____ 4. Easily palpable epitrochlear node
_____ 5. Warm feet
_____ 6. Positive Homan's sign
_____ 7. Symmetrical popliteal pulses
_____ 8. Yellow, thick toenails
_____ 9. Brachial pulse 102 in an adult
_____ 10. BP 102/62 on an 8-year-old

_____ 11. Regularly irregular rhythm
_____ 12. Capillary refill < 2 seconds
_____ 13. Non-palpable axillary nodes
_____ 14. Necrotic left great toe
_____ 15. Varicosities of the lower extremities
_____ 16. Non-palpable femoral pulse
_____ 17. +1 dorsalis pedis pulse
_____ 18. Lymphedema
_____ 19. Clubbing of fingernails
_____ 20. Unilateral swelling of the lower extremities

FACTORS THAT INFLUENCE PHYSICAL ASSESSMENT FINDINGS

Fill in the blank to complete each statement.

1. The _____ culture has the highest incidence of hypertension.

2. Individuals of Irish and _____ descent have a greater risk of varicose veins.

3. The arterial walls of an older adult will lose _____.

4. Pressure from the pregnant uterus on the lower extremities obstructs _____ _____.

5. A child over 1 year of age will have a systolic pressure in the thigh that is _____ than the arm.

6. Clients with jobs that require standing for most of the day are at greater risk for _____ _____.

7. Hypertension is known as the "silent killer" because it is often _____.

8. Obesity is a risk factor for _____ _____ disease.

9. The _____of peripheral vascular resistance as a client ages increases the risk of hypertension.

10. In a baby less than 1 year of age, the systolic pressure in the thigh should _____ that of the arm.

PULSE PREDICAMENTS

For the conditions listed below, select a pulse or pulses from the box that best describes anticipated findings. Some conditions may have more than one descriptor.

Normal	Pulsus Alternans	Pulsus Paradoxus	Weak/Thready
Absent	Pulsus Bigeminus	Unequal Pulses	Bounding

1. Aortic regurgitation_____

2. Cardiac tamponade_____

3. Shock_____

4. Dissecting aneurysm_____

5. Pericarditis_____

6. Anemia_____

7. Anxiety_____

8. Severe peripheral vascular disease_____

9. Cardiac arrest_____

10. Systemic hypertension_____

11. Pregnancy_____

12. Hyperthyroidism_____

13. Heart failure_____

EDEMA

1. Describe the assessment technique that should be used to stage edema.

2. Stage the levels of edema in the diagram below.

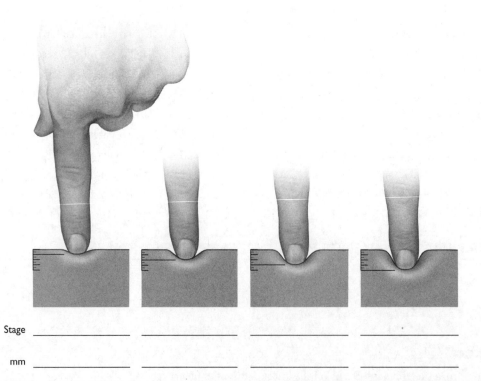

Stage _____ _____ _____ _____

mm _____ _____ _____ _____

3. Name three conditions that a client may have if edema is noted.

   1.

   2.

   3.

APPLICATION OF THE CRITICAL THINKING PROCESS

Read the scenario and answer the following questions.

Agnes is a 72-year-old female who was admitted to a medical-surgical unit for a non-healing wound of her right lateral malleolus. She states it began as a small circular discolored lesion that has slowly formed into a pale, non-bleeding, open-centered wound over the past 2 months.

Agnes has a medical history of diabetes, hypertension, obesity, and she has smoked one pack of cigarettes per day for the past 50 years. Her surgical history is 2 cesarean sections, a hysterectomy, coronary artery stent placements, and a femoral-popliteal bypass of the left leg 2 years ago that failed and lead to a left foot amputation.

Upon admission to the nursing unit, the initial assessment by the nurse notes cool, shiny, pale, hairless skin of both lower legs and thick, brittle, yellow toenails on the right foot. The pedal pulse in the right foot is non-palpable but faintly audible with the Doppler. The wound is circular, 2 cm in diameter, and has well-defined edges, and the wound bed is a pale yellow with no drainage noted. Agnes states she is in severe pain at an 8 on a scale of 1 to 10.

1. Determine if this wound is due to an arterial or venous problem.

2. Identify signs or symptoms that support your conclusion.

3. What is the best position for Agnes in order to help relieve her pain? Provide rationale.

4. What risk factors does Agnes have for this type of wound?

5. Is the wound assessment that has been provided complete? If not, what is missing?

6. List at least four questions that the nurse should ask to complete the pain assessment.

HEALTHY PEOPLE 2020

Please read the *Healthy People 2020* objective and answer the following questions.

A *Healthy People 2020* objective is:

Reduce stroke deaths.

1. Stroke is listed as the _____ leading cause of death in the United States.

2. List two risk factors for stroke that cannot be changed (non-modifiable).

1.

2.

3. List two risk factors for stroke that can be changed (modifiable).

1.

2.

4. Search the website of a health-related organization to identify the components of commonly used stroke scales.

1. Name of Scale:_____

Components of Scale

Site resource (website)

2. Name of Scale:_____

Components of Scale

Site resource (website)

5. Discuss which stroke scale you prefer. What are the advantages to this scale that helped you make the decision?

6. Discuss how a community health nurse can use this *Healthy People 2020* objective to promote and maintain health and function of the peripheral vascular system.

ASSESSMENT AND DOCUMENTATION

Perform a peripheral vascular assessment on your lab partner, and document your findings using the provided documentation form. You can download the form from the Pearson Student Resources site.

NCLEX®-STYLE REVIEW QUESTIONS

Read each question carefully. Choose the best answer for each question.

1. The nurse identifies which of the following statements as true about veins? Veins:
1. carry oxygenated blood.
2. have thicker walls than arteries.
3. have one-way intraluminal valves.
4. carry blood away from the heart.

2. Which of the following would the nurse consider an average blood pressure for a newborn?
1. 62/35
2. 120/80
3. 100/60
4. 50 palpable

3. Hypertension is called the "silent killer" because it is often asymptomatic. Which of the following does the nurse identify as symptoms that may be associated with hypertension? (Select all that apply)
   1. Headache
   2. Epistaxis
   3. Twitching of the eyelids
   4. Chest pain
   5. Palpitations

4. The nurse identifies which of the following clients as least likely to develop varicose veins?
   1. 32-year-old hairdresser
   2. 45-year-old trauma nurse
   3. 55-year-old administrative assistant
   4. 26-year-old pregnant female

5. Which one of the following questions would be inappropriate for the nurse to ask during a focused interview regarding the peripheral vascular system?
   1. Have you noticed a change in hair growth on your legs?
   2. Have you experienced any difficulty in achieving an erection?
   3. Do you smoke?
   4. Have you noticed any blood in your urine?

6. The nurse knows that the carotid pulse should be synchronous with:
   1. S1.
   2. S2.
   3. S3.
   4. S4.

7. A middle-aged client is assisted back to bed after 30 minutes of physical therapy on postoperative day 2 following a left total hip replacement. The client reports pain of 8 out of 10 on the pain scale. The nurse obtains a set of vital signs and notes a radial pulse of 104. The nurse's next step would be to:
   1. notify the doctor because the client is tachycardic.
   2. offer the client an analgesic and reassess the vital signs and pain later.
   3. notify physical therapy that the sessions should be shorter.
   4. allow the client to rest.

8. When assessing the carotid pulse of a client in fluid overload, the nurse would expect the amplitude to be:
   1. 0.
   2. 1.
   3. 2.
   4. 3.

9. Which of the following tests might the nurse perform if it is suspected that the client may have a deep vein thrombosis?
   1. Allen's test
   2. Manual compression test
   3. Homan's sign
   4. Trendelenburg's test

10. An older adult client has a history of venous insufficiency. The client has been admitted to the hospital with an ulcer on the right medial malleolus. The nurse assessing the wound notes which of the following common characteristics of a venous leg ulcer? (Select all that apply)
    1. Wound is moist and bleeds
    2. Temperature of the skin is cool to the touch
    3. Well-defined wound edges
    4. Presence of deep muscle pain
    5. Thickened skin around the ankles that may be darker in appearance

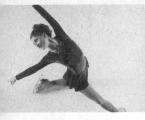

19 Abdomen

You don't understand anything until you learn it more than one way.
—Marvin Minsky

The abdomen contains organs associated with various body systems. Through a skillful focused interview and physical assessment, the nurse will be able to determine which body systems require further investigation. This chapter will focus on gathering both subjective and objective data related to the assessment of the abdomen, as well as analysis of the data collected.

OBJECTIVES

At the completion of these exercises you will be able to:

1. Define key terminology associated with the abdomen.
2. Review the anatomy and physiology of the abdomen.
3. Select the equipment necessary to complete the assessment of the abdomen.
4. Identify the correct assessment techniques.
5. Analyze data related to the assessment of the abdomen.
6. Recognize factors that can influence assessment findings.
7. Assess the abdomen on a laboratory partner.
8. Document an assessment of the abdomen.
9. Apply critical thinking in analysis of a case study.
10. Relate objectives in *Health People 2020* to the assessment of the abdomen.
11. Complete NCLEX®-style review questions related to the assessment of the abdomen.

RESOURCES

Pearson Nursing Student Resources
Find additional review materials at
nursing.pearsonhighered.com

Prepare for success with additional NCLEX®-style practice questions, interactive assignments and activities, Web links, animations and videos, and more!

Additional resources: *www.CDC.gov*
www.childcancerpain.org (assessment of pain)

CROSSWORD PUZZLE FOR KEY TERMS

Read each definition below and fill in the correct term on the puzzle grid. If the answer requires two or more words do not leave a blank space between the words. Use a pencil so you can erase easily.

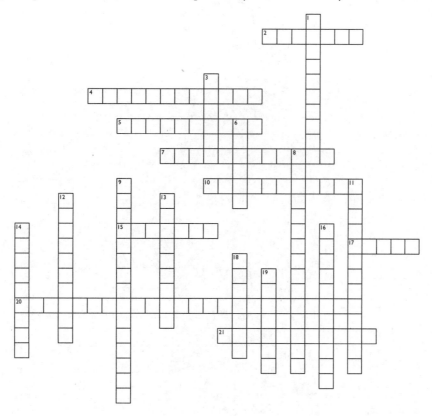

CLUES

Across

2. The largest cavity of the body that contains organs and structures belonging to various systems of the body
4. An imbalance, whether an excess or deficit, of the required nutrients of a balanced diet
5. A weight of 10% to 20% in excess of recommended body weight
7. Pain felt in a part of the body that is considerably removed or distant from the area actually causing the pain (**two words**)
10. A rough, grating sound caused by the rubbing together of organs or an organ rubbing on the peritoneum (**two words**)
15. The process of dividing the abdomen into quadrants or regions for the purpose of assessment
17. A loud blowing sound that is most often associated with a narrowing of an artery
20. The structures connected to the alimentary canal by ducts that contribute to the digestive process of foods (**three words**)
21. A local or generalized inflammatory process of the peritoneal membrane of the abdomen

Down

1. Stomach growling
3. Stretch marks
6. A protrusion of an organ or structure through an abnormal opening or weakened area in a body wall
8. A complex psychosocial and physiological problem characterized by a severely restricted intake of nutrients and a low body weight (**two words**)
9. A continuous, hollow, muscular tube that begins at the mouth and ends at the anus (**two words**)
11. The experience of sharp stabbing pain as the compressed area returns to a noncompressed state (**two words**)
12. A thin, double layer of serous membrane in the abdominal cavity
13. An inflammatory process of the liver
14. Difficulty swallowing
16. Inflammatory process of the esophagus, caused by a variety of irritants
18. An abnormal collection of fluid in the peritoneal cavity
19. Weight of 20% or more above the recommended body weight

ANATOMY & PHYSIOLOGY REVIEW

1. For each diagram below write the name of the structure indicated by each line.

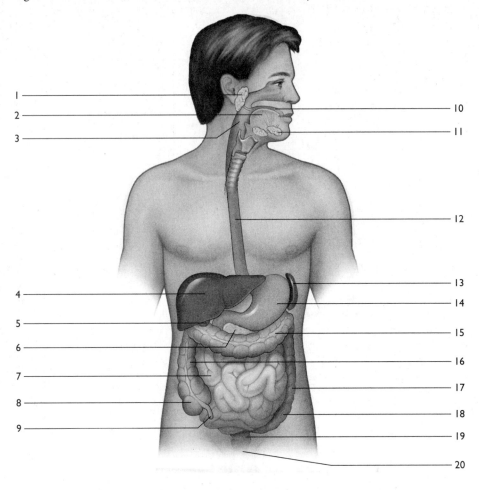

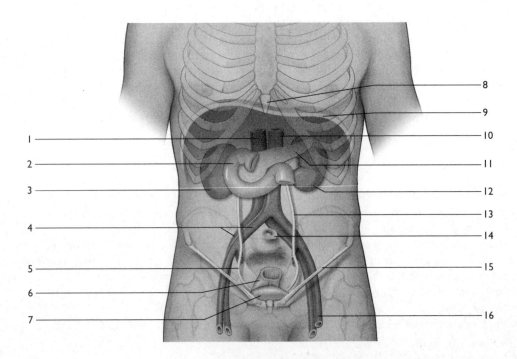

2. Draw lines to map Figure A into four quadrants and Figure B into nine regions. Label each quadrant and region.

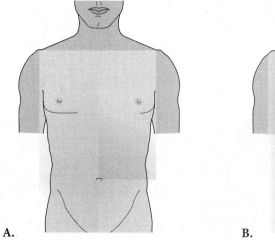

A.

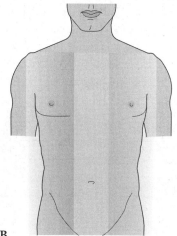

B.

3. Place the following structures involved in the digestive process in the correct order from 1 (the first structure involved) through 14 (the last structure involved).

_____ **a.** Anus

_____ **b.** Ascending colon

_____ **c.** Descending colon

_____ **d.** Duodenum

_____ **e.** Esophagus

_____ **f.** Hepatic flexure of the colon

_____ **g.** Ileum

_____ **h.** Jejunum

_____ **i.** Mouth

_____ **j.** Pharynx

_____ **k.** Rectum

_____ **l.** Splenic flexure of the colon

_____ **m.** Stomach

_____ **n.** Transverse colon

4. Identify the location of each of the structures by placing the letter from the provided key on the provided line.

RUQ = Right Upper Quadrant

RLQ = Right Lower Quadrant

LUQ = Left Upper Quadrant

LLQ = Left Lower Quadrant

_____ **1.** Head of the pancreas

_____ **2.** Sigmoid colon

_____ **3.** Stomach

_____ **4.** Right adrenal gland

_____ **5.** Pyloric sphincter

_____ **6.** Left ovary

_____ **7.** Duodenum

_____ **8.** Left ureter

_____ **9.** Hepatic flexure of colon

_____ **10.** Body of the pancreas

_____ **11.** Appendix

_____ **12.** Spleen

_____ **13.** Gallbladder

_____ **14.** Right spermatic cord

EQUIPMENT SELECTION

Prior to beginning the physical assessment of a client's abdomen, it is important to gather the appropriate equipment. Place a check mark next to each piece of equipment that you would need to perform this assessment.

EQUIPMENT					
	Cotton balls		Lubricant		Sphygmomanometer
	Cotton-tipped applicator		Nasal speculum		Stethoscope
	Culture media		Ophthalmoscope		Tape measure
	Dental mirror		Otoscope		Test tubes
	Doppler ultrasonic stethoscope		Penlight		Thermometer
	Drape sheet		Reflex hammer		Tissues
	Examination gown		Ruler		Transilluminator
	Examination light		Skinfold calipers		Tuning fork
	Gauze		Skin-marking pen		Vaginal speculum
	Gloves		Slides		Vision chart
	Goggles		Small pillow		Watch with second hand
	Goniometer		Specimen containers		Wood's lamp

ASSESSMENT TECHNIQUES

Review each assessment technique. If the technique is correct, circle the number. If the technique is incorrect, write the correct assessment technique on the line provided.

1. The client should be in a supine position with a small pillow placed behind the head for assessment of the abdomen.

   _____

   _____

2. The examination gown should cover the chest and the drape sheet should be placed 1–2 inches below the umbilicus.

   _____

   _____

3. The contour of the abdomen should be assessed at eye level with a light source.

   _____

   _____

4. The examiner should visualize imaginary horizontal and vertical lines delineating the abdominal quadrants while observing the abdomen.

   _____

   _____

5. The auscultation pattern for bowel sounds should begin with the right lower quadrant using the diaphragm of the stethoscope.

   _____

   _____

6. The auscultation pattern for vascular sounds should begin with the femoral arteries.

   _____

   _____

7. During the abdominal assessment, the examiner should auscultate over the liver and spleen for friction rubs.

_____

_____

8. When percussing the borders of the liver, the examiner should begin at the level of the umbilicus and move towards the rib cage along the extended left midclavicular line.

_____

_____

9. Palpation should occur prior to auscultation in order to avoid changing the natural sounds and movements of the abdomen.

_____

_____

10. Murphy's sign is assessed while the client is lying supine. The examiner can place the right hand above the client's knee. The client is then asked to raise the leg to meet the examiner's hand.

_____

_____

ASSESSMENT FINDINGS

Read each assessment finding. Identify if the finding is normal or abnormal. Write an A for abnormal and an N for normal on each line provided.

_____ 1. Guarded abdomen

_____ 2. Smooth and moist skin

_____ 3. Hyperactive bowel sounds

_____ 4. Tympany on percussion over the left lower quadrant

_____ 5. Friction rub over RUQ

_____ 6. Renal artery bruit

_____ 7. Rebound tenderness to the LLQ

_____ 8. Hypoactive bowel sounds throughout

_____ 9. Obesity

_____ 10. Venous hum auscultated below the xiphoid process

_____ 11. Rounded abdominal contour

_____ 12. Bulges

_____ 13. Borborygmi

_____ 14. Non-palpable spleen

_____ 15. Resonance on percussion over the RUQ

_____ 16. Non-palpable liver

_____ 17. Liver span of 5.5 cm RMCL

_____ 18. Ascites

_____ 19. Pain during the psoas sign

_____ 20. Displaced umbilicus in a 7-month-pregnant female

FACTORS THAT INFLUENCE PHYSICAL ASSESSMENT FINDINGS

Fill in the blank to complete each statement.

1. The umbilical cord consists of _____ artery(ies) and _____ vein(s).

2. Abdominal breathing is seen in the _____ age group.

3. Linea nigra is seen in _____ females.

4. Digestive enzymes _____ in the older adult.

5. Jewish Americans have a greater occurrence of _____ intolerance.

6. The _____ culture is at greater risk for gastric cancer.

7. During pregnancy the _____ enlarges and expands into the abdominal cavity.

8. The older adult and the pregnant female are at risk for _____.

9. Clients who have surgical scars on the abdomen may experience body _____ disturbances.

10. During pregnancy, the fundus of the uterus should be above the pubic bone by week _____.

APPLICATION OF THE CRITICAL THINKING PROCESS

Read the scenario and answer the following questions.

SCENARIO I

Yvonne is a 36-year-old African American female who delivered a baby boy at 34 weeks' gestation by cesarean section 2 months ago. As Yvonne is changing her baby's diaper, he begins to cry; she notices that he has a lump on his belly. Highly concerned, she calls the pediatrician's office for an appointment.

1. List three focused interview questions the nurse should ask Yvonne upon arrival to the office.

    1.

    2.

    3.

2. The baby's vital signs are BP 75/40, HR 122, RR 38, Temp 99.1°F. Are these stable vital signs for a 2-month-old baby?

3. Upon physical assessment, the nurse notices a ½-inch bulge just below the baby's umbilicus. She reports this finding to the physician. The baby is diagnosed with an umbilical hernia. List two other signs and/or symptoms that may be noted on assessment of the abdomen.

    1.

    2.

4. The baby appears to be comfortable and in no distress. What pain scale would be appropriate for the nurse to use to assess for pain? Provide a rationale.

5. Develop a nursing diagnosis for this baby from the data in the scenario.

SCENARIO 2

Alfonso is a 38-year-old male who arrives at the emergency department complaining of abdominal pain and mild nausea. He has a medical history of irritable bowel syndrome and asthma. He has no surgical history. He has smoked one pack of cigarettes per day for the last 10 years and drinks 2–3 beers on the weekend.

1. List three focused questions the nurse should ask during this initial interview.

    1.

    2.

    3.

The nurse completes a pain assessment and learns that the pain suddenly started 5 hours ago to the right lower quadrant, it is constant, and is a 7 on a numerical scale. He took three ibuprofen tablets 2 hours ago with no relief.

2. List four questions that should be asked to complete the pain assessment.

    1.

    2.

    3.

    4.

Further data collection reveals the following: BP 142/82, HR 98, RR 20, Temp 101.2°F. Alfonso states he has not had much of an appetite in the past few days. Upon physical assessment, the abdomen is soft and non-distended with positive bowel sounds in all four quadrants. Rebound tenderness is noted in the right lower quadrant, and pain is noted during the psoas test.

3. Alfonso is diagnosed with appendicitis. What assessment factors support this diagnosis?

4. Identify a learning need for this client in the above scenario.

HEALTHY PEOPLE 2020

A *Healthy People 2020* objective is:

Increase the percentage of persons aware they have a chronic hepatitis C infection.

1. List three signs or symptoms of hepatitis C.

   1.

   2.

   3.

2. Discuss how a community health nurse can use this objective to promote and maintain health.

ASSESSMENT AND DOCUMENTATION

Perform an assessment of the abdomen on your lab partner and document your findings on the provided documentation form. You can download the form from the Pearson Student Resources site.

NCLEX®-STYLE REVIEW QUESTIONS

Read each question carefully. Choose the best answer for each question.

1. The nurse is aware that the alimentary canal begins at the:
   1. mouth and ends at the anus.
   2. esophagus and ends at the large intestine.
   3. jejunum and ends at the rectum.
   4. small intestine and ends at the large intestine.

2. The nurse can refer to which of the following as accessory digestive organs? (Select all that apply)
   1. Liver
   2. Pancreas
   3. Spleen
   4. Gallbladder
   5. Cecum

3. When performing a physical assessment on a client's abdomen, the nurse will follow which sequence of techniques?
   1. Inspection, palpation, percussion, auscultation
   2. Auscultation, inspection, palpation, percussion
   3. Auscultation, inspection, percussion, palpation
   4. Inspection, auscultation, percussion, palpation

4. When obtaining health history data from a pregnant female, the nurse must be sure to ask questions about: (Select all that apply)
   1. hemorrhoids.
   2. constipation.
   3. frequent voiding.
   4. nausea and vomiting.
   5. heartburn.

5. A 32-year-old male enters the medical clinic for an annual physical. He states that he has lost 22 lb in the last 2 months. An appropriate follow-up question from the nurse would be:
   1. "Was the weight loss intentional or unintentional?"
   2. "Did you join a fitness center?"
   3. "How much more weight do you want to lose?"
   4. "Good for you! Are you proud of yourself?"

6. Prior to starting the assessment of the abdomen, the nurse should:
   1. provide a warm, comfortable, and private environment.
   2. ask the client not to void for at least 1 hour.
   3. perform a pain assessment because the nurse should examine the painful area first.
   4. stand on the left side of the client.

7. The nurse is caring for a second-day postoperative client following bowel surgery. The client has had a bowel movement or passed flatus since surgery. When the nurse auscultates the client's abdomen for bowel sounds, an expected finding would be:
   1. hyperactive.
   2. normal.
   3. hypoactive.
   4. borborygmi.

8. The nurse begins percussion at the level of the umbilicus and moves toward the rib cage along the right midclavicular line. The percussion sounds change from tympany to dullness. The nurse has now identified:
   1. the lower border of the liver.
   2. the lowest rib.
   3. the spleen.
   4. an abnormal finding.

9. The nurse is about to palpate the abdomen of his client. The nurse should keep in mind that it is best to:
   1. begin with a light palpation.
   2. slide his hand from each spot of the abdomen.
   3. use a bimanual technique for a cachexic client.
   4. use deep palpation if an abdominal aortic aneurysm is suspected.

10. The nurse is aware that referred pain from the liver may be to the:
    1. left flank.
    2. right shoulder.
    3. jaw.
    4. right groin.

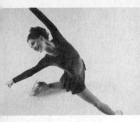

20 Urinary System

One may go a long way after one is tired.
—French Proverb

The elimination of waste products and toxins from the body is an important function of the urinary system. Without filtration by the kidneys, the accumulation of these products will affect the entire body. This chapter will focus on gathering both subjective and objective data related to the urinary system, as well as analysis of the data collected.

OBJECTIVES

At the completion of these exercises you will be able to:

1. Define key terminology associated with the urinary system.
2. Review the anatomy and physiology of the urinary system.
3. Select the equipment necessary to complete the urinary assessment.
4. Identify the correct techniques for assessment of the urinary system.
5. Analyze data related to assessment of the urinary system.
6. Recognize factors that can influence assessment findings.
7. Assess the urinary system on a laboratory partner.
8. Document an assessment of the urinary system.
9. Apply critical thinking in analysis of a case study.
10. Relate objectives in *Healthy People 2020* to the assessment of the urinary system.
11. Complete NCLEX®-style review questions related to the urinary assessment.

RESOURCES

Pearson Nursing Student Resources
Find additional review materials at
nursing.pearsonhighered.com

Prepare for success with additional NCLEX®-style practice questions, interactive assignments and activities, Web links, animations and videos, and more!

Additional resources: *www.CDC.gov*

WORD SEARCH

Find and circle the correct term in the word search puzzle for each of the definitions listed below. The word may be horizontal, vertical, or diagonal.

```
R R E A B K Z F G E D Y S R E F L E X I A W W
I Y Z Z N I H W I V A O W S D H W M R E I I L
Q A X F U I P J U U V U A J X W W X C N E U D
B X Y Y A U N T N O C T U R I A U O E K J E K
Q H U H J T D C Q D A J U B W X C S S I B Z Y
E D R S Z I U J O K Z U T R T Z U U A D K Z B
S Z I G F X L K P N W O S Z E H O O X N D B I
X B N U M W G H Q M T L R D O T X C B E Z T H
J W A M L T Y A T G X I H R C Y H C R Y K F O
E Y R X H O G T T E C H N M T N X R T S F M D
E J Y S C O S T O V E R T E B R A L A N G L E
Y E R M B U L A N R R T C R N G M U P O Q A P
O Q E Q B C Y V C Q C T F F P C M M U U R Z
R B T C R A W M A K V R Z V K H E G A G I D I
O L E R A Y Q A O L I G U R I A L R L R H C
H Z N B Z L R N Z J I O Y E U C L H U T D E Y
U E T L G L C O B D E K M V V U R S U T M C
Q A I R W A M U R E L C O J D Z E G I R A A L
D B O L V A C D L A H P O E C M B N R E S T O
B E N M U U B S O I P W M R O T I U G T U U L
P J I D U V D N U W A E S L T K I R O E Z R N
M L W D V U I S F J Q J G M J E D C X R A I I
Y Q E N J R E N U R E S I S J R X Y B S X A Q
```

CLUES

1. Stones that block the urinary tract _____
2. The outer portion of each kidney composed of over 1 million nephrons, which form urine _____
3. The area on the lower back formed by the vertebral column and the downward curve of the last posterior rib **(two words)**_____ _____
4. An alteration in urinary elimination that affects clients with spinal cord injuries at level T_7 or higher _____
5. Involuntary urination, such as bed-wetting, that occurs after age 4 _____
6. Tufts of capillaries of the kidneys that filter more than 1 liter of fluid each minute _____
7. Blood in urine _____
8. The inability to hold urine _____
9. Bean-shaped organs located in the retroperitoneal space on either side of the vertebral column _____
10. The inner portion of the kidney, composed of structures called pyramids and calyces _____
11. Nighttime urination _____
12. Diminished volume of urine _____
13. Mucous-lined narrow tubes whose major function is transporting urine from the kidney to the urinary bladder _____
14. Mucous-lined tube that transports urine from the urinary bladder to the exterior _____
15. A chronic state in which the client cannot fully empty his or her bladder **(two words)**_____ _____

ANATOMY & PHYSIOLOGY REVIEW

1. For each diagram below write the name of the structure indicated by each line.

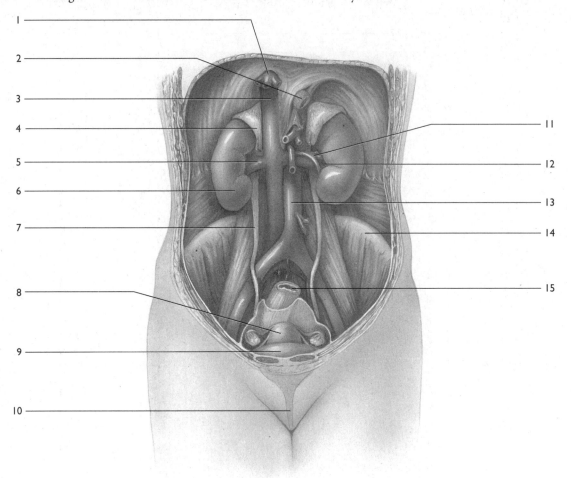

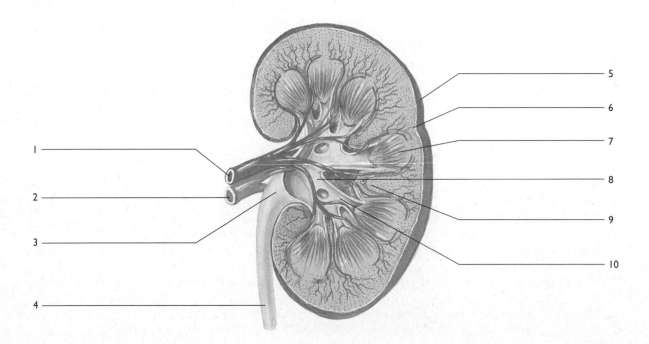

2. Read each statement. Place a K on the line that relates to a function of the kidney or place a B on the line if it is a function of the bladder. Write N/A if it does not relate to the function of either organ.

   _____ **1.** Produces erythropoietin

   _____ **2.** Regulates volume of blood

   _____ **3.** Filters lymph

   _____ **4.** Eliminates waste products

   _____ **5.** Contracts during micturition

   _____ **6.** Temporarily stores urine

   _____ **7.** Assists in the metabolism of vitamin D

   _____ **8.** Secretes cortisol

   _____ **9.** Produces renin

   _____ **10.** Maintains acid–base balance

EQUIPMENT SELECTION

Prior to beginning the physical assessment of a client's urinary system, it is important to gather the appropriate assessment equipment. Place a check mark next to each piece of equipment that you would need to perform this assessment.

EQUIPMENT					
Cotton balls		Lubricant		Sphygmomanometer	
Cotton-tipped applicator		Nasal speculum		Stethoscope	
Culture media		Ophthalmoscope		Tape measure	
Dental mirror		Otoscope		Test tubes	
Doppler ultrasonic stethoscope		Penlight		Thermometer	
Drape sheet		Reflex hammer		Tongue blade	
Examination gown		Ruler		Transilluminator	
Flashlight		Skinfold calipers		Tuning fork	
Gauze		Skin-marking pen		Vaginal speculum	
Gloves		Slides		Vision chart	
Goggles		Small towel		Watch with second hand	
Goniometer		Specimen containers		Wood's lamp	

ASSESSMENT TECHNIQUES

Review each assessment technique. If the technique is correct, circle the number. If the technique is incorrect, write the correct assessment technique on the line provided.

1. The examiner should instruct the client to report any pain or discomfort during the assessment process.

   _____

   _____

2. Assessment of the urinary system should begin with the client sitting upright on an examination table with legs dangling.

   _____

   _____

3. The examiner should visually inspect the client's suprapubic area.

   _____

   _____

4. The bell of the stethoscope should be placed over each renal artery at the midclavicular line about 1–2 cm above the level of the umbilicus.

   _____

   _____

5. The costovertebral angles are inspected while the client is in a supine position.

_____

_____

6. Palpation over the costovertebral angles should initially be done with deep pressure.

_____

_____

7. Indirect percussion is used by placing the palm of the examiner's nondominant hand over the left or right costovertebral angle and using the ulnar surface of the dominant hand to thump the back of the nondominant hand.

_____

_____

8. The client should take and hold a deep breath throughout the entire capture maneuver of a kidney.

_____

_____

9. The fundus of the bladder can be located easily with light palpation.

_____

_____

10. Percussion of the bladder should begin over the suprapubic area and proceed superiorly toward the umbilicus.

_____

_____

ASSESSMENT FINDINGS

Read each assessment finding. On the first line before each assessment finding, place an "N" before each normal assessment finding and an "A" before each abnormal finding. In addition, identify each finding as either subjective "S" or objective "O" by placing the appropriate letter on the line before the finding.

_____ 1. Non-palpable kidney

_____ 2. Dark cloudy urine

_____ 3. Burning at time of voiding

_____ 4. Oliguria

_____ 5. Puffiness in the face

_____ 6. CVA tenderness

_____ 7. Pruritus of the skin

_____ 8. Suprapubic tenderness

_____ 9. Calculi

_____ 10. Bladder distention

_____ 11. Incontinence of urine

_____ 12. Urethral discharge

_____ 13. Palpable smooth, round, firm kidney

_____ 14. Upper abdominal bruit in young adult

_____ 15. Colic

_____ 16. Hematuria

_____ 17. Frequency

_____ 18. Dry, scaly skin

_____ 19. Urgency to void

_____ 20. An elevation over the costovertebral angle

FACTORS THAT INFLUENCE PHYSICAL ASSESSMENT FINDINGS

Fill in the blank to complete each statement.

1. Fluid and electrolyte balance is very fragile in _____ and _____.

2. During the first trimester of pregnancy, changes in the body cause _____ in urination.

3. The ability to concentrate and _____ urine decreases slowly after 40 years of age.

4. Concentrations of renin and aldosterone _____ with advanced age.

5. Incomplete emptying of the bladder during the postpartum period can increase a client's risk for _____ _____ _____.

6. Bed-wetting during the night is not considered abnormal until after the age of _____.

7. Diaper rash is an indicator that the nurse should assess _____ practices of the family.

8. Postmenopausal females have a decrease in _____ that may affect the strength of the pubic muscles leading to urine leakage.

9. African Americans and Hispanics have higher rates of hypertension and diabetes that put them at greater risk for _____ _____.

10. People who live in the southwest United States are at higher risk for _____ _____ due to the high mineral content in the water.

APPLICATION OF THE CRITICAL THINKING PROCESS

Read the scenario and answer the following questions.

Romul is a 32-year-old male who is attending a family barbeque when he suddenly feels a sharp stabbing pain in his mid-back with a wave of nausea. The pain lasts approximately 20 min and resolves on its own. Unfortunately, 2 hours later the pain returns. It is more intense, and Romul begins to vomit. His brother becomes concerned and drives him to the emergency department.

Romul is 5′11″ and 325 lb. He has a history of a gastric bypass surgery 4 months ago. He has lost 42 lb since the surgery and had no complications during his recovery. He does 30 minutes of cardiovascular activity every day and participates in a weight training class three times per week. He takes a multivitamin daily and two types of antihypertensive medication to regulate his blood pressure. As the nurse begins to interview Romul, she finds that he has only had an instant breakfast drink for breakfast and a plate of salad and barbequed chicken for lunch. The pain continues to intensify, and he scales it as a 12 on a scale of 0 to 10. He rolls over onto his side and begins to scream out in agony. He states his groin is starting to hurt him. When asked for a urine sample, gross hematuria is noted.

1. How should the nurse proceed with the physical assessment?

2. Should the nurse consider medicating the client for the severe pain prior to performing the physical assessment? Support your answer.

After a complete assessment including diagnostic testing, it is determined that Romul has a 6-mm renal calculus. (Additional resources may be needed to answer the following questions.)

3. What risk factors did Romul have for a renal calculus?

Romul will require lithotripsy (a medical procedure that uses shock waves to break up a calculus).

4. Write two priority nursing diagnoses for this client.

    1.

    2.

5. Romul and his family are concerned that this could happen to him again. The nurse prepares to educate Romul on the prevention of renal calculi. Develop a teaching plan for this scenario.

Goal:			
Objectives:	Content:	Teaching Strategies:	Evaluation:

HEALTHY PEOPLE 2020

Please read the *Healthy People 2020* objective and answer the following questions.

A *Healthy People 2020* objective is:

Reduce the rate of new cases of end-stage renal disease (ESRD).

1. What conditions increase a client's risk for developing ESRD?

2. Discuss how a nurse can use this objective to promote and maintain health and function of the urinary system.

ASSESSMENT AND DOCUMENTATION

Perform an assessment of the urinary system on your lab partner and document your findings on the provided documentation form. You can download the form from the Pearson Student Resources site.

NCLEX®-STYLE REVIEW QUESTIONS

Read each question carefully. Choose the best answer for each question.

1. The nurse understands that females are more likely to develop urinary tract infections than males because:
   1. the length of the female urethra is longer than the male's.
   2. the proximity of the urethral meatus to the rectum is closer in females.
   3. females are more likely to take bubble baths.
   4. females and males are equally as likely to develop a urinary tract infection.

2. The nurse identifies the area of the lower back formed by the vertebral column and the downward curve of the last posterior rib as the:
   1. symphysis pubis.
   2. costovertebral angle.
   3. cortex.
   4. rectus abdominis.

3. The nurse knows that formation of kidney stones can be attributed to conditions that increase the client's level of
   _____.
   1. potassium
   2. sodium
   3. estrogen
   4. calcium

4. An older adult male presents to the emergency department complaining of blood in his urine. Which of the following questions would be appropriate for the nurse to include in assessing this client? (Select all that apply)
1. "Have you been passing any blood clots?"
2. "Tell me about any recent falls."
3. "Tell me about any pain you have had or may be having."
4. "Do you take a multivitamin every day?"
5. "Do you take aspirin every day?"

5. The nurse is beginning to assess the urinary system of a client. The best position for the client to be in is:
1. prone.
2. supine.
3. lithotomy.
4. High-Fowler's.

6. The nurse explains to a new graduate nurse that auscultation of the renal arteries for bruits is:
1. not necessary in the urinary assessment because it is performed during the abdominal assessment.
2. done by placing the bell of the stethoscope over the umbilical and epigastric areas.
3. performed last during the urinary assessment.
4. only necessary if the client complains of flank pain.

7. The nurse identifies which of the following conditions as those that put a client at higher risk for end-stage renal disease? (Select all that apply)
1. Hypertension
2. Obesity
3. Frequent kidney infections
4. Diabetes
5. Hydronephrosis

8. The nurse notes a distended bladder on physical assessment of a client. In describing this finding, the nurse uses which of the following terms?
1. Tender and firm
2. Smooth, round, and taut
3. Boggy
4. A distended bladder is not palpable.

9. An older adult female complains of leaking urine whenever she coughs, sneezes, or laughs hard. The nurse documents this finding as:
1. total incontinence.
2. functional incontinence.
3. stress incontinence.
4. reflex incontinence.

10. When developing a teaching plan for a client who develops frequent renal calculi, the nurse should include the following:
1. Drink enough fluids to produce 2,000 ml of urine per day.
2. Drink large amounts of caffeinated beverages.
3. Drink lots of milk.
4. Drink enough fluids to produce 4,800 ml of urine per day.

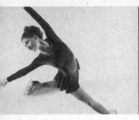

21 Male Reproductive System

The difference between the impossible and the possible lies in a person's determination.
—Tommy Lasorda

The male reproductive system consists of multiple organs that are responsible for the production of hormones and male reproductive cells. The system has a great impact on male sexual behavior and requires a comprehensive assessment that will include psychosocial, self-care, and environmental factors. This chapter will focus on gathering both subjective and objective data related to the male reproductive system, as well as analysis of the data collected.

OBJECTIVES

At the completion of these exercises you will be able to:

1. Define key terminology associated with the male reproductive system.
2. Review the anatomy and physiology of the male reproductive system.
3. Select the equipment necessary to complete the male reproductive assessment.
4. Identify the correct techniques for assessment of the male reproductive system.
5. Analyze data related to assessment of the male reproductive system.
6. Recognize factors that can influence assessment findings.
7. Assess the male reproductive system on a model.
8. Document an assessment of the male reproductive system.
9. Apply critical thinking in analysis of a case study.
10. Relate objectives in *Healthy People 2020* to the male reproductive system.
11. Complete NCLEX®-style questions related to the assessment of the male reproductive system.

RESOURCES

Pearson Nursing Student Resources

Find additional review materials at
nursing.pearsonhighered.com

Prepare for success with additional NCLEX®-style practice questions, interactive assignments and activities, Web links, animations and videos, and more!

Additional resources: *www.pilonidal.org*
www.CDC.gov

CROSSWORD PUZZLE FOR KEY TERMS

Read each definition below and fill in the correct term on the puzzle grid. If the answer requires two words do not leave a blank space between the words. Use a pencil so you can erase easily.

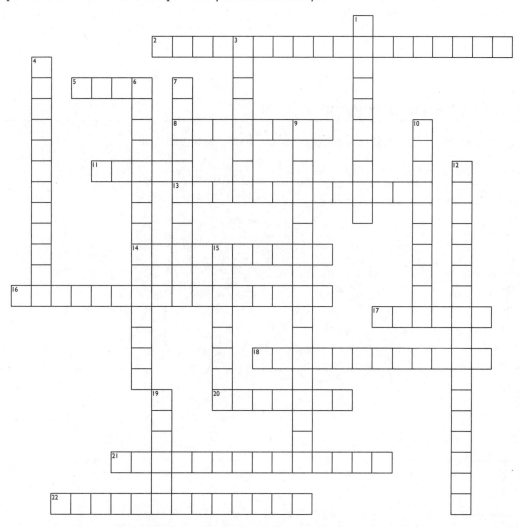

Across

2. Cowper's glands that are located just below the prostate **(two words)**
5. The terminal end of the large intestines exiting the body
8. The space between the scrotum and the anus
11. The male organ used for both elimination of urine and ejaculation of sperm during reproduction
13. Organ that borders the urethra near the lower part of the bladder; it lies just anterior to the rectum **(two words)**
14. A condition in which the urethral meatus is located on the superior aspect of the glans
16. Disease that causes the shaft of the penis to be crooked during an erection **(two words)**
17. Two firm, rubbery, olive-shaped structures that manufacture sperm and are thus the primary male sex organs
18. A common infection in males characterized by a dull, aching pain
20. A loosely hanging, pliable, pear-shaped pouch of darkly pigmented skin located behind the penis that houses the testes, which produce sperm
21. When a separation of the abdominal muscle exists, the weak points of these canals afford an area for the protrusion of the intestine into the groin region **(two words)**
22. A cord that forms a protective sheath around the nerves, blood vessels, lymphatic structures, and muscle fibers associated with the scrotum **(two words)**

Down

1. A varicose enlargement of the veins of the spermatic cord causing a soft compressible mass in the scrotum
3. Inflammation of the testicles

4. A cyst located in the epididymis
6. A pair of saclike glands, located between the bladder and rectum, that are the source of 60% of the semen produced **(two words)**
7. A condition in which the urethral meatus is located on the underside of the glans
9. Condition indicated by pinpoint appearance of the urinary meatus **(two words)**
10. A crescent-shaped system of ductules emerging posteriorly from the testis which holds the sperm during maturation
12. A reflexive action that may cause the testicles to migrate upward temporarily **(two words)**
15. Condition in which the foreskin of a penis cannot be fully retracted
19. A white, cheesy sebaceous matter that collects between the glans of the penis and the foreskin

ANATOMY & PHYSIOLOGY REVIEW

1. For each diagram below write the name of the structure indicated by each line.

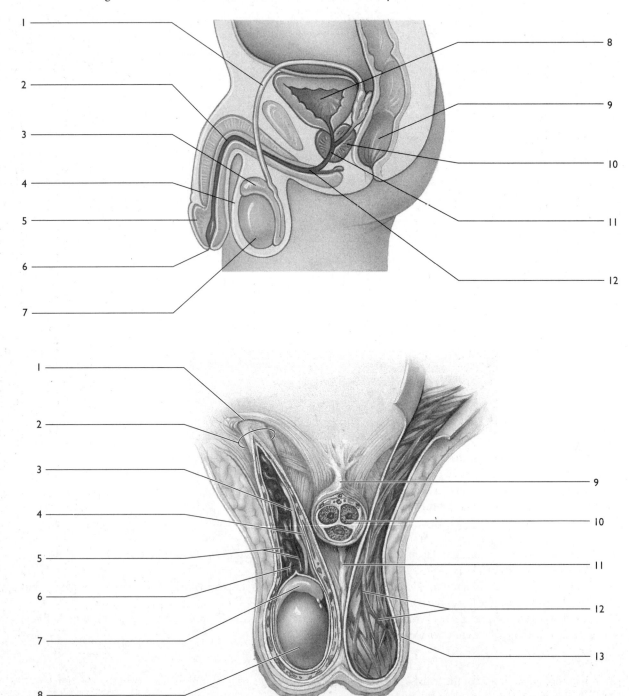

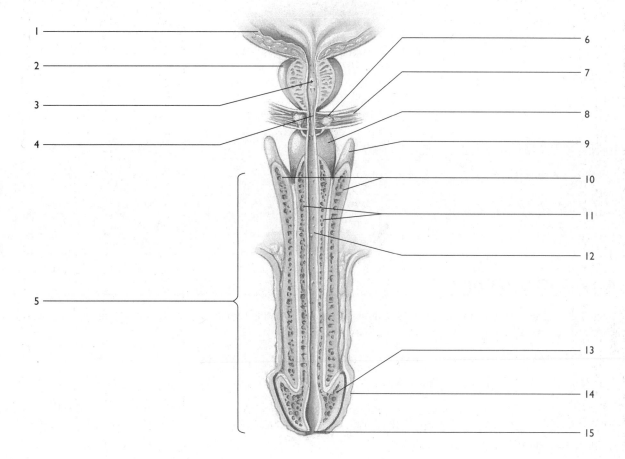

2. The following are structures involved in the pathway for sperm. Place them in correct order from origin to ejaculation by placing the number from 1 to 6 on the line corresponding to the structure.

_____ Spermatic cord

_____ Ductus deferens

_____ Epididymis

_____ Seminiferous tubules

_____ Ejaculatory duct

_____ Seminal vesicles

EQUIPMENT SELECTION

Prior to beginning the physical assessment of a male client's reproductive system, it is important to gather the appropriate equipment. Place a check mark next to each piece of equipment that you would need to perform this assessment.

EQUIPMENT		
Cotton balls	Lubricant	Sphygmomanometer
Cotton-tipped applicator	Nasal speculum	Stethoscope
Culture media	Ophthalmoscope	Tape measure
Dental mirror	Otoscope	Test tubes
Doppler ultrasonic stethoscope	Penlight	Thermometer
Drape sheet	Reflex hammer	Tongue blade
Examination gown	Ruler	Transilluminator
Flashlight	Skinfold calipers	Tuning fork
Gauze	Skin-marking pen	Vaginal speculum
Gloves	Slides	Vision chart
Goggles	Small towel	Watch with second hand
Goniometer	Specimen containers	Wood's lamp

ASSESSMENT TECHNIQUES

Review each assessment technique. If the technique is correct, circle the number. If the technique is incorrect, write the correct assessment technique on the line provided.

1. The client should be instructed to empty his bladder and bowel prior to the assessment.

   _____

   _____

2. Explain to the client that if an erection occurs during the assessment that this is normal and has no sexual connotation.

   _____

   _____

3. The client should be in the supine position for the first portion of this assessment.

   _____

   _____

4. If the client is uncircumcised, it is inappropriate for the examiner to ask the client to retract the foreskin.

   _____

   _____

5. Position of the urinary meatus should be assessed during the inspection of the penis.

   _____

   _____

6. To allow adequate visualization of the scrotum, the examiner should hold the penis firmly in the left hand and lift.

   _____

   _____

7. Transillumination of the scrotum can be performed by placing a lighted flashlight behind the scrotum in a well-lit room.

   _____

   _____

8. The client should breathe normally at first when inspecting the right and left inguinal areas.

_____

_____

9. The finger pads should be used to palpate the anterior side of each testicle to locate the epididymis.

_____

_____

10. When palpating the bulbourethral gland, the examiner's index finger should gently be inserted into the anus with the thumb gently pressing against the perianal area. The examiner's index finger should gently press away from the thumb.

_____

_____

ASSESSMENT FINDINGS

Read each assessment finding. Determine if the finding is normal or abnormal. Write an A for abnormal and an N for normal on each line provided.

_____ 1. Firm prostate

_____ 2. Heavy distribution of hair at the symphysis pubis on the adult

_____ 3. Smegma

_____ 4. Hard and beaded spermatic cord

_____ 5. Non-palpable inguinal lymph nodes

_____ 6. Negative occult blood

_____ 7. Soft and boggy scrotal sac

_____ 8. Pinpoint-size meatus

_____ 9. Genital itching

_____ 10. Phimosis

_____ 11. Pain upon palpation of the bulbourethral gland

_____ 12. Prostate extends ½ cm into rectal area

_____ 13. Walnut-sized testis in the adult

_____ 14. A bulge at the external ring

_____ 15. Darker skin around the anus

_____ 16. Nits

_____ 17. Hypospadias

_____ 18. Decreased libido

_____ 19. Torsion of the testicle

_____ 20. Decreased ability to maintain an erection

FACTORS THAT INFLUENCE PHYSICAL ASSESSMENT FINDINGS

Fill in the blank to complete each statement.

1. Cultural and religious beliefs may influence a family's decision to _____ a newborn male.

2. Dense pubic hair and penile and testicular enlargement in a male under the age of 10 is characterized as _____ _____.

3. Testicular cancer occurs more frequently in _____ than in any other ethnic group.

4. Drugs and alcohol may _____ a client's sexual drive.

5. During puberty, elevated _____ levels will cause the development of adult sexual characteristics.

6. The most common type of cancer in males between the ages of 20 and 35 is _____.

7. Cryptorchidism, also known as _____ testicles, is common in preterm male infants.

8. Diminished libido may occur in the older adult male because of decreased level of _____.

9. Sexual interests and urges that are acted upon prior to counseling of safe sex practices can put an adolescent at risk for _____ _____ _____.

10. Some signs of _____ _____ in male children may be depression, eating disorders, and swelling of the genitalia.

THE TESTICULAR EXAM

Use the words in the Word Bank to complete each statement regarding the self-testicular exam.

Word Bank

Monthly	Cold	Gentle Pressure
Shower	Epididymis	Firm
Smooth	Lumps	Round
Adolescence		

1. The self-testicular exam should be performed _____.

2. Males should begin doing self-testicular exams during _____.

3. Do not perform the self-testicular exam if your hands are _____.

4. The best time to perform the self-testicular exam is during a _____.

5. Feel each testicle by applying _____.

6. The contour of the testicle should be _____, _____, and _____.

7. You will feel the _____ on top of and behind each testicle.

8. The testicle should not have any _____.

APPLICATION OF THE CRITICAL THINKING PROCESS

Read the scenario and answer the following questions.

SCENARIO 1

Hugh is a 32-year-old male that is 5′9″ who weighs 250 lb. He is the author of several best-selling novels and spends a great deal of time using his laptop. He has been riding his bike 10–15 miles per day in order to lose some weight. He began having a constant pain in his rectal area 4 days ago. He assumed the pain was from the bicycle seat being hard and the bounce from some of his trail rides. Today he is being seen in the clinic for "pain in the rectal area." He states the pain is "very sharp and so bad he can barely sit down"; he prefers to stand during the interview. The pain is now a 7 on a scale of 0 to 10. He admits to sitting in a hot bath and taking Tylenol for the pain, which has resulted in minimal relief.

The physical assessment yields the following information: BP 130/82, P 104, RR 20, T 100.7. His general skin color is pale. In the sacrococcygeal area, there is dimpling noted with erythema, moderate edema, and warmth to the area. In the center of the dimpling, a small coarse hair is noted with a small amount of yellow, foul-smelling drainage.

1. Using the information in the scenario, complete the OLDCART & ICE pain assessment.

   O

   L

   D

   C

   A

   R

   T

I

C

E

2. Are additional questions needed to complete the pain assessment? Explain.

3. List three focused questions related to sexuality that may be asked.

    1. _____

    2. _____

    3. _____

4. The nurse suspects that Hugh has a pilonidal cyst. What data support this suspicion?

5. The client asks the nurse "How did this happen and how can I make sure this doesn't happen again?" The nurse explains the risk factors for developing a pilonidal cyst as: (additional resources may be needed to answer this question)

The nurse reports her findings to the doctor. She assists him in an incision and drainage (I&D) procedure to clean out the infected wound. The doctor than sends the client home with a dressing and a prescription for an antibiotic and analgesic. The client returns to the clinic in 5 days. He states "I have no pain; I feel so much better!" His vital signs are BP 110/62, HR 72, RR 12, Temp 97.8°. During inspection of the wound there is a mild amount of erythema at the incision and no edema or drainage present.

6. Document an APIE note using the information provided in the scenario.

A

P

I

E

SCENARIO 2

Felix is a 73-year-old male being examined in the clinic for testicular discomfort. He has been widowed for 10 years and has never had any children. He was told he was infertile when he was 28 years old after trying to have children with his wife for almost 5 years. His doctor told him his infertility was probably related to his history of cryptorchidism as an infant. The nurse is gathering subjective data:

1. List three focused questions the nurse should ask this client.

    1.

    2.

    3.

2. Felix is uncircumcised. Discuss additional measures that must be taken during the assessment of the penis of an uncircumcised male.

3. Upon completion of the physical assessment, the health care provider discusses the findings with the nurse and states, "The finding of a large palpable mass is suggestive of testicular cancer." List two risk factors for testicular cancer that may be revealed in a health history.

    1.

    2.

4. Transillumination of the scrotum is performed. Describe the anticipated findings of transillumination of the scrotum when a mass is present.

HEALTHY PEOPLE 2020

Please read the *Healthy People 2020* objective and answering the following questions.

A *Healthy People 2020* objective is:

Reduce gonorrhea rates.

1. List four signs or symptoms of gonorrhea.

    1. _____

    2. _____

    3. _____

    4. _____

2. Discuss how a nurse on a college campus can use this objective to promote and maintain health of the students.

ASSESSMENT AND DOCUMENTATION

Perform an assessment of the male reproductive system. Complete the subjective data collection on a lab partner (answers may be fabricated) and complete the objective data collection on an anatomical model. Document your findings on the provided documentation form. You can download the form from the Pearson Student Resources site.

NCLEX®-STYLE REVIEW QUESTIONS

Read each question carefully. Choose the best answer for each question.

1. Which of the following statements is true about the scrotum?
    1. The right side extends lower than the left.
    2. The temperature is about 3 degrees warmer than core temperature.
    3. A vertical septum divides it into two sections.
    4. It is housed by the testes.

2. Upon inspection of the newborn male's penis, which of the following would require further investigation?
    1. A hypospadias
    2. A penis size of 2.7 cm
    3. Scrotum color–deep red
    4. Undescended testicles

3. During a focused interview, the nurse asks the client if he is aware if his mother received diethylstilbestrol (DES) treatment during pregnancy. This is important because sons that are born to mothers who have had DES are at higher risk for: (Select all that apply)
   1. testicular cancer.
   2. low sperm counts.
   3. hypospadias.
   4. cryptorchidism.
   5. polycystic kidney disease.

4. A 78-year-old male presents to the medical clinic with multiple questions about his fertility. He has recently married a 42-year-old female, and together they would like to have a child. The nurse must consider which of these age-related changes when discussing the possibility of reproduction with the client?
   1. The older male may produce viable sperm throughout his entire life span.
   2. Sexual libido increases with age.
   3. Older men who are on multiple types of medication should not try to attempt to reproduce.
   4. Ejaculation in the older adult male does not change throughout the life span.

5. A 41-year-old male presents to the medical clinic complaining of difficulty achieving an erection. Which of the following focused interview questions would be appropriate for the nurse to ask? (Select all that apply)
   1. Do you have a history of genitourinary surgery?
   2. What medications are you taking?
   3. Were you born with undescended testicles?
   4. At what age did you begin having sexual intercourse?
   5. Did you have chickenpox as a child?

6. The best position for the male client to be in at the beginning of the physical assessment of the male reproductive structures is:
   1. supine.
   2. semi-Fowler's.
   3. standing upright.
   4. left side-lying.

7. During inspection of the male genitalia, the nurse notices small bluish-gray spots at the base of the pubic hairs. This finding can be indicative of:
   1. crab or pubic lice.
   2. cryptorchidism.
   3. smegma.
   4. syphilitic lesions.

8. The cremasteric reflex can occur in which type of an environment?
   1. Cold
   2. Hot
   3. Moist
   4. Stressful

9. Which instruction by the nurse is most appropriate to give a client while assessing for an inguinal hernia?
   1. "Cough or bear down."
   2. "Take a deep breath in."
   3. "Stand on one leg."
   4. "Bend over at the waist."

10. A 17-year-old lacrosse player suddenly develops severe unilateral testicular pain. His mother brings him to the pediatrician's office for an evaluation. Upon the initial assessment, the nurse suspects a testicular torsion. The nurse's next step should be to:
    1. inform the client the healthcare provider is running behind and it may be about a 30-minute wait.
    2. apply ice to the scrotum for 20 minutes while the client waits.
    3. administer an analgesic because a torsion can be extremely painful.
    4. call for the healthcare provider; the client might require immediate surgical intervention.

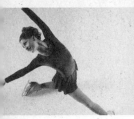

22 Female Reproductive System

Our greatest glory is not in never failing, but in rising up every time we fail.
—Ralph Waldo Emerson

The female reproductive system consists of multiple organs that are responsible for the production of hormones and female reproductive cells. The system has a great impact on sexual behavior and requires a comprehensive assessment that will include psychosocial, self-care, and environmental factors. This chapter will focus on gathering both subjective and objective data related to the female reproductive system, as well as analysis of the data collected.

OBJECTIVES

At the completion of these exercises you will be able to:

1. Define key terminology associated with the female reproductive system.
2. Review the anatomy and physiology of the female reproductive system.
3. Select the equipment necessary to complete the female reproductive assessment.
4. Identify the correct techniques for assessment of the female reproductive system.
5. Analyze data related to assessment of the female reproductive system.
6. Recognize factors that can influence assessment findings.
7. Assess the female reproductive system on a model.
8. Document an assessment of the female reproductive system.
9. Apply critical thinking in analysis of a case study.
10. Relate objectives in *Healthy People 2020* to the female reproductive system.
11. Complete NCLEX®-style review questions related to the assessment of the female reproductive system.

RESOURCES

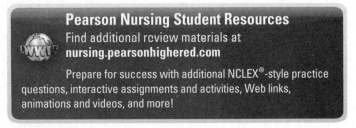

Pearson Nursing Student Resources
Find additional review materials at
nursing.pearsonhighered.com

Prepare for success with additional NCLEX®-style practice questions, interactive assignments and activities, Web links, animations and videos, and more!

Additional resources: *www.CDC.gov*

WORD SEARCH

Find and circle the correct term in the word search puzzle for each of the definitions listed below. The word may be horizontal, vertical, or diagonal.

```
O  D  K  A  M  X  K  H  C  N  K  M  J  K  K  A  T  W  P  B  A  K  R  O  L
R  A  U  S  K  T  X  Q  G  Q  R  U  C  E  Y  W  S  R  Y  I  Z  Z  L  W  C
Z  X  Y  I  J  W  V  I  I  X  R  R  E  C  T  O  C  E  L  E  M  L  E  X  W
Z  R  W  N  U  E  Q  E  F  X  E  C  N  E  X  U  J  C  Y  J  P  Q  Y  U  A
X  E  A  Q  Z  A  Q  K  N  K  Z  Q  I  R  C  I  T  K  Q  M  D  V  P  R  M
C  X  R  V  A  N  C  U  G  I  C  K  G  V  L  I  H  E  I  C  D  S  A  Y  R
V  G  E  N  I  T  A  L  W  A  R  T  S  I  R  H  E  G  R  X  I  N  R  I  A
V  P  Q  C  K  E  B  H  R  J  F  O  V  C  Z  Z  N  A  G  U  T  A  A  I  U
X  K  S  H  B  V  I  W  E  Y  W  B  T  A  P  Y  T  V  Q  B  S  E  U  F  G
K  A  L  A  K  E  X  V  T  N  A  W  F  L  N  J  P  O  P  A  G  E  R  R  O
E  O  O  D  H  R  V  M  R  M  V  B  R  O  K  Z  N  N  K  R  M  Z  E  B  J
L  H  G  W  F  S  W  R  O  M  T  X  P  S  M  V  O  R  R  T  O  Z  T  E  C
P  Z  O  I  J  I  S  P  V  C  V  B  S  T  Y  I  U  F  G  H  H  A  H  G  W
Z  H  O  C  Z  O  M  D  E  R  J  A  I  O  X  S  J  M  G  O  L  L  R  T  L
L  T  D  K  K  N  A  S  R  O  M  E  L  E  E  K  H  D  Y  L  X  A  A  W  C
D  O  E  S  P  S  V  P  S  G  M  V  L  B  L  Z  Y  J  K  I  Z  A  L  X  Y
Y  S  L  S  K  N  A  R  I  T  Y  F  U  S  R  Q  M  I  K  N  X  Y  G  X  S
I  I  L  I  O  K  P  L  O  R  E  T  G  W  D  P  E  N  C  S  H  B  L  V  T
C  F  S  G  V  S  E  S  N  T  E  K  D  L  C  M  N  T  L  G  C  V  A  A  O
E  L  S  N  A  F  R  G  N  N  S  D  U  D  B  D  B  R  I  L  E  S  N  G  C
R  A  I  P  R  N  I  A  I  P  Z  O  P  W  J  K  K  O  T  A  R  U  D  I  E
V  B  G  D  I  H  N  R  R  E  T  R  O  F  L  E  X  I  O  N  T  H  S  N  L
I  I  N  M  E  D  E  W  S  R  X  K  A  R  A  F  N  T  R  D  W  N  C  A  E
X  A  A  E  S  T  U  T  X  B  K  R  V  G  S  J  C  U  I  S  J  P  S  J  O
L  I  C  O  U  K  M  I  D  P  O  S  I  T  I  O  N  S  S  B  A  K  Z  R  U
```

CLUES

1. Abnormal variations of uterine position in which the uterus is folded forward at about a 90-degree angle, and the cervix is tilted downward _____
2. Normal uterine position in which the uterus is tilted forward, cervix tilted downward _____
3. Glands located posteriorly at the base of the vestibule that produce mucus, which is released into the vestibule and actively promotes sperm motility and viability **(two words)** _____ _____
4. The vaginal end of the canal **(two words)** _____ _____
5. Portion of the uterus that projects 2.5 cm into the vagina _____
6. Vascular congestion that occurs during pregnancy creating a bluish-purple blemish or change in cervical coloration **(two words)** _____ _____
7. The primary organ of sexual stimulation, it is a small, elongated mound of erectile tissue located at the anterior of the vestibule _____
8. A hernia that is formed when the urinary bladder is pushed into the anterior vaginal wall _____
9. Raised, moist cauliflower-shaped papules **(two words)** _____ _____
10. An increase in cervical vascularity that contributes to softening of the cervix during pregnancy **(two words)** _____ _____
11. A thin layer of skin within the vagina _____

12. The vaginal opening _____
13. A dual set of liplike structures lying on either side of the vagina _____
14. Uterine position that lies parallel to the tailbone, with the cervix pointed straight _____
15. Almond-shaped glandular structures that produce ova, as well as estrogen and progesterone _____
16. Glands located just posterior to the urethra that open into the urethra and secrete a fluid that lubricates the vaginal vestibule during sexual intercourse **(two words)** _____ _____
17. The space between the vaginal opening and anal area _____
18. A hernia that is formed when the rectum pushes into the posterior vaginal wall _____
19. Abnormal variation of uterine position in which the uterus is folded backward at about a 90-degree angle, cervix tilted upward _____
20. Normal variation of uterine position in which the uterus is tilted backward, cervix tilted upward _____
21. Ducts on either side of the fundus of the uterus **(two words)** _____ _____
22. A pear-shaped, hollow, muscular organ that is located centrally in the pelvis between the neck of the bladder and the rectal wall _____
23. A long, tubular, muscular canal that extends from the vestibule to the cervix at the inferior end of the uterus _____

ANATOMY & PHYSIOLOGY REVIEW

1. For each diagram below write the name of the structure indicated by each line.

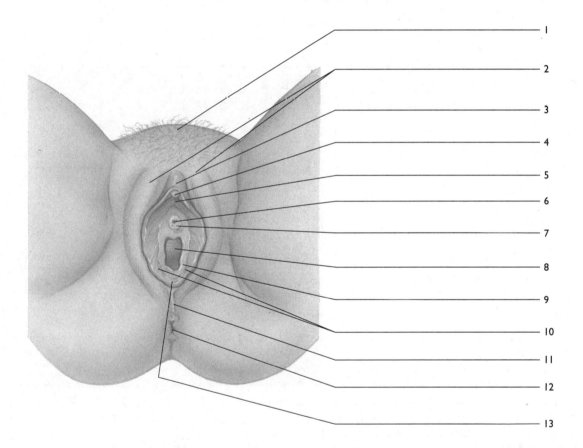

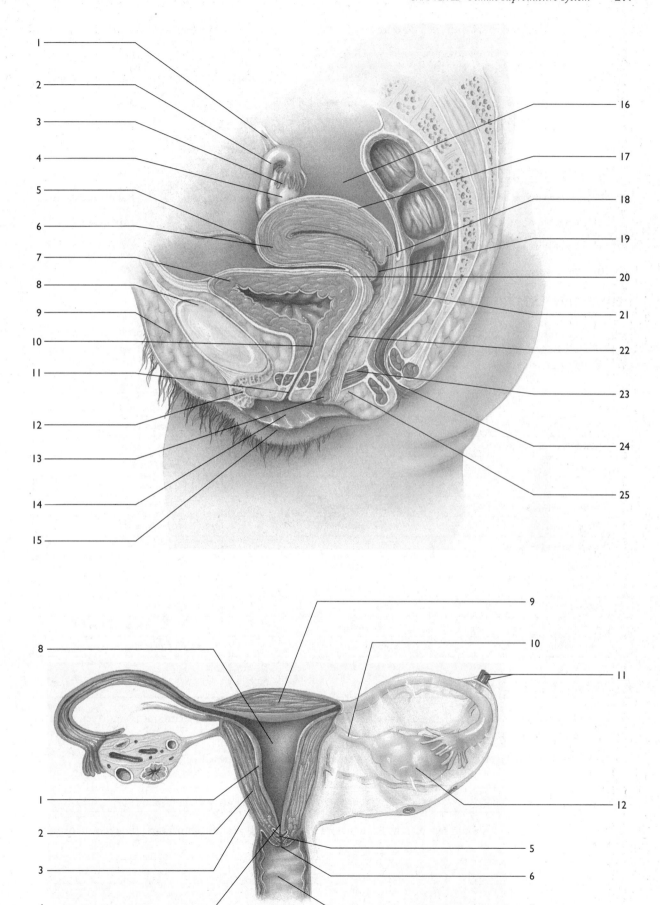

2. Circle the organ associated with each descriptor.

1.	Channel for menstrual flow	**Uterus**	**Vagina**	**Fallopian tubes**
2.	Produce ova	**Ovaries**	**Bartholin's glands**	**Fallopian tubes**
3.	The "birth canal"	**Fallopian tubes**	**Mons pubis**	**Vagina**
4.	Produce estrogen	**Ovaries**	**Skene's glands**	**Bartholin's glands**
5.	Produce(s) vaginal lubricant	**Vagina**	**Skene's glands**	**Bartholin's glands**
6.	Site of fertilization of the ovum	**Fallopian tubes**	**Ovaries**	**Uterus**
7.	Produce progesterone	**Ovaries**	**Skene's glands**	**Bartholin's glands**
8.	Protective sac for fetus	**Ovaries**	**Uterus**	**Introitus**
9.	Site of implantation of fertilized ovum	**Ovaries**	**Fallopian tubes**	**Uterus**
10.	Primary organ of sexual stimulation	**Introitus**	**Clitoris**	**Vagina**

EQUIPMENT SELECTION

Prior to beginning the physical assessment of a female client's reproductive system, it is important to gather the appropriate assessment equipment. Place a check mark next to each piece of equipment that you would need to perform this assessment.

EQUIPMENT					
	Cotton balls		Lubricant		Sphygmomanometer
	Cotton-tipped applicator		Nasal speculum		Stethoscope
	Culture media		Ophthalmoscope		Tape measure
	Dental mirror		Otoscope		Test tubes
	Doppler ultrasonic stethoscope		Pap smear equipment		Thermometer
	Drape sheet		Reflex hammer		Tongue blade
	Examination gown		Ruler		Transilluminator
	Flashlight		Skinfold calipers		Tuning fork
	Gauze		Skin-marking pen		Vaginal speculum
	Gloves		Slides		Vision chart
	Goggles		Small towel		Watch with second hand
	Handheld mirror		Speculum		Wood's lamp

ASSESSMENT TECHNIQUES

Review each assessment technique. If the technique is correct, circle the number. If the technique is incorrect, write the correct assessment technique on the line provided.

1. The client should be placed in the lithotomy position for the female reproductive assessment.

_____

_____

2. The hand of the nurse should separate the labia majora in order to inspect the clitoris and the urethral orifice.

_____

_____

3. The nurse should ask the client to bear down in order to inspect for any protrusions from the vagina.

   _____

   _____

4. When palpating the vaginal walls, the nurse should begin with the right palm facing down toward the floor.

   _____

   _____

5. When palpating for the Skene's glands, the nurse's right index finger should apply gentle pressure downward against the vaginal wall and a stroking movement should milk the gland.

   _____

   _____

6. Prior to insertion, the vaginal speculum should be placed in the nurse's nondominant hand.

   _____

   _____

7. A closed vaginal speculum should be inserted slowly at a 45-degree angle.

   _____

   _____

8. A slide or specimen container should be labeled and ready for specimen collection during the vaginal exam.

   _____

   _____

9. The nurse should remain seated during bimanual palpation.

   _____

   _____

10. The nurse should insert one finger into the vagina and one finger into the rectum to perform the rectovaginal exam.

    _____

    _____

ASSESSMENT FINDINGS

Read each assessment finding. Determine if the finding is normal or abnormal. Write an A for abnormal and an N for normal on each line provided.

_____ 1. Moist dark anus

_____ 2. Heavy distribution of hair at the mons pubis and sparse at the labia

_____ 3. Pink introitus

_____ 4. 30-day menstrual cycle

_____ 5. Discharge from the Skene's gland

_____ 6. 1-cm long clitoris

_____ 7. Cervical polyp

_____ 8. Uterus slightly tilted upward

_____ 9. Genital itching

_____ 10. Non-tender uterine wall

_____ 11. Pain upon palpation of the Bartholin's glands

_____ 12. Firm perineum

_____ 13. Cystocele

_____ 14. Smooth and pink labia minora

_____ 15. Pink moist cervix

_____ 16. Bluish-gray spots at the base of pubic hair

_____ 17. Clear vaginal discharge

_____ 18. Decreased libido

_____ 19. Non-palpable ovary

_____ 20. Candidiasis

FACTORS THAT INFLUENCE PHYSICAL ASSESSMENT FINDINGS

Fill in the blank to complete each statement.

1. Female genital mutilation is a cultural practice in _____, _____, and _____ countries.

2. The uterine capacity of a pregnant female can increase to _____ liters.

3. The female child reaches puberty _____ the male child.

4. Lesbian experimentation is developmentally _____ in adolescents.

5. The observed/palpated softening of the cervix during pregnancy is called _____ _____.

6. Human papillomavirus (HPV) increases a female's risk for _____ cancer.

7. Roman Catholicism forbids _____ _____.

8. Hydrocarbons polychlorinated biphenyls (PCBs) found in _____ manufacturing are associated with low birth weight, spontaneous abortion, hyperpigmentation of infants, and microcephaly.

9. Human papillomavirus quadrivalent (Gardisil) is a _____ that may protect females against most cervical cancers.

10. Nurses working in _____ and exposed to antineoplastic drugs may have a higher risk of irregular menstrual cycles and spontaneous abortions.

APPLICATION OF THE CRITICAL THINKING PROCESS

Read the scenario and answer the following questions.

Shannon is a 23-year-old female college student. During a health and wellness fair on campus, she stopped at a booth set up by students in the nursing department to provide information about human papillomavirus (HPV). The booth was very crowded but Shannon was very anxious to learn if she was at risk for this virus.

1. List three focused questions that the student nurse should ask Shannon to assess her risk factors for HPV:

   1. _____

   2. _____

   3. _____

2. Shannon feels that she is at risk for HPV after speaking with a nursing student. She is now worried about how she can go about finding out if she has it. The nursing student explains that the HPV screening includes:

3. Shannon asks the nursing student where she could find out more information on HPV. The nursing student provides various resources to learn more.

   1. Name one campus resource:

   2. Name one website (provide address):

   3. Name one community-based (off-campus) resource:

4. Shannon decides to make an appointment with a women's health practitioner on her campus. What signs and symptoms may be noted during the physical assessment that would support the presence of HPV.

HEALTHY PEOPLE 2020

Read the *Healthy People 2020* objective and answer the following questions.

A *Healthy People 2020* objective is:

> **Reduce the proportion of females aged 15 to 44 years who have ever required treatment for pelvic inflammatory disease (PID).**

1. List four signs and symptoms of PID.

    1. _____
    2. _____
    3. _____
    4. _____

2. Discuss how a nurse at a women's health clinic can use this objective to promote and maintain health of the clients.

ASSESSMENT AND DOCUMENTATION

Perform an assessment of the female reproductive system. Complete the subjective data collection on a lab partner (answers may be fabricated) and complete the objective data collection on an anatomical model. Document your findings on the provided documentation form. You can download the form from the Pearson Student Resources site.

NCLEX®-STYLE REVIEW QUESTIONS

Read each question carefully. Circle the letter that best answers each question.

1. The nurse uses the word introitus to identify the:
    1. clitoris.
    2. vaginal opening.
    3. perineum.
    4. cervix.

2. The menstrual cycle is:
    1. defined by the first day of one period until the first day of the next.
    2. defined by the last day of one period until the first day of the next.
    3. defined by the first day of a period until the last day of the same period.
    4. 28 days long.

3. A 31-year-old female presents to the women's health clinic complaining of premenstrual syndrome (PMS). The nurse conducts a focused interview to gather more data. Which of the following symptoms would be expected during PMS?
    1. Weight loss
    2. A relaxed feeling
    3. Breast engorgement
    4. Nipple discharge

4. When preparing a client for the assessment of the female reproductive system, it is important for the nurse to explain to the client:
    1. what will happen during the exam.
    2. that the exam may be painful.
    3. that the nurse will conduct the exam as quickly as possible.
    4. that it is best to have a full bladder during the exam.

5. During a pelvic examination, the nurse notes a client has raised, moist, cauliflower-shaped lesions on the labia majora. The nurse correctly documents these lesions as:
    1. a normal finding.
    2. yeast infection.
    3. genital warts.
    4. pubic lice.

6. The nurse identifies a young female client with sparse, dark, visibly pigmented, curly pubic hair on the labia as in Tanner's stage _____ of maturation.
    1. 2
    2. 3
    3. 4
    4. 5

7. When preparing to perform the speculum examination in a female client, the nurse should:
    1. prewarm the speculum with warm water.
    2. lubricate the speculum with petroleum jelly.
    3. use the appropriate-sized speculum for the size of the client.
    4. hold the speculum in the nondominant hand.

8. A 19-year-old female recently went for her annual gynecological examination. During the examination the physician mentioned briefly that her uterus is retroverted. When the physician left the room, she immediately asked the nurse if this is something she should be worried about. The nurse explains retroversion means the uterus is:
    1. tilted forward and can be a normal variation.
    2. tilted backward and can be a normal variation.
    3. parallel to the tailbone and can cause difficulty during childbirth.
    4. tilted backward and can cause difficulty during childbirth.

9. In order to obtain a gonorrhea culture, the nurse should insert:
    1. a saline-moistened cotton applicator into the cervical os.
    2. the paddle end of a spatula into the fornix and rotate.
    3. a dry cotton applicator into the cervical os and leave in place for 1 full minute.
    4. a saline-moistened cotton applicator into the fornix.

10. A 21-year-old female has been experiencing lower back pain and pelvic pain for 3 days. After careful examination, it is found that she has a small ovarian cyst. The nurse explains to the client that:
    1. she will need to have immediate surgery before it ruptures.
    2. it may spontaneously reabsorb within several months.
    3. this most likely will lead to ovarian cancer.
    4. ovarian cysts are common in females with sexually transmitted diseases.

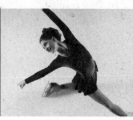

Musculoskeletal System 23

The way I see it, you can either run from it, or learn from it.
—Rafikki to Simba *(The Lion King)*

Enjoying a quality life may depend on a client's ability to participate in routine and daily activities. Muscles, bones, and joints must all be functioning properly for the human body to move. Throughout the life span, many changes occur in the musculoskeletal system. This chapter will focus on gathering both subjective and objective data related to the musculoskeletal system, as well as analysis of the data collected.

OBJECTIVES

At the completion of these exercises you will be able to:

1. Define key terminology associated with the musculoskeletal system.
2. Review the anatomy and physiology of the musculoskeletal system.
3. Select the equipment necessary to complete the musculoskeletal assessment.
4. Identify the correct techniques for assessment of the musculoskeletal system.
5. Analyze data related to assessment of the musculoskeletal system.
6. Recognize factors that can influence assessment findings.
7. Assess the musculoskeletal system on a lab partner.
8. Document an assessment of the musculoskeletal system.
9. Apply critical thinking in analysis of a case study.
10. Relate objectives in *Healthy People 2020* to the musculoskeletal system.
11. Complete NCLEX®-style review questions related to the assessment of the musculoskeletal system.

RESOURCES

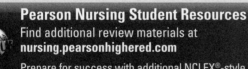

Pearson Nursing Student Resources

Find additional review materials at
nursing.pearsonhighered.com

Prepare for success with additional NCLEX®-style practice questions, interactive assignments and activities, Web links, animations and videos, and more!

CROSSWORD PUZZLE FOR KEY TERMS

Read each definition below and fill in the correct term on the puzzle grid. If the answer requires two words do not leave a blank space between the words. Use a pencil so you can erase easily.

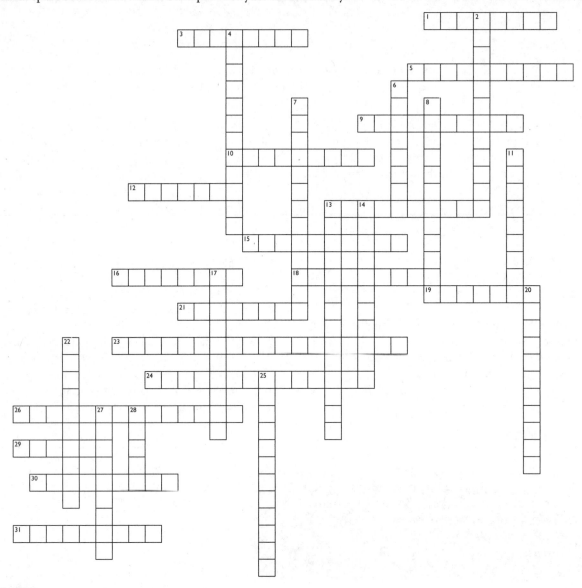

CLUES

Across

1. An exaggerated lumbar curve of the spine that compensates for pregnancy, obesity, or other skeletal changes
3. An exaggerated thoracic dorsal curve that causes asymmetry between the sides of the posterior thorax
5. The movement of touching the thumb to the tips of the other fingers of the same hand
9. A rounded cavity on the right and left lateral sides of the pelvic bone
10. A movement of a limb away from the midline
12. One flat bone surface slips over another similar surface
13. Movement of the forearm so that the palm faces up, anteriorly or superiorly
15. A tarsal bone of the foot, the heel bone
16. A partial or complete break in the continuity of the bone from trauma
18. A movement in which the sole of the foot is turned medially or inward
19. Tough fibrous bands that attach muscle to bone, or muscle to muscle
21. The turning movement of a bone around its own long axis
23. Bones joined by cartilage (**two words**)
24. Extension of the ankle away from the body (**two words**)
26. A bending of a joint beyond 180 degrees

29. Small, synovial-fluid-filled sacs that protect ligaments from friction
30. Movement of the forearm so that the palm faces down, posteriorly or inferiorly
31. A lateral curvature of the lumbar or thoracic spine that is more common in children with neuromuscular deficits

Down

2. Flexion of the ankle so that the superior aspect of the foot moves in an upward direction
4. The great toe is abnormally adducted at the metatarsophalangeal joint (**two words**)
6. A movement in which the sole of the foot is turned laterally
7. The movement in which the limb describes a cone in space
8. A palpation technique used to detect fluid
11. A movement of a limb toward the body midline
13. Bones separated by a fluid-filled joint cavity (**two words**)
14. A nonangular anterior movement in a transverse plane
17. A nonangular posterior movement in a transverse plane
20. A partial dislocation of the bones in a joint
22. A movement in which the elevated part is moved downward to its original position
25. Bones joined by fibrous tissue (**two words**)
27. Lifting or moving superiorly along a frontal plane
28. Gout-related hard nodules that may appear over the joint

ANATOMY & PHYSIOLOGY REVIEW

1. For each diagram below write the name of the structure indicated by each line.

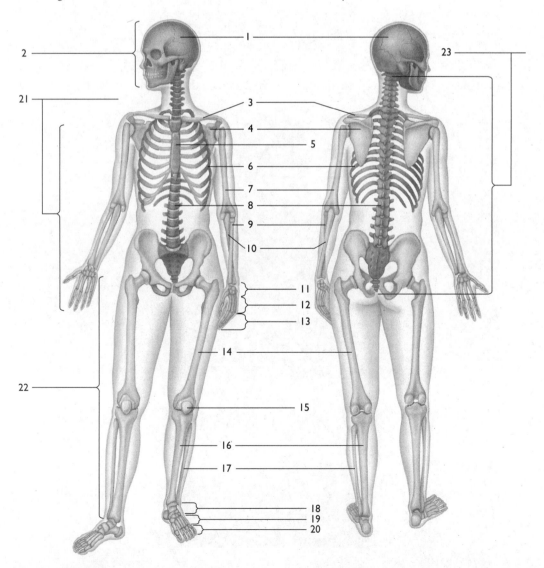

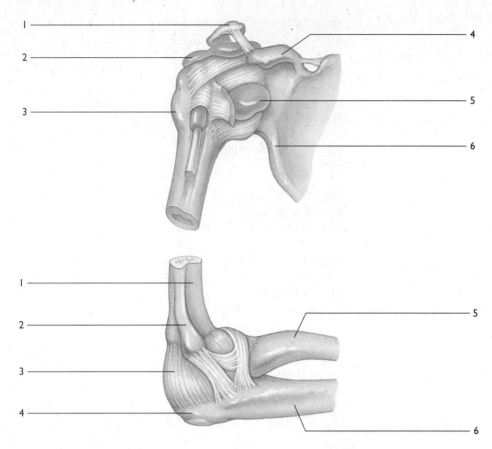

2. Read each statement, follow the instruction, and place the action on the diagram provided.

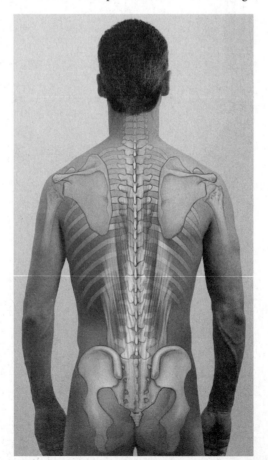

1. Connect the left iliac crest to the right iliac crest
2. Connect the spinous process T_1 to the right posterior superior iliac spine
3. Connect the spinous process C_7 to the left posterior superior iliac spine
4. Draw a line between L_5 and S_1
5. Circle the coccyx bone

3. For each picture below list the type of movement that is being displayed.

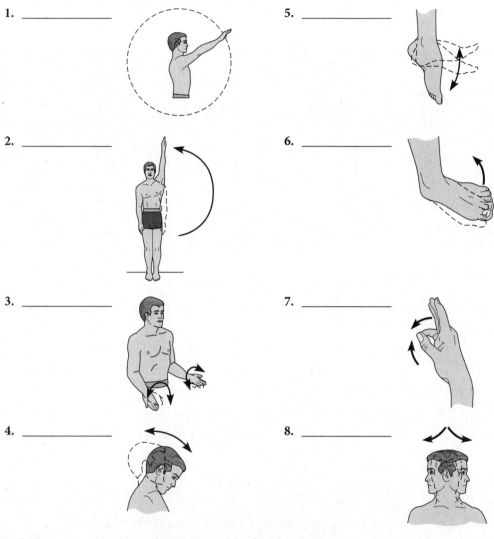

1. _____

2. _____

3. _____

4. _____

5. _____

6. _____

7. _____

8. _____

4. Circle the movements that each joint is capable of performing.

1. Shoulder	**Abduction**	**External rotation**	**Hyperextension**
2. Wrist	**Flexion**	**Supination**	**Radial deviation**
3. Hip	**Extension**	**Internal rotation**	**Pronation**
4. Knee	**Pronation**	**Extension**	**Hyperextension**
5. Elbow	**Supination**	**Flexion**	**Circumduction**
6. Thumb	**Radial deviation**	**Extension**	**Opposition**
7. Ankle	**Plantar flexion**	**Eversion**	**Lateral flexion**
8. Spine	**Rotation**	**Supination**	**Lateral flexion**
9. Toe	**Abduction**	**Adduction**	**Inversion**
10. Finger	**Circumduction**	**External rotation**	**Extension**

EQUIPMENT SELECTION

Prior to beginning the physical assessment of a client's musculoskeletal system, it is important to gather the appropriate assessment equipment. Place a check mark next to each piece of equipment that you would need to perform this assessment.

EQUIPMENT		
Cotton balls	Lubricant	Sphygmomanometer
Cotton-tipped applicator	Nasal speculum	Stethoscope
Culture media	Ophthalmoscope	Tape measure
Dental mirror	Otoscope	Test tubes
Doppler ultrasonic stethoscope	Penlight	Thermometer
Drape sheet	Reflex hammer	Tongue blade
Examination gown	Ruler	Transilluminator
Flashlight	Slkinfold calipers	Tuning fork
Gauze	Skin-marking pen	Vaginal speculum
Gloves	Slides	Vision chart
Goggles	Small towel	Watch with second hand
Goniometer	Specimen containers	Wood's lamp

ASSESSMENT TECHNIQUES

Review each assessment technique. If the technique is correct, circle the number. If the technique is incorrect, rewrite the correct assessment technique on the line provided.

1. The index and middle fingers of the nurse should be positioned in front of the tragus when palpating the client's temporomandibular joint.

_____

_____

2. When assessing internal rotation of the shoulders, the nurse should ask the client to clasp his or her hands behind the head.

_____

_____

3. Abduction at the shoulder should be 50 degrees as demonstrated by extension of the arm.

_____

_____

4. When assessing for muscle strength, the nurse should provide opposing force while the client puts a joint through range of motion.

_____

_____

5. In order to palpate the olecranon process, the nurse must palpate the junction between the acromion and the clavicle.

_____

_____

6. Auscultation is not a technique used in the musculoskeletal assessment.

_____

_____

7. During Phalen's test, the client's wrists should be bent with hands palm to palm.

   _____

   _____

8. Light percussion over the median nerve is used to assess Tinel's sign.

   _____

   _____

9. Range of motion of the spine begins with the neck.

   _____

   _____

10. Hyperextension of the spine should never be attempted.

    _____

    _____

ASSESSMENT FINDINGS

Read each assessment finding. Determine if the finding is normal or abnormal. Write an A for abnormal and an N for normal on each line provided.

_____ 1. Symmetrical joints

_____ 2. Crepitus

_____ 3. Muscle Strength 1

_____ 4. Ganglion

_____ 5. Dupuytren's contracture

_____ 6. Convex thoracic curve

_____ 7. Inversion of the foot 30°

_____ 8. Convex cervical curve

_____ 9. Ulnar deviation 55°

_____ 10. Hyperextension of the neck

_____ 11. Non-tender masseter muscle

_____ 12. Shoulder internal rotation 90°

_____ 13. Warm hands for the nurse

_____ 14. Wrist extension 70°

_____ 15. Firm and stable hip joint

_____ 16. Hallux valgus

_____ 17. Muscle Strength 5

_____ 18. Genu varum

_____ 19. Elbow flexion 160°

_____ 20. Fluid collected in the suprapatellar bursa

FACTORS THAT INFLUENCE PHYSICAL ASSESSMENT FINDINGS

Fill in the blank to complete each statement.

1. Arches in the feet develop during the _____ years.

2. Lordosis of the _____ progresses in the pregnant female to compensate for the growing fetus.

3. Osteoarthritis develops more frequently in _____ _____ than in Caucasians.

4. The nurse should consider _____ _____ if a client has a history of frequent fractures or musculoskeletal trauma.

5. Longitudinal bone growth ends at _____ years of age.

6. Asians and Caucasians have a higher incidence of _____.

7. The average person's height decreases by _____ to _____ inches from age 20 to 70.

8. Glucocorticoids may _____ bone density.

9. Estrogen and other hormones may _____ cartilage in the pregnant female.

10. The _____ _____ position stresses the hips, knees, and ankle joints of children.

MUSCLE STRENGTH

Match the Muscle Strength Rating in Column A with its characteristic in Column B. You may use each answer more than once.

Column A (Rating)

A. Five

B. Four

C. Three

D. Two

E. One

F. Zero

Column B (Characteristics)

_____ **1.** Full range of motion against gravity with moderate resistance

_____ **2.** Trace

_____ **3.** No muscle contraction

_____ **4.** Full range of motion against gravity with full resistance

_____ **5.** Fair

_____ **6.** Full range of motion without gravity (passive) motion

_____ **7.** Full range of motion with gravity

_____ **8.** Palpable muscle contraction but no movement

_____ **9.** Normal

_____ **10.** Good

ABNORMAL FINDINGS

Write the name of each musculoskeletal disorder on the first line next to each illustration. On the second line, write one associated characteristic.

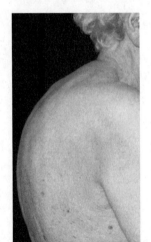

1. _____

_____

Dr. P. Marazzi/Photo Researchers, Inc.

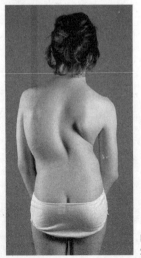

2. _____

_____

Princess Margaret Rose Orthopaedic Hospital, Edinburgh,
Scotland/Science Photo Library/Photo Researchers, Inc.

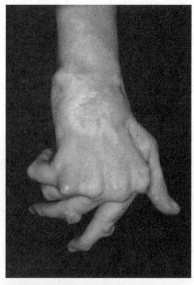

3. _____

_____

Princess Margaret Rose Orthopaedic Hospital/Photo Researchers, Inc.

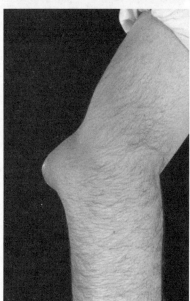

4. _____

_____

Medical-On-Line Ltd.

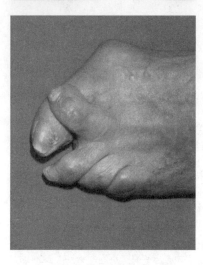

5. _____

_____

Dr. P. Marazzi/Photo Researchers, Inc.

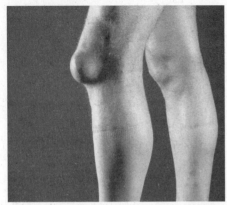

6. _____

_____

Princess Margaret Rose Orthopaedic Hospital/
Photo Researchers, Inc.

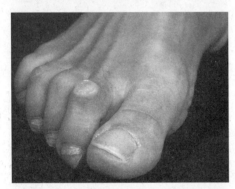

7. _____

_____

M. English/Stockphoto.com/Medichrome/
The Stock Shop, Inc.

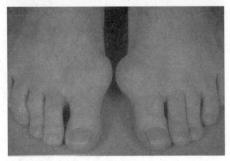

8. _____

_____

Biophoto Associates/Science Source/
Photo Researchers, Inc.

APPLICATION OF THE CRITICAL THINKING PROCESS

PART I

Read the scenario and answer the following questions.

Michelle is an 18-year-old girl who plays varsity basketball and volleyball at her high school. She has been playing sports since she was 5 years old. During a championship volleyball game, Michelle jumped up to block the ball and landed hard on her right knee. She states she felt her knee "pop" when she landed. She complained of extreme pain and difficulty with movement. She had to be removed from the game and brought to the school nurse because of edema at the injury site. Michelle begins to cry because it is too painful to move or bear weight on the right leg and states my leg feels "wobbly."

Michelle's past medical history is two sprained left ankles and a fractured right wrist. She has just completed her menstrual period 2 days ago. She takes a multivitamin daily.

Physical assessment reveals a well-developed female 5'9", weighing 129 lb. The skin on her right knee is warm and dry. The color is consistent with the rest of her body. Her gait is unsteady, and she appears to hop on the left foot to avoid weight bearing on the right leg. She has limited ROM because of the pain. She states when she is not moving her right knee the pain is a 4 to 5 on a scale 0 to 10, but when she moves it the pain increases to a 9 to 10.

The nurse suspects that Michelle has injured her right anterior cruciate ligament (RACL). The nurse calls for an ambulance to take her to the emergency department.

1. List three pieces of subjective data provided in this scenario.

    1. _____

    2. _____

    3. _____

2. List three pieces of objective data provided in this scenario.

    1. _____

    2. _____

    3. _____

3. What further information should be collected in order to complete the pain assessment for this client?

4. List two reasons why it is important to assess this client's last menstrual period if her injury is musculoskeletal.

    1. _____

    2. _____

5. List two risk factors for an ACL injury for this client.

    1. _____

    2. _____

6. The client is told that she will need to ambulate with crutches until she has a surgical repair. The nurse will need to teach her how to use the crutches with no weight bearing on the right foot. Write a goal and three objectives that would be appropriate for this teaching plan.

    Goal—

    Objectives

    1. _____

    2. _____

    3. _____

APPLICATION OF THE CRITICAL THINKING PROCESS

PART 2

View the following picture and answer the following questions.

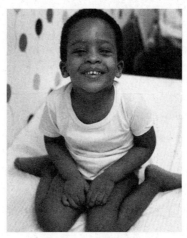

© Judy Braginsky

1. What is the name of this position? _____

2. The nurse notices a 2-year-old sitting in this position while playing a game.
   What should the nurse tell the parents regarding this finding? Provide a rationale.

HEALTHY PEOPLE 2020

Please read the *Healthy People 2020* objective and answer the following questions.

A *Healthy People 2020* objective is:

Reduce the proportion of adults with osteoporosis.

1. List five focused questions that should be asked to determine a client's risk for osteoporosis.

   1. _____
   2. _____
   3. _____
   4. _____
   5. _____

2. A client with osteoporosis is at a great risk for fractures. A fall assessment may be necessary to prevent such injury. Perform a search to find a Fall Assessment Tool (you may use the Internet, health-related databases, etc.).

   1. State the name of the Fall Assessment Tool: _____

   2. State the source: _____

   3. What are the elements that put a client at higher risk for falls according to your tool? _____

   4. How can a home health nurse utilize this tool in order to prevent falls in the elderly? _____

   5. How can a staff nurse in a postsurgical unit utilize this tool in order to prevent falls on a client who is recovering from surgery? _____

3. Discuss how an occupational nurse can use this objective to promote and maintain the health of the client.

ASSESSMENT AND DOCUMENTATION

Perform an assessment of the musculoskeletal system on your lab partner and document your findings on the provided documentation form. You can download the form from the Pearson Student Resources site.

NCLEX®-STYLE REVIEW QUESTIONS

Read each question carefully. Choose the best answer for each question.

1. The head of the femur placed into the acetabulum forms the:
   1. hip joint.
   2. shoulder.
   3. elbow.
   4. knee.

2. A middle-aged client seeks clarification from the nurse between a muscle strain and a muscle sprain. The nurse explains that: (Select all that apply)
   1. a strain includes the partial tear or overstretching of a muscle or tendon.
   2. a sprain includes the tear or overstretching of a ligament.
   3. a strain is medical terminology for a fatigued muscle.
   4. a sprain is medical terminology for a ruptured tendon.
   5. a strain is a term for inflammation and weakness in skeletal muscles.

3. When one articulating bone has a concave area and the other a convex area, a _____ joint is formed.
   1. hinge
   2. saddle
   3. pivot
   4. condyloid

4. Inversion and eversion refer to movements of the:
   1. hand.
   2. arm.
   3. thumb.
   4. ankle.

5. While assessing the back of a newborn, the nurse sees a tuft of hair at the base of the spine. This may indicate:
   1. Allis sign.
   2. genu valgum.
   3. spina bifida.
   4. genu varum.

6. A 62-year-old male reports to the clinic complaining of a flare-up of his gout. Which signs and symptoms does the nurse anticipate to find during an assessment? (Select all that apply)
   1. Swelling in the affected joint
   2. Inflammation in the affected joint
   3. A yellow discoloration to the skin
   4. A gritty texture to the skin
   5. Pain in the affected joint

7. When performing the musculoskeletal assessment, the nurse must remember to:
   1. use as many client position changes as possible.
   2. work distal to proximal.
   3. attempt to move a joint about 5 degrees farther when pain is elicited.
   4. demonstrate the movements.

8. When rating muscle strength as a 4 on a scale from 0 to 5, the nurse can express to the client that this is:
   1. poor.
   2. fair.
   3. good.
   4. excellent.

9. The nurse performs the Phalen's test on a client with carpal tunnel syndrome. Pain will radiate to the:
   1. legs.
   2. knees.
   3. shoulder.
   4. spine.

10. A nurse who suspects a client may have carpal tunnel syndrome may decide to use which of the following assessment techniques? (Select all that apply)
    1. Phalen's test
    2. The Bulge test
    3. Tinel's sign
    4. The Ballottement test
    5. The straight leg raise test

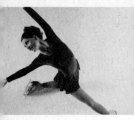
The mind, once expanded to the dimensions of larger ideas, never returns to its original size.

—Oliver Wendell Holmes

The neurologic system includes reflexes, movements, sensations, and the senses. The nurse must have knowledge of the ways in which the neurologic system affects human function in order to determine if an assessment indicates abnormalities within this system. This chapter will focus on gathering both subjective and objective data related to the neurologic system, as well as analysis of the data collected.

OBJECTIVES

At the completion of these exercises you will be able to:

1. Define key terminology associated with the neurologic system.
2. Review the anatomy and physiology of the neurologic system.
3. Select the equipment necessary to complete the assessment of the neurologic system.
4. Identify the correct techniques for assessment of the neurologic system.
5. Analyze data related to assessment of the neurologic system.
6. Recognize factors that can influence assessment findings.
7. Assess the neurologic system on a lab partner.
8. Document an assessment of the neurologic system.
9. Apply critical thinking in analysis of a case study.
10. Relate objectives in *Healthy People 2020* to the neurologic system.
11. Complete NCLEX®-style review questions related to the assessment of the neurologic system.

RESOURCES

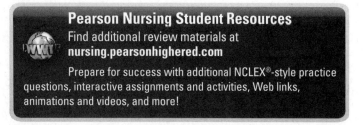

Pearson Nursing Student Resources
Find additional review materials at
nursing.pearsonhighered.com

Prepare for success with additional NCLEX®-style practice questions, interactive assignments and activities, Web links, animations and videos, and more!

Additional resources: *www.strokeassociation.org*
www.stroke.org
www.CDC.gov

WORD SEARCH

Find and circle the correct term in the word search puzzle for each of the definitions listed below. The word may be horizontal, vertical, or diagonal.

```
N Y S T A G M U S C X V R N D L E K U E C H E C A J M Z C V
X J B I R G Q M Y L E O B U Z U H G X M I Z N W G E S A D S
K L B E U K D E R M A T O M E B I E E S M C W N T P H M E H
H A F S X H O J V M R J R O L U Y T H D F D Q S H A Q X Y Y
B A B I N S K I R E S P O N S E S P L T R R Y P S A E J Q P
W K L V E W C K A J X F Z N K Y R J A M P S U X M L T A Y E
K Q X P C R W X T W Z L P U S U G N O P S V M H F Y A N I R
C O R M C Z D Y C Y Q F A S L X X Y M U I C L E I I Q E M E
B Q J U P Q G M E H J I U M E S Z V O H D L R K G B B S R S
K K W T H I X F R W Y O P X S E E V P G F K L A R Y F T Z T
W H W A U W S X E Z V W Z O M E R I K A C G H E I D K H M H
Q I V C H V B R B R P N V G P E S L Z V D P C M D L K E J E
I C G Q J K M C E O X S I I N T B P V U S I Y F G E T S S S
H X M A G A W N L W F T U L J W I F J Y R S P A P S M I M I
K H J C I M L G L Q O D A J R J B C D I F E U L N U X A K A
W M W L A A A Z U O Y R L K R U G L A C R Z S I O O Z J Y Z
B E Q D R T X T M S E O H C X O G A Y T C O A T B P S G M S
I B D T S C P K D H G M Z J F A V G N A R R Q Q P A I M D N
C B N D M T K Y P B D B H A Y W W J I A B O A Q I C D A I P
O E U E J S Q I Z D K E B V O C R J G X L Q P S B D M Y H A
C E J G U Y R T R Y X R A K P O W I Z D J G E H B I X N T J
V H F N A E G O E N S G T T O S O L M G J G E G Y J A M N U
D L O S P L C C Z N J S D U A W R H W P L Z T S A X S E X J
M L F I M L N K J L Y T Y H Y E S H A A L R I X I P Y N S F
C Y O F A D A Y V O W E B Q F X P Y P T V C D L M A N I E A
L N P N C M D F D T J S Z H E I L Y G L D F O U K U C N W V
R U I B F O B N Z Y R T T H L R H H T H A L A M U S O G E H
P P G W S O M P F Q W M S J F L S G L T U H G A M C P E Q F
S B T C R J B A I F W D O K S D H D M S G E Q X E W E S A M
C E R E B R U M V O A X L N U C H A L R I G I D I T Y T U K
```

CLUES

1. The absence of pain sensation _____
2. The inability to perceive the sense of touch _____
3. The absence of the sense of smell _____
4. The fanning of the toes with the great toe pointing toward the dorsum of the foot (**two words**) _____ _____
5. Contains the midbrain, pons, and medulla oblongata and connects pathways between the higher and lower structures (**two words**) _____ _____
6. Nervous system of the body that consists of the brain and the spinal cord (**three words**) _____ _____ _____
7. Coordinates stimuli from the cerebral cortex to provide precise timing for skeletal muscle coordination and smooth movements _____
8. The largest portion of the brain, responsible for all conscious behavior _____
9. Rhythmically alternating flexion and extension _____
10. A prolonged state of unconsciousness, with pronounced and persistent changes _____
11. An area of skin innervated by the cutaneous branch of one spinal nerve _____
12. Double vision _____
13. Difficulty swallowing _____
14. Decreased pain sensation _____
15. An increased sensation _____
16. Three connective tissue membranes that cover, protect, and nourish the central nervous system _____
17. Stiffness of the neck (**two words**) _____ _____
18. Rapid fluttering or constant involuntary movement of the eyeball _____
19. Degeneration of the optic nerve resulting in a change in the color of the optic disc and decreased visual acuity (**two words**) _____ _____

20. Swelling and protrusion of the blind spot of the eye caused by edema _____
21. System of the body that consists of the cranial nerves and spinal nerves (**three words**) _____
_____ _____
22. An automatic stimulus-response that involves a nerve impulse passing from a peripheral nerve receptor to the spinal cord and then outward to an effector muscle without passing through the brain _____
23. A test that assesses coordination and equilibrium (**two words**) _____ _____
24. Sudden and rapid physical manifestations, resulting from excessive discharges of electrical energy in the brain _____
25. A continuation of the medulla oblongata that has the ability to transmit impulses to and from the brain via the ascending and descending pathways (**two words**) _____ _____
26. Brief loss of consciousness, usually sudden _____
27. The largest subdivision of the diencephalon, which is the gateway to the cerebral cortex _____

ANATOMY & PHYSIOLOGY REVIEW

1. For each diagram below write the name of the structure indicated by each line.

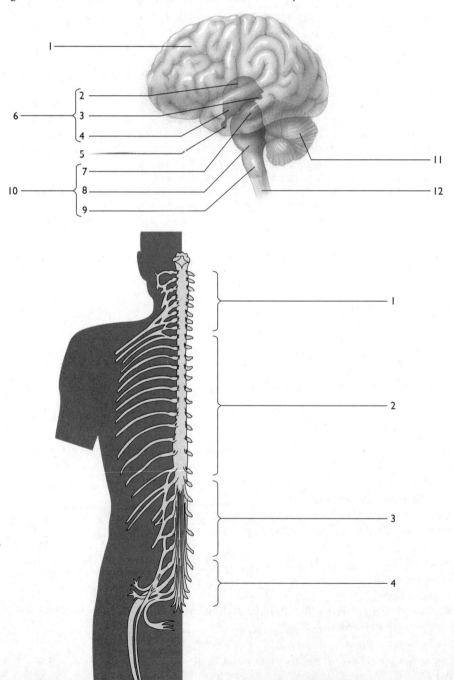

2. Match each lobe of the cerebrum in Column B to its function in Column A. Some lobes will be used more than once.

<u>Column A</u>   <u>Column B</u>

_____ 1. Creation of abstract ideas   **A.** Frontal lobe
_____ 2. Interprets visual stimuli   **B.** Parietal lobe
_____ 3. Awareness of sensation   **C.** Temporal lobe
_____ 4. Concern for others   **D.** Occipital lobe
_____ 5. Contains the olfactory cortex
_____ 6. Awareness of somatosensory stimuli
_____ 7. Controls intellect
_____ 8. Interprets auditory stimuli
_____ 9. Controls speech
_____ 10. Controls reasoning

3. Read the scenario and answer the questions.

   A 3-year-old boy touches the hot oven while his mother is baking cupcakes. He quickly pulls his hand away and begins to cry. The mother jumps up from her seat and runs to her son in a panic.

   1. List the components of the reflex arc that occurred when the boy touched the stove.

   2. What portion of the brain is responsible for the boy's emotional response of crying?

   3. List four physiological changes that may be noted during the fight-or-flight response of the mother.

       1.

       2.

       3.

       4.

4. Identify the cranial nerve(s) responsible for each activity by placing the name and corresponding number next to the activities below. More than one nerve may be responsible for an activity.

   1. Sticking out the tongue   **4.** Rolling of the eyes

       Name_____   Name_____

       Number_____   Number_____

   2. Swallowing lunch   **5.** Singing a song

       Name_____   Name_____

       Number_____   Number_____

   3. Seeing a rainbow   **6.** Feeling a sharp object on the right cheek

       Name_____   Name_____

       Number_____   Number_____

7. Listening to music

   Name_____

   Number_____

8. Raising of the eyebrows

   Name_____

   Number_____

9. Smelling a flower

   Name_____

   Number_____

10. Shrugging of the shoulders

    Name_____

    Number_____

11. Constricting of pupils

    Name_____

    Number_____

12. Walking on a balance beam

    Name_____

    Number_____

13. Clenching of the teeth

    Name_____

    Number_____

14. Tasting a strawberry

    Name_____

    Number_____

15. Smiling at a friend

    Name_____

    Number_____

16. Gagging

    Name_____

    Number_____

EQUIPMENT SELECTION

Prior to beginning the physical assessment of a client's neurologic system, it is important to gather the appropriate assessment equipment. Place a check mark next to each piece of equipment that you would need to perform this assessment.

EQUIPMENT					
	Cotton balls (sterile)		Lubricant		Specimen containers
	Cotton-tipped applicator		Nasal speculum		Sphygmomanometer
	Culture media		Ophthalmoscope		Stethoscope
	Dental mirror		Otoscope		Test tubes
	Doppler ultrasonic stethoscope		Penlight		Thermometer
	Drape sheet		Percussion hammer		Tongue blade
	Examination gown		Ruler		Transilluminator
	Flashlight		Sharp object		Tuning fork
	Gauze		Skinfold calipers		Vaginal speculum
	Gloves		Skin-marking pen		Vision chart
	Goggles		Slides		Watch with second hand
	Goniometer		Small towel		Wood's lamp

Other Neurologic Assessment–SpecificObjects (*List 4*):

ASSESSMENT TECHNIQUES

Review each assessment technique. If the technique is correct, circle the number. If the technique is incorrect, rewrite the correct assessment technique on the line provided.

1. In order to assess the client's sensorium, the nurse should ask the client to determine the date, time, place, and reason for today's visit.

   _____

   _____

2. The client should close both eyes and one nare when having cranial nerve II (two) assessed.

_____

_____

3. When testing motor function of cranial nerve V (five), the client should be asked to tightly clench teeth.

_____

_____

4. Convergence and accommodation should be assessed for sensory function of cranial nerve V.

_____

_____

5. When assessing the client's gait, the nurse must be sure the client is looking straight ahead and not at the floor.

_____

_____

6. The nurse should stand in front of the client when performing the Romberg test.

_____

_____

7. A rapid alternating action can be assessed by asking the client to touch the thumb to each finger in sequence with increasing pace.

_____

_____

8. When testing for graphesthesia the client should keep both eyes open.

_____

_____

9. When assessing the brachioradialis reflex, the nurse should briskly strike the tendon toward the radius about 1 inch above the wrist.

_____

_____

10. The flat end of the reflex hammer is used to assess the Babinski reflex.

_____

_____

ASSESSMENT FINDINGS

Read each assessment finding. Determine if the finding is normal or abnormal. Write an A for abnormal and an N for normal on each line provided.

_____ 1. Asymmetrical facial movements

_____ 2. Hoarseness of voice

_____ 3. Glasgow Coma Scale 3

_____ 4. Dysphagia

_____ 5. +4 triceps reflex

_____ 6. Short-term memory intact

_____ 7. Nuchal rigidity

_____ 8. Ataxic gait

_____ 9. Dystonia

_____ 10. Two-point discrimination at 10 cm in the lower leg

_____ 11. Vertigo

_____ 12. Articulate speech

_____ 13. Anosmia

_____ 14. Negative Romberg

_____ 15. 20/15 vision

_____ 16. Auditory hallucinations

_____ 17. Glasgow Coma Scale 14

_____ 18. +2 brachioradialis reflex

_____ 19. Anesthesia

_____ 20. Monotone voice

FACTORS THAT INFLUENCE PHYSICAL ASSESSMENT FINDINGS

Fill in the blank to complete each statement.

1. Hyperactive reflexes may indicate _____ _____ _____ in the pregnant female.

2. African Americans have a higher incidence of hypertension, thus increasing their risk for _____.

3. During pregnancy, as the uterus enlarges it may exert pressure on the pelvic nerves causing pain, numbness, or tingling to travel to the _____.

4. Cerebral disease should be considered if a newborn has a _____cry.

5. The growth of the nervous system is very _____ during the fetal period.

6. The Moro and sucking reflexes are considered _____ reflexes in the newborn.

7. Peripheral neuropathy and encephalopathy may be caused by _____ poisoning.

8. In the United States, _____ _____ have higher rates of Alzheimer's disease than Caucasians.

9. The senses tend to _____ in the older adult.

10. Research suggests that toxins such as carbon monoxide may cause some cases of_____ _____.

APPLICATION OF THE CRITICAL THINKING PROCESS

Read each scenario and answer the following questions.

SCENARIO I

Melanie is a 32-year-old female who is in the intensive care unit after a drug overdose with suicidal intent. When the nurse enters the room to assess her, the nurse notes Melanie's eyes are closed. When the nurse calls her name, it is noted that Melanie opens her lids but does not focus on any specific object. The nurse informs Melanie that her intravenous site is due to be changed. She asks if she can move her left arm closer to the edge of the bed, Melanie does not respond. When the nurse attempts to insert the angiocatheter into the basilic vein, Melanie pulls back her arm and groans. The nurse asks Melanie if she is feeling pain. Melanie again just moans and closes her eyes.

1. List the three areas of the Glasgow Coma Scale.

    1.

    2.

    3.

2. Use the Glasgow Coma Scale to assess Melanie's level of consciousness.

3. What are the implications of your findings?

SCENARIO 2

Mrs. Sharon Sanchez, a 42-year-old Hispanic female, has been married for 15 years and has a 10-year-old son. She suffered a head injury 20 years ago in a motor vehicle accident as an unbelted passenger. She was treated and released after 2 days of observation for a concussion. At this time she works as a hairstylist in a local beauty salon. She takes no medications except for an occasional Excedrin for the migraine headaches she has been having for the past 3 weeks. She denies the use of alcohol and tobacco.

Mrs. Sanchez's chief complaint is a sharp pain above and behind her right eye. Her husband states "her face just doesn't look right to me." Upon physical assessment, the nurse notes ptosis of the right eyelid and mild unilateral right facial weakness. Her speech is articulate and the motor movements of her upper extremities are symmetrical and strong.

1. Use OLDCART & ICE to identify five focused interview questions that the nurse should ask this client.

2. Perform a web search through the National Institutes of Health for the NIH stroke scale. List the performance indicators for this scale.

3. Perform a web search for the Cincinnati Stroke Scale. List the performance indicators for this scale.

4. Evaluate the two scales in relationship to ease of use and the healthcare setting.

5. After careful assessment and diagnostic testing, an unruptured brain aneurysm has been detected. Name at least three other signs or symptoms that may be noted for this diagnosis. (Additional resources may be necessary)

   1.

   2.

   3.

6. Identify and prioritize two nursing diagnoses for this client.

   1.

   2.

HEALTHY PEOPLE 2020

Please read the *Healthy People 2020* objective and answer the following questions. (Additional resources may be necessary)

A *Healthy People 2020* objective is:

Reduce traumatic brain injury morbidity and mortality.

1. A concussion is considered a mild traumatic brain injury. List five signs and symptoms of a concussion.

   1. _____

   2. _____

3. _____

4. _____

5. _____

2. According to the Centers for Control and Prevention, children between the ages of 0 and 19 years of age are at highest risk for traumatic brain injury. List three reasons that support this risk.

1. _____

2. _____

3. _____

3. Discuss how a nurse can use this objective to promote and maintain the health of the client.

ASSESSMENT AND DOCUMENTATION

Perform an assessment of the neurologic system on your lab partner and document your findings on the provided documentation form. You can download the form from the Pearson Student Resources site.

NCLEX®-STYLE REVIEW QUESTIONS

Read each question carefully. Choose the best answer for each question.

1. The nurse identifies which portion of the brain as the one responsible for all conscious behavior?
   1. Cerebellum
   2. Brain stem
   3. Cerebrum
   4. Central nervous system

2. The nurse understands that a positive Babinski reflex is a normal finding in:
   1. all clients.
   2. an infant.
   3. an adult client.
   4. a pregnant client.

3. The nurse notes which of the following neurologic findings as part of the normal aging process in the older adult client. (Select all that apply)
   1. Increased deep tendon reflexes
   2. Decreased visual acuity
   3. Decreased reaction time
   4. Erect posture
   5. Tremor

4. The nurse will use which of the following questions during the focused neurologic interview of the client? (Select all that apply)
   1. "Have you ever experienced a seizure?"
   2. "Do you have numbness or tingling in your arms or legs?"
   3. "Have you ever had an injury to your head?"
   4. "Have you experienced any redness or swelling to your eyes?"
   5. "Do you consume alcohol?"

5. Which of the following is true about the physical assessment of the neurologic system? (Select all that apply)
   1. The nurse should proceed cephalocaudal and proximal to distal.
   2. It begins after the focused interview.
   3. Several assessments may occur at one time.
   4. It will always require three sessions with an elderly client.
   5. The nurse will use inspection, palpation, auscultation, and percussion in the neurologic assessment of a client.

6. When assessing the Achilles tendon reflex, the expected response would be:
   1. plantar flexion of the foot.
   2. dorsiflexion of the foot.
   3. fanning of the toes, with dorsiflexion of the great toe.
   4. no response.

7. The components of the Glasgow Coma Scale are: (Select all that apply)
   1. eye response.
   2. sensory response.
   3. motor response.
   4. verbal response.
   5. reflexes.

8. When assessing for cortical disease in a client, the nurse should perform which of the following tests?
   1. Deep tendon reflex testing
   2. Stereognosis
   3. Rapid alternating actions of the upper extremity
   4. Romberg's test

9. An older adult female client is brought to the medical clinic by her daughter. The client's daughter states, "I think my mother is showing signs of Alzheimer's disease." Based on the daughter's statement, the nurse would expect that the client is showing which group of signs and symptoms?
   1. A flat affect, diplopia, and memory loss
   2. Memory loss, confusion, and periods of disorientation
   3. Disorientation, shuffled gait, and dystonia
   4. Tics and tremors, confusion, and diplopia

10. When assessing the deep tendon reflexes on a client, the nurse notes they are brisk. The nurse documents this finding as:
    1. 1+
    2. 2+
    3. 3+
    4. 4+

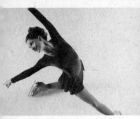

25 Infants, Children, and Adolescents

We must teach our children to dream with their eyes open.
—Harry Edwards

The assessment of infants, children, and adolescents differs from that of the adult in many ways. Assessment techniques and findings will vary according to the growth and developmental stage of the client. Parents or legal guardians must be considered in an assessment that involves a minor. This chapter will focus on gathering both subjective and objective data related to assessments involving infants, children, and adolescents as well as analysis of the data collected.

OBJECTIVES

At the completion of these exercises you will be able to:

1. Define key terminology associated with the assessment of infants, children, and adolescents.
2. Describe the anatomical and physiological differences between the various age groups.
3. Identify variations in assessment technique that are appropriate during various stages of growth and development.
4. Identify assessment findings that are consistent with growth and development milestones.
5. Identify assessment findings that are consistent with various diagnoses related to infants, children, and adolescents.
6. Review cultural considerations that apply in assessment of infants, children, and adolescents.
7. Apply critical thinking skills to a case study.
8. Relate *Healthy People 2020* objectives to various age groups.
9. Document assessment findings.
10. Complete NCLEX®-style questions related to the assessment of infants, children, and adolescents.

RESOURCES

Pearson Nursing Student Resources
Find additional review materials at
nursing.pearsonhighered.com

Prepare for success with additional NCLEX®-style practice questions, interactive assignments and activities, Web links, animations and videos, and more!

Additional resources: *www.healthypeople.gov*
www.childwelfare.gov
www.childhelp.org
www.preventchildabuse.org
www.nationaleatingdisorders.org

CROSSWORD PUZZLE FOR KEY TERMS

Read each definition below and fill in the correct term on the puzzle grid. If the answer requires two words do not leave a blank space between the words. Use a pencil so you can erase easily.

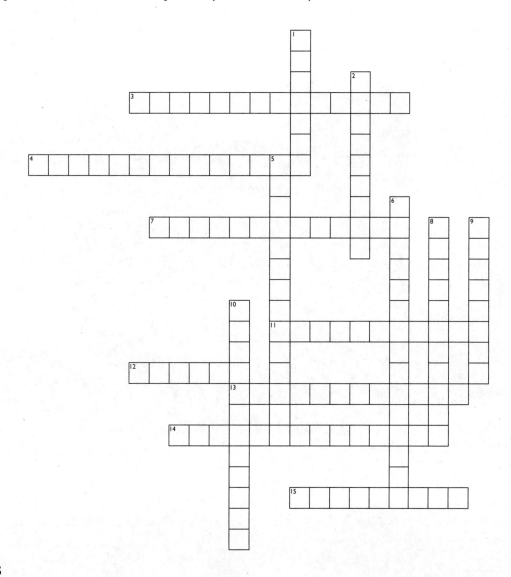

CLUES

Across

3. Congenital defect of the cartilage in the larynx
4. Gray, blue, or purple spots in the sacral and buttocks area of newborns that fade during the first year of life (**two words**)
7. The failure of one or both testicles to descend through the inguinal canal during the final stages of fetal development
11. The period between 11 and 21 years of age
12. Atopic dermatitis
13. Any child whose head circumference is above the 95th percentile
14. Palpable gaps between the bones of the skull (**two words**)
15. Bowlegs (**two words**)

Down

1. Children 1 month of age through 11 months of age
2. A lateral curvature of the lumbar or thoracic spine that is more common in children with neuromuscular deficits
5. Congenital defect of the cartilage in the trachea
6. A protrusion at the umbilicus, visible at birth (**two words**)
8. Comparisons of various measurement values used to assess growth rate and healthy weights versus heights

9. Child who is at least 1 year old but who has not yet reached 3 years of age

10. The second shunt in fetal circulation prior to birth that connects the fetal right atrium to the fetal left .atrium **(two words)**

ANATOMY & PHYSIOLOGY REVIEW

1. For each diagram below write the name of the structure indicated by each line.

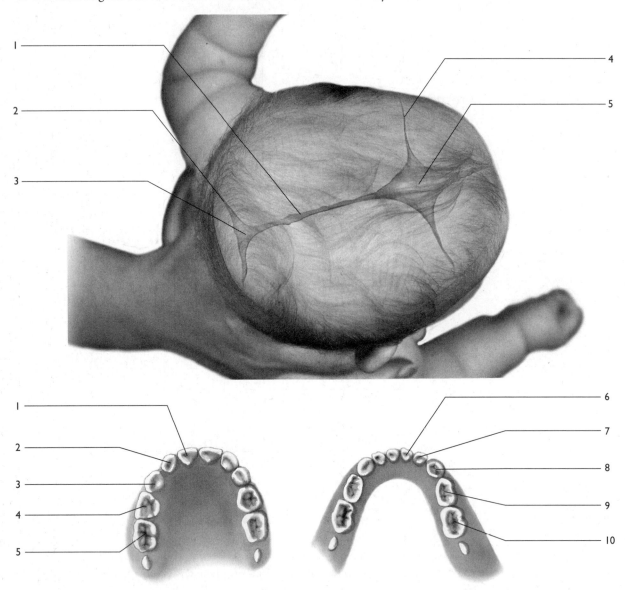

2. Provide a rationale for each statement in the space provided.

Integumentary

1. It is not advisable to apply topical medications to the skin of infants under 6 months of age.

Rationale _____

2. Infants are at a greater risk of heat intolerance than the young adult.

Rationale _____

Head, Eyes, Ears, Nose, and Throat

3. It is imperative that a newborn with craniosynostosis receive treatment as soon as possible.

Rationale _____

4. Children under the age of 5 years are prone to minor head injuries related to falls.

Rationale _____

5. The nurse explains to a mother of a 3-year-old that there is no need to worry about a "shotty" lymph node that is palpated on the child's neck.

Rationale _____

6. A mother is concerned that her 2-year-old has a sinus infection. The nurse explains that this is unlikely.

Rationale _____

7. Ear infections are more common in infants and children than adults of any age.

Rationale _____

Respiratory System

8. The nurse should carefully assess children under the age of 6 years for early signs of respiratory distress when nasal congestion is present.

Rationale _____

Cardiovascular

9. Children have louder heart sounds than young adults.

Rationale _____

10. The nurse explains to a new mother that her 1-year-old child has an innocent heart murmur that was noted when the child was hospitalized for pneumonia.

Rationale _____

Breasts

11. A milky-white discharge may be noted from the nipples of a newborn.

Rationale _____

Abdomen

12. A student nurse is concerned because she believes she can palpate an infant's liver approximately 0.5 cm below the costal margin. Her clinical instructor explains that this is an expected finding.

Rationale _____

Genitourinary and Reproductive

13. Males with undescended testicles past 6 months of age should have a surgical evaluation.

Rationale _____

14. A visiting nurse calms a new mother who is concerned over the bloody vaginal discharge she noted during the diaper change of her 1-week-old daughter. The visiting nurse knows this is an expected finding.

Rationale _____

Musculoskeletal

15. A 5-year-old falls off the monkey bars in a playground and fractures his left leg. The mother expresses concern that the left leg will be shorter when he is an older adult.

Rationale _____

Neurologic

16. In the infant, gross motor skills will develop before fine motor skills.

Rationale _____

INFANT AND EARLY CHILDHOOD REFLEXES

Match the name of each reflex in Column A with its description in Column B. Place the letter on the line provided.

Column A

_____ 1. Tonic Neck
_____ 2. Babinski
_____ 3. Moro
_____ 4. Plantar
_____ 5. Rooting
_____ 6. Stepping
_____ 7. Palmar

Column B

A. Infant will flex the leg and take steps if the infant is upright with the feet touching a surface.
B. Infant will grasp fingers or objects placed in the palm of the hand.
C. Infant will extend the arms with the fingers spread and flex the legs with loud sounds or if the infant's body drops suddenly.
D. Gently stroke the plantar surface of the foot from heel to toe. Infants will extend and fan the toes and flex the foot.
E. Lightly stroke the infant's cheek. Infant will turn the head with the mouth open toward the stroked side.
F. Turn the infant's head to one side while the infant is supine. The infant will extend the arms and legs on the side the head is turned to while flexing the opposite arm and leg.
G. Infant will curl toes when the base of the toes is touched.

DEVELOPMENTAL MILESTONES

Circle the average age that the child is expected to achieve each developmental milestone.

1. Pulls self to standing position

   5 months   8 months   12 months

2. Goes up and down stairs alternating feet

   12 months   2 years   3 years

3. Smiles socially

   2 weeks   2 months   5 months

4. Places objects in mouth

   1½ months   3½ months   5½ months

5. Babbles and coos

   Birth   2 months   4 months

6. Walks independently

   9 months   13 months   18 months

7. Prints name

   1 year   3 years   5 years

8. Plays "peekaboo" and "pat-a-cake"

   4 months   10 months   18 months

9. Says one word

   11 months   18 months   22 months

10. Transfers objects from one hand to another

    3 months   6 months   10 months

11. Sits without support

    5 months   7 months   11 months

12. Cruises

    5 months   10 months   18 months

CALCULATIONS FOR BLADDER CAPACITY AND URINE OUTPUT

Bladder Capacity

Calculate the bladder capacity in ounces for each child.

1. Age— 3 years _____ oz

2. Age— 5 years _____ oz

3. Age— 7 years _____ oz

4. Age— 8 years _____ oz

Urine Output

Calculate the normal urine output in ml per hour for each child.

1. 14-lb child _____ ml/hr

2. 25-lb child _____ ml/hr

3. 32-lb child _____ ml/hr

4. 55-lb child _____ ml/hr

5. 78-lb child _____ ml/hr

6. 90-lb child _____ ml/hr

VITAL SIGNS

Circle the vital sign result that would be considered normal for each client.

1. Blood pressure of an 8-year-old
   90/40   **110/70**   **120/90**

2. Respiratory rate of a 4-year-old
   12   **22**   **34**

3. Heart rate of a 2-year-old
   58 bpm   **110 bpm**   **155 bpm**

4. Heart rate of a 10-year-old
   60 bpm   **84 bpm**   **140 bpm**

5. Blood pressure of a 2-month-old
   60/40   **70/30**   **95/55**

6. Respiratory rate of a newborn
   25   **45**   **65**

7. Blood pressure of a 15-year-old
   90/50   **110/65**   **125/90**

8. Respiratory rate of a 10-year-old
   16   **20**   **28**

EATING DISORDER FINDINGS

Identify each assessment finding that is consistent with anorexia, bulimia, or both disorders. On the line provided, place an A for anorexia, B for bulimia, and the number 2 for both disorders. Leave the line blank if the assessment finding is not consistent with either disorder.

_____ 1. Hoarse voice

_____ 2. Positive psoas

_____ 3. Dental erosion

_____ 4. Loss of muscle tone

_____ 5. Ruptured tympanic membrane

_____ 6. Pedal edema

_____ 7. Leukoplakia

_____ 8. Enlarged cervical chain lymph nodes

_____ 9. Decreased gag reflex

_____ 10. Enlarged thyroid

_____ 11. Ventricular hypertrophy

_____ 12. Swollen parotid glands

_____ 13. Clubbing

_____ 14. Bloodshot eyes

FACTORS THAT INFLUENCE PHYSICAL ASSESSMENT FINDINGS

Read each sentence and write the scrambled word correctly on the line provided.

1. African American infants should be tested for _____ _____ _____ at birth.

2. Asian children may find direct eye contact to be _____.

3. Chinese parents or caregivers may use _____ to draw illness out of the skin of a child.

4. Many Mexicans view it as bad luck to touch a child's _____.

5. Many Hispanics view a child being overweight as a sign of being _____.

6. Hair texture is _____ in African American infants.

7. Native Americans are more likely to develop a _____.

8. Middle Eastern children are more likely to develop _____.

9. Native Americans may find it to be bad luck to purchase baby _____ or _____ before a baby is born.

10. Asian, African American, and Native American infants commonly have _____ _____ on the sacral or buttock areas.

APPLICATION OF THE CRITICAL THINKING PROCESS

Read the scenario and answer the following questions.

Liam is a 6-year-old boy in kindergarten. He often comes to school wearing the same clothes he wore the previous day. His fingernails are in need of trimming, and his hair is often uncombed. He causes lots of mischief in the classroom and is often sent to the principal's office. His teacher and principal have called his mother multiple times, and her reply is "boys will be boys." Today, his teacher sent him to the principal's office because he exposed his genitalia to a little girl on the playground. The principal has requested the help of the school nurse for assessment and counseling for Liam. The school nurse notices what appears to be bite marks on Liam's arm. Liam states that he is unsure how they got there. She also notices bruises that have a shape similar to a belt buckle on his lower back. Liam becomes silent when asked about the markings.

1. What may the nurse suspect is happening to Liam?

2. List all assessment findings discussed in the scenario that may support your answer in Question 1.

3. List additional assessment findings for each category of abuse.

    1. Physical:

    2. Sexual:

    3. Neglect:

    4. Emotional:

4. What is the responsibility of the school nurse in this situation?

5. Identify a *Healthy People 2020* objective that relates to this scenario.

6. Describe the role of the school nurse in relation to this HP objective.

DOCUMENTATION SCENARIOS

Read each scenario and answer the following questions.

SCENARIO 1

Josepina is a 24-year-old new mother who brings her 2-week-old daughter to the well-baby clinic for a routine visit. Josepina received prenatal care and took a prenatal vitamin once per day. She gained 28 lb during her pregnancy. She delivered her child by normal vaginal delivery at 38 weeks' gestation. She has been breast-feeding without any difficulties. The baby weighs 10 lb 4 oz and is 23 inches long with a head circumference in the 50th percentile. A 0.5-cm red circular birthmark is noted on the child's left anterior thigh consistent with a port-wine stain. Tiny white facial papules are noted across the nose.

1. Fill in the collected data from the above scenario using the documentation tool below.

Birth History (for the mother of the child)

Did you receive prenatal care? _____

How much weight did you gain during pregnancy? _____

Describe any complications during the pregnancy: _____

Did you use any medications, alcohol, drugs, or herbal/complementary medicines during pregnancy? _____

Describe your labor and delivery: _____

How many weeks' gestation was your child born at? _____

Describe your child's health immediately after delivery: _____

Is your child breast fed or formula fed? _____

2. State the purpose of the birth history from the mother during a well-baby visit:

_____

3. List four pieces of objective data that have been collected in this scenario:

   1. _____

   2. _____

   3. _____

   4. _____

4. In the space provided, use a narrative format to document the assessment findings of the skin lesions noted.

SCENARIO 2

Raul is a 6-year-old boy who is brought to the emergency room by his parents. The father states he is concerned that Raul may have pneumonia because he has been "coughing a lot and spiked a fever an hour ago." He states his son did not want to go to his baseball game this afternoon because he was too tired. The nurse begins to assess the child and learns that the coughing began 2 weeks ago, is nonproductive, and tight. His fever 1 hour ago was 102.7°F (tympanic) and the parents gave him ibuprofen. Raul has a history of seasonal allergies resulting in coughing and watery eyes during the spring season. These symptoms are controlled by an over-the-counter antihistamine that is administered daily. Raul had surgery as an infant to repair a hypospadias. He is up to date with all his immunizations. During the assessment the child is extremely quiet and shy. He appears fatigued and pale. The vital signs are BP 92/52, HR 135, RR 48, Temperature 102.3°F using a digital tympanic thermometer. Chest expansion is symmetrical, substernal and intercostal retractions are noted, ronchi are auscultated with an inspiratory and expiratory wheeze throughout the bilateral lower lobes. All other fields remain clear.

1. Fill in the collected data from the above scenario using the documentation tool below.

General Questions

Reason for today's visit: _____

Describe any recent illness your child has experienced: _____

Describe any recent changes in your child's behavior: _____

Allergies: _____

Past medical conditions: _____

Past surgeries: _____

Immunizations: _____

Describe sports, clubs, or activities that your child engages in: _____

2. State the importance of focused questions regarding a child's social interaction.

3. In the space provided, use a narrative format to document the assessment findings of the respiratory system.

NCLEX®-STYLE REVIEW QUESTIONS

Read each question carefully. Circle the letter that best answers each question.

1. When obtaining a nutritional history from a 10-year-old, it is best to:
   1. ask the questions directed to the parents or caregiver.
   2. ask the questions directed to the child.
   3. separate the parents or caregiver and the child to question individually and then compare answers for consistency.
   4. ask the questions directed to the child and defer to the parents only when the answer is not known.

2. After a comprehensive physical assessment of a 3-year-old, the nurse calculates that the child can be categorized as obese according to her BMI. In regard to nutritional education, the nurse suggests to the mother:
   1. limit snacking to 4–5 times per day.
   2. limit fruit juice intake to 12 oz per day.
   3. use food as a reward for good behavior.
   4. allow the child to eat in front of the television to distract her from smaller portions.

3. The nurse realizes education must be initiated to the mother of 14-month twin girls when a focused interview reveals she:
   1. has introduced cow's milk to the girls.
   2. puts the girls to sleep with a bottle of 2% milk in the crib.
   3. puts a small drop of honey in their morning cereal.
   4. continues to occasionally offer breast milk.

4. A 16-year-old girl is on the cheerleading squad at her high school. She has just completed her sports health clearance assessment. The nurse would be concerned with which of the following findings? (Select all that apply)
   1. A BMI that has dropped from the 25th percentile to the 5th percentile
   2. The student admitting to dieting in order to stay fit for the squad by limiting her calories to 1800–2000 calories per day
   3. The student drinking about 3–4 energy drinks per day
   4. The student has become a vegan and avoids all carbohydrates in order to lose weight quickly
   5. The student admitted to running 3 miles a day to keep fit for the squad

5. Iron deficiency is found in up to 9% of all children. Which of the following are good sources of iron? (Select all that apply)
   1. Raisins
   2. Cocoa
   3. Oatmeal
   4. Spinach
   5. Cows' milk

6. A 6-week-old baby boy has been brought to the emergency department for vomiting and fever. The baby cried during the entire assessment. The nurse notes that the anterior fontanelle is bulging slightly. The nurse's next step would be to:
   1. palpate the fontanelle again when the baby stops crying.
   2. begin IV therapy for obvious signs of dehydration.
   3. explain to the mother that the anterior fontanelle should have closed up by now.
   4. continue to assess for any other signs of decreased intracranial pressure.

7. A mother brought her 1-year-old son to the pediatrician's office because she felt a small growth on the back of her son's head. The nurse palpates the growth and finds it to be pea-size, mobile, and non-tender. She reports her findings to the doctor as a:
   1. palpable cervical lymph node.
   2. pilonidal cyst.
   3. palpable occipital lymph node.
   4. infected sebaceous cyst.

8. A child is excited because he lost his first tooth and learned that the "tooth fairy" may be leaving him a special treat. The child's age is most likely:
    1. 3 years old.
    2. 6 years old.
    3. 8 years old.
    4. 10 years old.

9. A 16-year-old female is having her annual physical today. The nurse knows that it is important to obtain a sexual history from her because many adolescents are sexually active. The best way for the nurse to obtain reliable information from this client is to:
    1. question the girl with her mother present so her mother can help educate her about safe sexual practices.
    2. ask her to fill out a questionnaire.
    3. question the girl in a private examination room while her mother waits in the waiting area.
    4. do nothing, since a sexual history is not required until the adolescent is 18 years old.

10. When assessing a young child, it is important for the nurse to:
    1. begin with more invasive or uncomfortable procedures first to get them over with.
    2. save more invasive or uncomfortable procedures until last.
    3. avoid using toys, puppets, or other childlike distracters.
    4. avoid letting the child sit on the lap of a parent or caregiver.

The Pregnant Female 26

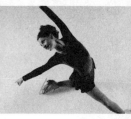

> *A mother is she who can take the place of all others but whose place no one else can take.*
> —Cardinal Mermillod

This chapter is designed to help you develop the skills needed for the assessment of the pregnant female. The data collected provide a basis for the planning of nursing care.

OBJECTIVES

At the completion of these exercises you will be able to:

1. Define key terminology regarding the pregnant female.
2. Describe anatomical and physiological variations in the pregnant client.
3. Write focused interview questions related to pregnancy.
4. Using Nagle's rule and last menstrual period, calculate estimated date of delivery.
5. Describe uterine size and fetal position of the pregnant female.
6. Explain abnormal findings associated with pregnancy.
7. Identify risk factors concerning pregnancy for women of various age groups.
8. Describe the health promotion and education topics necessary in the care of the pregnant female.
9. Apply critical thinking in analysis of a case study.
10. Respond to NCLEX®-style questions related to assessment of pregnant and postpartum females.

RESOURCES

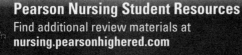

Pearson Nursing Student Resources
Find additional review materials at
nursing.pearsonhighered.com

Prepare for success with additional NCLEX®-style practice questions, interactive assignments and activities, Web links, animations and videos, and more!

WORD SEARCH

Find and circle the correct term in the word search puzzle for each of the definitions listed below. The word may be horizontal, vertical, or diagonal.

```
Z Q C Q C T R M Z L B Q O W A B M N Y U U H Q K I
G Y H R I P E N I N G A N R T U R S Y C M P A O X
D I R D Q I G R O Q R C L H E G A R S S I G N H R
B S F B S S L A D P J X Z L V I A B I L I T Y A L
V J T U L G Y H N G R L U O O D O Q O E N Q A M F
M Q E M I W J K M I F K E G V T W J R X N N S N L
N M R O G O O D E L L S S I G N T E M B R Y O I P
X N A N K K L H V Z G U L X T H D E P Z F V O O I
I V T Q A W D O N R I U K P J F E Y M G L S Y T S
O C O L O S T R U M L X O N N J J J R E I F W I K
W Q G U B G V X D P Z U Q J X M W X H V N G A C A
E Q E V G D K F E T O S C O P E H I E D E T W F C
M G N J U E P D S F K C F L P N S C N R A N F L E
Q U N L S O Q E W Q J G L I G H T E N I N G A U K
I J K V N E Z U E Q R O K I F I U X X M I Q D I S
M U L T I G R A V I D A S A Y O D B W W G U X D S
K M Q D Q L S W L H U S W O K P M P L T R I O N I
M U C O U S P L U G K S K S J Q K Z I X A C F O G
F B J J A A Y P E C H J I L Q P B X S H M K G M N
T F K W Q B X W I B Z G R M A P D Z W J I E G L G
U H G I F T C W Z I U A K I C N V B G F U N D U S
J Z U W H M D Q B C O D C T G O G C J G N I R R F
K D R E W A U E F F A C E M E N T V Z S B N J X D
E B Y B H M C D O N A L D S R U L E J F V G Y D D
S E Q C Y Y X K M R X B J Z J S H I I L R K S L S
```

CLUES

1. A clear, slightly yellowish liquid that surrounds the fetus during pregnancy (**two words**) _____ _____

2. A rule for estimating fetal growth that states after 20 weeks in pregnancy, the weeks of gestation approximately equal the fundal height in centimeters (**two words**) _____ _____

3. A protective covering of the cervix that develops during pregnancy due to progesterone (**two words**) _____ _____

4. Thinning of the cervix occurring near the end of pregnancy in preparation for labor _____

5. The point at which the fetus can survive outside the uterus _____

6. Softening of the cervix near the end of pregnancy in anticipation of birth _____

7. A female who has been pregnant two or more times _____

8. An agent that causes birth defects, such as a virus, a drug, a chemical, or radiation _____

9. The top of the uterus _____

10. An increase in cervical vascularity that contributes to the softening of the cervix during pregnancy (**two words**) _____ _____

11. A palpation technique used to detect fluid or examine floating body structures by using the hand to push against the body _____

12. Thick yellow discharge that may leak from breasts in the month prior to birth in preparation for lactation _____

13. The softening of the uterus and the region that connects the body of the uterus and cervix that occurs throughout pregnancy (**two words**) _____ _____

14. A specialized stethoscope for listening to fetal heart sounds, beginning at approximately 18 weeks' gestation

    _____

15. A dark line running from the umbilicus to the pubic area (**two words**) _____ _____

16. Child during any development stage of pregnancy prior to birth _____

17. The descent of the fetal head into the pelvis _____

18. Vascular congestion that creates a bluish-purple blemish or change in cervical coloration (**two words**)

    _____ _____

19. The irregular shape of the uterus due to the implantation of the ovum (**two words**) _____

    _____

20. The fluttery initial sensations of fetal movement perceived by the mother _____

ANATOMIC AND PHYSIOLOGIC CHANGES OF PREGNANCY

List anatomic and physiologic changes seen in a pregnant female for the following categories.

1. Weight: _____

   _____

   _____

2. Skin, Hair, and Nails: _____

   _____

   _____

3. Cardiovascular System: _____

   _____

   _____

4. Respiratory System: _____

   _____

   _____

5. Gastrointestinal System: _____

   _____

   _____

6. Urinary System: _____

   _____

   _____

7. Reproductive System: _____

   _____

   _____

FOCUSED INTERVIEW

1. Write five focused interview questions related to assessing a pregnant female at the first visit to the obstetric office.

   1. _____

   2. _____

   3. _____

   4. _____

   5. _____

2. Write five focused interview questions at the next or follow-up visit.

   1. _____

   2. _____

   3. _____

   4. _____

   5. _____

ASSESSMENT OF FETAL GROWTH

1. Calculate the estimated date of delivery using Nägele's rule for the following LMPs.

   1. July 20: _____

   2. January 3: _____

   3. November 12: _____

2. Describe the height of the uterus in the following weeks of gestation.

   1. 20 weeks of gestation: _____

   2. 28 weeks of gestation: _____

   3. 36 weeks of gestation: _____

FETAL LIE, PRESENTATION, AND POSITION

Answer the following questions that support the fetus in the uterus.

1. Define Leopold's maneuvers. _____

   _____

   _____

2. Match the data in Column A with the Leopold's maneuvers found in Column B.

   Column A

   _____ 1. A longitudinal lie will find the head of the fetus in the fundus of the uterus

   _____ 2. Identifies the depth of the presenting part in the pelvis

   _____ 3. Location of the fetal back

   _____ 4. Nothing in the fundus of the uterus indicates transverse lie

   _____ 5. Soft irregular mass in fetal breech

   _____ 6. A hard round independently movable mass is palpated in the pelvis

   _____ 7. Fetal back against mother's back is a posterior position

   _____ 8. Identification of the presenting part of the uterus

   _____ 9. During palpation of the mother's abdomen, the fingers of the nurse come together above the superior edge of the symphysis pubis, the presenting part is floating

   _____ 10. Identification of fetal small parts on the left side of the mother

   Column B

   A. First

   B. Second

   C. Third

   D. Fourth

3. Identify fetal position in the following diagrams by using the accepted abbreviations.

1.

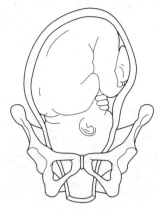

Answer _____

4.

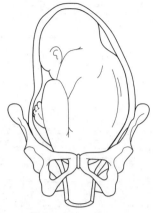

Answer _____

2.

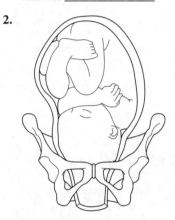

Answer _____

5.

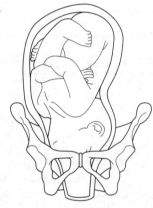

Answer _____

3.

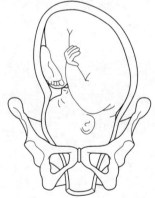

Answer _____

Source: Courtesy of Abbott Nutrition, Columbus, OH

RISK FACTORS AND ABNORMAL FINDINGS

1. Describe five risk factors associated with pregnancy.

1. _____

2. _____

3. _____

4. _____

5. _____

2. List or describe signs and symptoms of the following abnormal findings associated with pregnancy.

    1. Preeclampsia: _____

_____

_____

    2. Gestational diabetes: _____

_____

_____

    3. Preterm labor: _____

_____

_____

    4. Mood disorders: _____

_____

_____

APPLICATION OF THE CRITICAL THINKING PROCESS

Read each scenario and answer the following questions.

SCENARIO 1

A nurse in an obstetric clinic is caring for Ms. K. B., a 36-year-old with an obstetric history of spontaneous abortions at age 30 and 32, a preterm vaginal delivery at 35 weeks 2 years ago, and is pregnant again. Ms. K. B. states that her LMP was 2 months ago on 12/21. Ms. K. B. is a single mom to a toddler and works full time. Ms. K. B. reports to the nurse that her BP was elevated, and she had swelling of face, arms, and legs during the pregnancy 2 years ago.

1. Document Ms. K. B.'s Gravidity and Parity in obstetrical terms.

2. Using Nägele's rule, calculate the expected date of confinement (EDC).

3. Identify four risk factors associated with Ms. K. B.'s pregnancy.

    1.

    2.

    3.

    4.

4. Identify three educational topics Ms. K. B. can benefit from.

    1.

    2.

    3.

5. State five objectives presented in *Healthy People 2020* that would apply to this client.

    1.

    2.

    3.

    4.

    5.

6. Explain the following signs of pregnancy.

    1. Presumptive: _____

    2. Probable: _____

    3. Positive: _____

SCENARIO 2

The nurse is caring for D. K., a 23-year-old on the second postpartum day after a normal vaginal delivery and giving birth to a healthy newborn. D. K. had a second-degree vaginal tear during childbirth. D. K.'s obstetrical history is Gravida 1 and Para 1. D. K. states that she is a single mother and that her mother agreed to help with the baby for a few weeks.

1. During assessment on the second postpartum day, the nurse observes that the fundal height is above the umbilicus and displaced to the right side of the abdomen. The nurse concludes that this may be the result of:

    _____

2. What should be the nurse's next assessment, based on the above conclusion?

3. Based on D. K.'s obstetrical history, identify three teaching-learning needs for this client.

4. When caring for this client, the nurse understands that the two most important causes of postpartum infection are

    _____ and _____.

NCLEX®-STYLE REVIEW QUESTIONS

Read each question carefully. Choose the best answer for each question.

1. For a woman with a 28-day menstrual cycle, ovulation begins on the:
    1. first day of the menstrual cycle.
    2. seventh day of the menstrual cycle.
    3. 14th day of the menstrual cycle.
    4. 28th day of the menstrual cycle.

2. An emergency department nurse is talking to a young female who states that she was sexually assaulted by a friend during a party the day before. The woman stated that "I felt so ashamed and dirty that I ran home and took a shower." The initial response of the nurse in this situation is:
    1. "You may have destroyed the evidence by taking a shower."
    2. "Do you remember exactly what happened? Were you drunk?"
    3. "I understand that it was important for you to take a shower after what happened."
    4. "Do you have the clothes you were wearing at the time and have you washed them?"

3. The nurse assessing an antenatal client determines that the presumptive signs of pregnancy are: (Select all that apply)
    1. breast tenderness.
    2. amenorrhea.
    3. uterine enlargement.
    4. increased urinary frequency.
    5. quickening.

4. Which of the following would be included when performing a postpartum assessment on a client who is first-day postpartum after a vaginal delivery? (Select all that apply)
    1. Assess the breasts
    2. Assess the perineum
    3. Assess extremities
    4. Check vaginal discharge
    5. Assess fundal height

5. During the postpartum period, which of the hormones will sharply increase in a client that will aid in breast milk production?
    1. prolactin
    2. estrogen
    3. human chorionic gonadotropin
    4. human placental lactogen

6. A Muslim client who has just delivered states that she is hungry and requests food. The nurse should ensure that the following products are avoided in the meal.
    1. beef
    2. pork
    3. milk
    4. poultry

7. Place the different stages of fetal development in chronological order.
    1. Vernix caseosa is seen.
    2. Blastocyst development is complete.
    3. Testes have descended into scrotal sac.
    4. Development of chambers of the heart.

8. A client showed up in the clinic and raises concern that she might be pregnant. Which of the hormone level elevations will confirm her doubts?
    1. human chorionic gonadotropin
    2. pitocin
    3. estrogen
    4. luteinizing hormone

9. Cardiac output in a pregnant female:
   1. increases along with stroke volume.
   2. decreases significantly.
   3. remains the same.
   4. increases with no change in stroke volume.

10. A woman who is 18 weeks pregnant and is complaining of lower abdominal pain may be experiencing:
    1. appendicitis.
    2. urinary tract infection.
    3. constipation.
    4. stretching of round ligament.

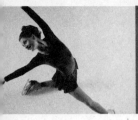

27 The Older Adult

About the only thing that comes to us without effort is old age.
—Gloria Pitzer

The population of adults over the age of 65 is growing at a tremendous rate. There are many normal changes that occur with the aging process. This chapter will focus on gathering both subjective and objective data related to the assessment of the older adult, as well as analysis of the data collected.

OBJECTIVES

At the completion of these exercises you will be able to:

1. Define key terminology associated with the older adult.
2. Review selected theories of aging.
3. Describe age-related changes in anatomy and physiology in the older adult.
4. Describe data-gathering techniques for the older adult.
5. Identify assessment findings that are consistent with various diagnoses related to the older adult.
6. Explore ways to promote health for the older adult.
7. Apply critical thinking skills to a case study.
8. Explore the role of the nurse in relation to *Healthy People 2020* objectives for the older adult.
9. Complete NCLEX®-style review questions related to the assessment of the older adult.

RESOURCES

Pearson Nursing Student Resources

Find additional review materials at
nursing.pearsonhighered.com

Prepare for success with additional NCLEX®-style practice questions, interactive assignments and activities, Web links, animations and videos, and more!

Additional resources: *www.healthypeople.gov*
www.ncea.aoa.gov
www.cdc.gov
www.aarp.org

CROSSWORD PUZZLE FOR KEY TERMS

Read each definition below and fill in the correct term on the puzzle grid. If the answer requires two words do not leave a blank space between the words. Use a pencil so you can erase easily.

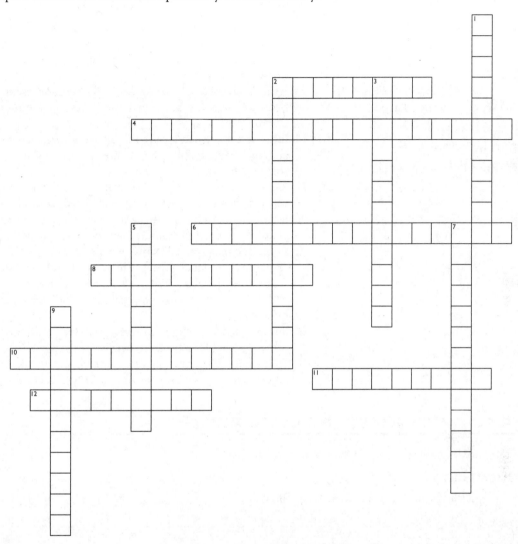

CLUES

Across

2. A condition in which the lens of the eye continues to thicken and yellow
4. Benign, greasy, wart-like lesions that are yellow-brown in color **(two words)**
6. Normal aging growths that can be considered precancerous **(two words)**
8. High-frequency hearing loss that occurs over time
10. Liver spots **(two words)**
11. An opacity of the bulbar conjunctiva that can grow over the cornea and block vision
12. Inflammation of the lip

Down

1. Yellowish nodules that are thickened areas of the bulbar conjunctiva caused by prolonged exposure to sun, wind, and dust
2. Nonsignificant tiny red spots that can be either macules or papules **(two words)**
3. Skin tags
5. Decreased ability of the eye lens to change shape to accommodate for near vision
7. A vascular lesion that can occur spontaneously or in response to minimal trauma in the very old client with fragile blood vessels **(two words)**
9. Soft, yellow plaques on the lids at the inner canthus that are sometimes associated with high cholesterolemia

THEORIES OF AGING

Match the theory of aging in Column A with its description in Column B.

Column A

_____   1. Disengagement Theory

_____   2. Theory of Individualism

_____   3. Theory of Thriving

_____   4. Functional Consequence Theory

_____   5. Age Stratification Theory

_____   6. Continuity Theory

_____   7. Activity Theory

_____   8. Lifespan Development Paradigm

Column B

A. Functioning in aging is impacted by psychobiological, sociocultural, and environmental factors. The impact of the factors creates changes in the individual and increased risk for functional limitations.

B. Aging is characterized by mutual withdrawal or disengagement between the aging individual and others in the individual's environment.

C. Life stages are structured according to roles, connections, values, and goals. Successful aging requires adjustment to changes in roles, relationships, and goals.

D. Successful aging requires achievement of the task of ego-integrity versus despair. Life is viewed as satisfying, death as completion of life.

E. Successful aging occurs when harmony exists among the aging individual, the physical environment, and the individual's relationships.

F. In old age the personality is stable. Personality patterns predict responses to the changes of age including health, socioeconomic status, and the activities in which one participates. Differing and varied responses to aging result from individual personality differences.

G. Successful adjustment to aging requires the individual to remain physically active and socially involved.

H. Successful aging encompasses acceptance of the past and adjustment to loss accompanying functional decline.

PHYSIOLOGICAL CHANGES IN THE OLDER ADULT

Provide a rationale for each statement in the space provided.

INTEGUMENTARY

1. As adults age, they begin to develop wrinkles on the skin.

    Rationale _____

2. As adults age, their hair color changes to grayish white.

    Rationale _____

HEAD, EYES, EARS, NOSE, AND THROAT

3. An older adult father tells his daughter that the meal she prepared is very bland. The daughter defends her work by explaining she used many fresh herbs and spices. Her father then states "now that I think of it, most foods I eat nowadays seem very bland."

    Rationale _____

4. An older adult is straining her eyes to read a new best-selling novel. She states "I guess I have hit the age that I need reading glasses."

    Rationale _____

5. An older adult is having a difficult time hearing consonants when being spoken to by the nurse.

    Rationale _____

RESPIRATORY SYSTEM

6. The nurse encourages the older adult to receive influenza and pneumonia vaccines.

    Rationale _____

CARDIOVASCULAR

7. The nurse explains to the older adult client that a gradual rise in his blood pressure has been noted throughout the years during the annual assessments.

Rationale_____

ABDOMEN

8. A father comments to his son that he is not able to eat the amount of food he used to; he feels fuller quicker now.

Rationale_____

9. Constipation can be a major problem for the older adult.

Rationale_____

GENITOURINARY

10. The nurse requests that the doctor decrease the dosage of an antibiotic for an older adult client to prevent drug toxicity.

Rationale_____

ENDOCRINE

11. An older adult male is experiencing erectile dysfunction and is very concerned.

Rationale_____

MUSCULOSKELETAL

12. The orthopedic nurse is explaining to a family how their grandmother fractured her arm by just having her 2-year-old grandson tug on it.

Rationale_____

13. An older adult male tries on a pair of pants from years ago and they are too long. He states "is it possible I am shrinking?"

Rationale_____

NEUROLOGIC

14. A middle-aged son tells his older adult father that he is not safe to drive a car anymore. He states "Dad, you just can't respond quickly anymore."

Rationale_____

ASSESSMENT FINDINGS

Circle each assessment finding that can be described as an age-related change.

Liver spots	Vitiligo
Decreased sense of taste	Thin skin
Thick skin	Pendulous earlobes
Dry skin	Increased sense of smell
Oily skin	Yellow plaque on the inner canthus
Red ring around the iris	Decreased sense of hearing
Increased chest wall expansion	Use of accessory muscles for breathing
Narrow pulse pressure	Slower gastric emptying times
Decline in muscle strength	Diminished deep tendon reflexes
Elongation of the spine	Penile swelling
Splenomegaly	Soft or boggy eyeballs

THE OLDER ADULT

Read each statement. Determine if each statement is true or false by circling the term. Rewrite all false statements to reflect the truth on the line provided.

1. Older adults require less sleep than younger adults.

   True   **False**

   _____

2. The older adult male has the same sperm production as a younger adult male.

   True   **False**

   _____

3. Many symptoms that older adults complain of may be a sign of thyroid dysfunction.

   True   **False**

   _____

4. Approximately 10% of muscle mass is lost by the age of 80.

   True   **False**

   _____

5. Only 20% of all older adults engage in sexual activity.

   True   **False**

   _____

6. Older adults should be assessed for psychological distress caused by multiple losses they may experience (e.g., a spouse, retirement, ability to drive, etc.).

   True   **False**

   _____

7. Older adults may have increased vitamin B_{12} levels due to increased acid production in the stomach.

   True   **False**

   _____

8. A decline in the older adult's functional status may cause poor nutrition.

   True   **False**

   _____

9. The older adult may be at risk for dehydration because they do not feel thirst when it is appropriate to drink.

   True   **False**

   _____

10. Medication side effects may cause a decrease in the production of female vaginal lubricant leading to an uncomfortable and dissatisfying sexual history.

    True   **False**

    _____

11. Older adults cannot learn new things.

    True   **False**

    _____

THE HOSPITALIZED OLDER ADULT

Read the scenario and answer the following questions.

Edward is a 91-year-old male who is hospitalized for pneumonia. Edward is awake, alert, and oriented. He has good long- and short-term recall. His son Hector accompanies him as he is admitted to the medical-surgical unit. The nurse plans to complete a health history and physical assessment. The nurse uses the SPICES method to collect data in order to help her develop a plan of care.

1. List the categories when using the SPICES acronym to assess the older adult.

S

P

I

C

E

S

2. Is it necessary for Hector to be present during the initial health history and physical assessment? Provide a rationale.

3. List one focused interview question that would be appropriate for the nurse to ask Hector about his father.

HEALTH PROMOTION AND THE OLDER ADULT

1. List three ways to encourage health promotion in the older adult.

1.

2.

3.

2. Perform a search (online, newspaper, telephone, etc.) to find an existing program in your community that promotes the health of older adults.

Name of program: _____

Location of program: _____

Sponsor of program: _____

Goal of program: _____

Cost of program: _____

3. Find a research article that supports one of your health promotion activities identified in Part 1 above. Describe how you can use this article to develop a program to improve the health of older adults in your community.

Research article reference:

Program description:

APPLICATION OF THE CRITICAL THINKING PROCESS

Read the scenarios and answer the questions provided.

SCENARIO I

Mildred is an 82-year-old widowed female who lives alone in a two-story colonial house. She has lived in this house for 45 years with her husband of 47 years. Together they raised their family, two sons and one daughter. It is a large home with many staircases, hardwood floors, ceramic tile floors, and area rugs. Mildred's son Gregory is very concerned about his mother's safety now that she has become increasingly frail through the years. He encourages her to walk with a cane but she refuses. She is relatively steady on her feet but does tire easily getting around such a large home. Her bedroom is on the second floor and the laundry is in the basement. The lighting in the house is old. Mildred does not have a nightstand lamp next to her bed because there is no nearby electric outlet. Gregory is concerned that she will fall in the dark if she gets up during the night to go to the bathroom. Last year Mildred did suffer a minor injury to her right wrist when she tripped over the electrical cord of the vacuum. She stated "if all I did was sprain my wrist with this fall, my bones must be made of steel"!

1. List at least four safety hazards that you have identified in the above scenario.

1.

2.

3.

4.

2. Search the Internet for a website that can provide Gregory with information on home safety and the elderly so he can help his mother.

List a website here:

Information provided:

Why is this website useful for Gregory?

3. Find a *Healthy People 2020* objective that will support this scenario.

4. Describe the nurse's role in relation to this *Healthy People 2020* objective.

SCENARIO 2

Ethel is an 82-year-old who lives with her son (William) and daughter-in-law (Victoria). She has a small bedroom in the basement that does not have any windows. She has a very good relationship with her son, but he travels for business most of the time. Ethel is left home alone with her daughter-in-law who has little patience for her and her increased daily needs. Ethel has been having trouble getting up the basement stairs and has had frequent episodes of incontinence and requires assistance with her diaper. She has also been quite forgetful. Today Ethel presents to the emergency department with a possible fractured humerus. As the nurse is gathering subjective data on the mechanism of the injury, she notes that Victoria is doing all the talking. Ethel is lying quietly on the stretcher staring down at her hands. When the nurse attempts to assess Ethel's pain, Victoria jumps in and says "how much pain can she be in, she is not crying or anything; I don't think it hurts her that bad." As the nurse continues to attempt to gather more information from Ethel, Victoria makes comments such as "old people can be a real pain in the behind sometimes" and "when you die you better leave me all your money to make up for all the time I have had to spend taking care of you." The nurse then asks Victoria to step out of the room so she can physically assess Ethel. Victoria becomes very agitated and is hesitant to leave her mother-in-law alone to be assessed.

The nurse is becoming more and more convinced that there may be some type of elder abuse.

1. What evidence does the nurse have at this point to support her assumption?

2. List five types of elder abuse.

3. Write a *Healthy People 2020* objective that supports this scenario.

4. Describe what the nurse's role may be in relation to this *Healthy People 2020* objective.

NCLEX®-STYLE REVIEW QUESTIONS

Read each question carefully. Circle the letter that best answers each question.

1. By the year 2030 the older population is expected to account for what percentage of the total population?
    1. 10
    2. 20
    3. 40
    4. 50

2. The nurse is aware that the older adult may experience which of the following changes regarding the integumentary system?
    1. Decrease in the number of sweat glands
    2. Increase in skin elasticity
    3. Increased coarse facial hair
    4. Decreased sebum production

3. A 76-year-old male had a Weber test performed by a nurse at the neighborhood clinic. It revealed conductive hearing loss. The next step for the nurse to proceed with would be:
    1. a referral to a specialist.
    2. measurement for a hearing aid.
    3. checking for earwax buildup.
    4. assessing for perforation of the tympanic membrane.

4. The Centers for Disease Control and Prevention recommend a pneumococcal vaccine for all adults 65 years and older. The nurse is aware that a booster should be given:
    1. every year.
    2. every 5 years.
    3. every 10 years.
    4. A booster is not necessary.

5. An older adult with an elevated BMI and a waist-hip ratio greater than 0.95 is at high risk for:
    1. hypothyroidism.
    2. coronary artery disease.
    3. liver cancer.
    4. kidney failure.

6. When assessing for orthostatic hypotension in the older adult, the nurse must:
    1. have the client go from a standing position to a sitting position.
    2. wait 5 minutes between each blood pressure reading.
    3. assist the client from the reclining position to a sitting position and then a standing position.
    4. look for a drop of 10% in pressure with each position change.

7. The nurse is aware that the older adult requires:
    1. more sleep than all other age groups.
    2. less sleep than all other age groups.
    3. an equal amount of sleep as younger age groups.
    4. Sleep need not be considered when assessing the older adult.

8. When assessing sexuality in the older adult, the nurse must keep in mind that:
    1. the majority of older adults do not engage in sexual relations.
    2. medications for chronic conditions may alter sexual function.
    3. it is not appropriate to question the older adults' sexuality unless it is brought up by the client.
    4. older adults may experience an increased libido.

9. An appropriate question for the nurse to include when assessing functional ability in the older adult would be:
    1. Do you need assistance when bathing?
    2. Are you able to walk a mile without becoming short of breath?
    3. Can you touch your toes?
    4. Have you experienced nocturia?

10. A 79-year-old male who lost his wife to cancer 3 months ago has now been diagnosed with prostate cancer and is refusing all treatments. Which of the following tools should the nurse utilize to further assess this client?
    1. Denver Developmental Screening Tool
    2. Mini-Mental State Exam
    3. The Geriatric Depression Scale
    4. The Elder Assessment Instrument

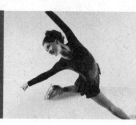
*Many of the great achievements of the world were accomplished
by tired and discouraged men who kept on working.*
—Author Unknown

This chapter is designed to help the student integrate all the information learned in order to be successful when conducting a complete health assessment.

OBJECTIVES

At the completion of these exercises you will be able to:

1. Define terms related to health and assessment.
2. Describe the elements of a complete health assessment.
3. Describe communication techniques.
4. Describe the components of the client interview.
5. Apply the concepts of communication process.
6. Describe the sources of information used by the nurse to obtain client data.
7. Apply client data to the components of the health history.
8. Write focused interview questions related to the neurologic system in selected age groups.
9. Identify expected findings from the assessment of the integumentary system in selected age groups.
10. Categorize assessment techniques and findings by systems.
11. Apply critical thinking in analysis of a case study.
12. Respond to NCLEX®-style questions related to the complete health assessment.

RESOURCES

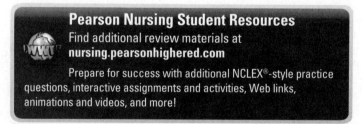

Pearson Nursing Student Resources
Find additional review materials at
nursing.pearsonhighered.com

Prepare for success with additional NCLEX®-style practice questions, interactive assignments and activities, Web links, animations and videos, and more!

HEALTH ASSESSMENT

KEY TERMS

Define the following terms.

1. Health

2. Wellness

3. Illness

4. Comprehensive health assessment

CHARACTERISTICS

1. Identify three component parts of the comprehensive health assessment.

    1.

    2.

    3.

2. Identify the type of data collected by the nurse when obtaining data in each of the component parts.

    1.

    2.

    3.

COMMUNICATION

THERAPEUTIC COMMUNICATION

Explain how therapeutic communication techniques will be helpful throughout nursing practice.

INTERVIEW

1. Define the interview process.

2. List the three phases of the interview process.

    1.

    2.

    3.

3. Indicate when each of the phases will be used by the nurse.

TECHNIQUES

Describe the following techniques and provide an example of each. Indicate by circling if the example will enhance or hinder the communication process.

1. Attending _____

   Example _____

   Enhance / Hinder

2. Paraphrasing _____

   Example _____

   Enhance / Hinder

3. Use of medical and technical terms _____

   Example _____

   Enhance / Hinder

4. Focusing _____

   Example _____

   Enhance / Hinder

5. Passing judgment: _____

   Example _____

   Enhance / Hinder

6. Reflecting _____

   Example _____

   Enhance / Hinder

7. False reassurance _____

   Example _____

   Enhance / Hinder

8. Summarizing _____

   Example _____

   Enhance / Hinder

9. Direct leading _____

   Example _____

   Enhance / Hinder

10. Questioning _____

    Example _____

    Enhance/Hinder

FOCUSED INTERVIEW

Read the scenario and answer the questions that follow.

A middle-aged adult male is married and has two school-aged sons. He works as a department supervisor in the office of a large construction firm and is a busy family man. His father died when he was in high school and now his paternal uncle is in the hospital for a myocardial infarction commonly known as a heart attack. His cousin, who is 2 years older than him, has coronary artery disease. Because he is overweight and has an elevated cholesterol level and a stressful job, he decides to visit the nurse practitioner in the Health and Wellness Center at work. The following is an excerpt from the focused interview between the nurse and this client.

Nurse: "Good afternoon, what brings you here today?"

Client: "I'm concerned. My uncle is in the hospital with a heart attack. His son, my cousin, also has heart problems. I'm afraid I might be next. My doctor told me my cholesterol level is high. I'm not sure what that means."

Nurse: "You seem to be concerned."

Client: "Yes, I am. I have two young sons and a wife, and I need to keep working. I can't afford any health problems."

Nurse: "Well, if you would lose 30 or more pounds your cholesterol level will drop and you would have nothing to worry about." (This is said with a sharp tone of voice.)

Client: "Oh!"

1. Review the first statement made by the nurse.

   a. What technique is the nurse using?

   b. Will this enhance or hinder the communication process?

    c. Provide a rational for your decision.

2. Review the second statement made by the nurse.

    a. What technique is the nurse using?

    b. Will this technique encourage or hinder the communication process?

    c. Provide a rational for your decision.

    d. Is there a need for the nurse to use a different strategy?

3. Review the third statement made by the nurse.

    a. Identify the three strategies used by the nurse in this statement.

        1.

        2.

        3.

    b. Do these strategies encourage the communication process?

        1.

        2.

        3.

4. Write three focused interview questions that the nurse could use that would enhance the communication process.

    1.

    2.

    3.

SOURCE OF INFORMATION

1. Define the sources of information used by the nurse to obtain client data.

    1. Primary source:

    2. Secondary source:

2. Read the list of data obtained by the nurse. On the line provided indicate if the data are from the primary source or secondary source. Use a P for primary and an S for secondary.

_____ **1.** My leg hurts		_____ **4.** I am always tired
_____ **2.** Seems to have trouble breathing		_____ **5.** BP 156/90
_____ **3.** Complete blood count within normal limits		_____ **6.** Recorded urinary output of 300 ml

HEALTH HISTORY

Match the data found in Column A with the component part of the health history in Column B by placing the letter or letters on the line provided. The component part might be used once, more than once, or not at all.

Column A Client Data

_____ 1. African American

_____ 2. Presence of yellow phlegm

_____ 3. MMR 3 months ago

_____ 4. Appendectomy age 7

_____ 5. Father died of MI

_____ 6. High school diploma

_____ 7. Young adult

_____ 8. No current health complaints

_____ 9. Exercises 3 times/week

_____ 10. Eats breakfast daily

_____ 11. Menstrual period every 28 days

_____ 12. Sister has asthma

_____ 13. Has trouble breathing when lying down

_____ 14. Can distinguish odors

Column B Component Part

A. Review of Systems

B. Biographical Data

C. Family History

D. Medical History

E. Surgical History

F. Current Health Status

G. Psychosocial Data

FOCUSED INTERVIEW QUESTIONS

Write four focused interview questions you would use for a given topic and age.

1. Older adult: Activities of Daily Living (ADL)

   1. _____.

   2. _____.

   3. _____.

   4. _____.

2. School-aged child: A 7-year-old falls on the playground at school and comes to the school nurse crying and has blood on his shirt.

   1. _____.

   2. _____.

   3. _____.

   4. _____.

EXPECTED FINDINGS

For each of the selected age groups, identify expected physical assessment findings for the assessment of the skin, hair, and nails.

1. Newborn

   1. _____.

   2. _____.

   3. _____.

   4. _____.

   5. _____.

2. Children

    1. _____.

    2. _____.

    3. _____.

3. Pregnant female

    1. _____.

    2. _____.

    3. _____.

4. Adult

    1. _____.

    2. _____.

    3. _____.

    4. _____.

5. Older Adult: Describe the anticipated physical assessment findings of the skin regarding:

    1. Turgor: _____.

    2. Moisture: _____.

    3. Texture: _____.

    4. Color: _____.

    5. Temperature: _____.

BODY SYSTEMS

Match the assessment technique in Column A with the body system found in Column B. The body system may be used once, more than once, or not at all.

Column A

_____	**1.** Apical pulse 68
_____	**2.** Turgor resilient
_____	**3.** Palpation of Skene's glands
_____	**4.** Diaphragmatic excursion
_____	**5.** Romberg test positive
_____	**6.** Capillary refill
_____	**7.** Phalen's test
_____	**8.** Palpating the spleen
_____	**9.** Confrontation test
_____	**10.** Babinski test
_____	**11.** Tactile fremitus
_____	**12.** Tinel's sign
_____	**13.** Palpating the tragus
_____	**14.** Ability to calculate
_____	**15.** CVA tenderness
_____	**16.** Rebound tenderness
_____	**17.** Whisper pectoriloquy
_____	**18.** Whisper test
_____	**19.** Cardinal fields
_____	**20.** Palpation of the axillae

Column B

A. Skin, hair, nails
B. Head, neck, and related lymphatics
C. Eye
D. Ear, nose, mouth, throat
E. Respiratory
F. Breast and axillae
G. Cardiovascular
H. Peripheral vascular
I. Abdomen
J. Urinary
K. Male reproductive
L. Female reproductive
M. Musculoskeletal
N. Neurologic

APPLICATION OF THE CRITICAL THINKING PROCESS

Read the scenario and answer the following questions.

> A middle-aged male reports to the healthcare provider's office for his yearly physical examination. He is 55 years old and has done the same type of job for the past 25 years. The company is going through an economic crisis, and the client is concerned about losing his job. He reports to the nurses, "I feel healthy except an occasional heartburn or pressure right here (pointing to the left side of his chest) and sometimes I feel my heart racing." The following is an excerpt from the focused interview.

Between the nurse and this client:

Nurse: "Good morning! I see that you were here last year for your physical."

Client: "Yes, that is correct."

Nurse: "Tell me how your health has been the past year."

Client: "I consider myself a really healthy person. I haven't been out sick from work all year. It is just the pressure that I get right here." Again, the client points to the left side of his chest.

Nurse: "Tell me more about this heartburn and the pressure on your chest."

Client: "It is just here, and not all the time."

Nurse: "Does the heartburn and pressure get worse before or after you eat?"

Client: "I have not noticed any change when I eat."

Nurse: "When do you notice the change?"

Client: "When I am at work either during or after our management meetings."

1. Based on the information obtained from the client, what subjective data could be the contributing factor for his "pressure in the chest area"?

2. When interviewing the client, what familial tendencies should be included in the interview?

3. What medical conditions could contribute to the client's risk of heart disease?

4. What other questions would be helpful to the nurse regarding the type of pain the client is experiencing?

5. How would you proceed with the physical assessment of the client?

NCLEX®-STYLE REVIEW QUESTIONS

Read each question carefully. Choose the best answer for each question.

1. The mother of a 12-month-old child tells the nurse, "I can see his belly rumbling. Is this normal?" Which of the following can be the response from the nurse?
   1. You need to bring him to a good pediatric gastroenterologist.
   2. This means that the gallbladder is digesting fats.
   3. No. This is not normal.
   4. The muscles of the abdomen are thin in babies. So, you will see this.

2. The client asks the nurse, "Is it normal to have a stomachache almost every day?" Which of the following could be the nurse's response to this client?
   1. That's not good at all.
   2. I would suggest that you see a specialist.
   3. No one can have a stomachache every day.
   4. Maybe we can talk about your diet.

3. A 14-year-old male client expresses concern over his "misshaped private parts." Upon examination, the nurse learns the client is concerned about his scrotum. Which of the following can the nurse explain to this client?
   1. You are right. The testicles should be even.
   2. This is completely normal.
   3. I think you should see a specialist.
   4. Well, your left testicle is lower than your right.

4. A client with a head injury is demonstrating difficulty swallowing and talking. Which cranial nerve might be adversely affected with this head injury?
   1. Glossopharyngeal
   2. Vagus
   3. Hypoglossal
   4. Accessory

5. A client is recovering from a cardiac catheterization where the right femoral artery was accessed. Which of the following pulses can the nurse use to assess the patency of this artery?
   1. Brachial
   2. Radial
   3. Posterior tibial
   4. Ulnar

6. The nurse hears a heart sound right before S1 on an 80-year-old male client. What can this finding suggest to the nurse?
   1. Nothing. This is normal.
   2. This is an atrial gallop and can mean that something is wrong.
   3. This is an atrial kick and helps the heart beat better.
   4. This is a ventricular gallop and is heard in healthy people.

7. An elderly client wants to know when she can stop doing breast exams. What can the nurse say to this client?
   1. You should have stopped right after menopause.
   2. You can probably stop in a month or two.
   3. Breast cancer can still develop when you get older.
   4. It's not recommended at your age.

8. While teaching, the nurse instructs a client about immunizations. What level of prevention does immunizations fall into?
   1. Tertiary
   2. Secondary
   3. Restorative
   4. Primary

9. After completing the health history on a client during assessment, the nurse begins to ask more questions about specific information. This portion of the health assessment is:
   1. documentation follow-up.
   2. focused interview.
   3. physical assessment.
   4. interpretation of findings.

10. A nurse is observed talking rudely to a client of a non-American culture. When approached about this behavior, the nurse responds, "These people have no right to be in the United States." This nurse is demonstrating:
    1. material culture.
    2. nonmaterial culture.
    3. competent culture care.
    4. ethnocentrism.

The Hospitalized Client 29

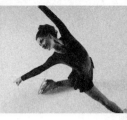

Accomplishment is easiest when we work the hardest, and it is hardest when we work the least.
—Author Unknown

This chapter is developed to help the student apply the principles of assessment to an individual in a state of health reflecting illness in a hospital setting. These principles could be applied across the age span and in any area of care.

OBJECTIVES

At the completion of these exercises you will be able to:

1. Apply the nursing process to a client situation.
2. Apply three assessment types the nurse will use when assessing a hospitalized client.
3. Identify expected findings from physical assessment of the respiratory status of a client across the age span.
4. Apply critical thinking in analysis of a case study.
5. Respond to NCLEX®-style questions related to assessment of a hospitalized client.

RESOURCES

Pearson Nursing Student Resources
Find additional review materials at
nursing.pearsonhighered.com

Prepare for success with additional NCLEX®-style practice questions, interactive assignments and activities, Web links, animations and videos, and more!

NURSING PROCESS

Read the scenario and answer the following questions.

Maggie Crumb, an 82-year-old female with a history of emphysema, is brought to the Emergi-Center by her niece. The niece became concerned when her aunt did not phone her for 3 days. The niece reports her aunt has been vomiting and has had severe diarrhea for 5 days. She has not eaten and is having difficulty with her speech. The niece says to the nurse, "my aunt looks terrible, she looks very thin to me. She must be dehydrated. I know she is not a big lady and weighs about 110 pounds—but now, I just do not know." Maggie Crumb responds with the statement, "I am so tired, it is an effort to do anything. I feel very weak. I do not think my legs will hold me up."

1. Write five focused interview questions the nurse should ask this client or the niece.

   1.

   2.

3.

4.

5.

2. The nurse begins the physical assessment by performing a rapid assessment. What data should the nurse gather?

3. Identify the anticipated findings for each of the following as the nurse proceeds with the physical assessment. Place your response on the line provided.

    1. Skin turgor _____   5. Serum sodium _____

    2. Skin color _____   6. Level of consciousness _____

    3. Mucous membranes _____   7. Behavior _____

    4. Weight _____   8. Serum potassium _____

The primary care provider makes a diagnosis of acute gastroenteritis with dehydration (hyperosmolar imbalance). It is decided the client needs to stay at the center to initiate fluid replacement.

The following nursing diagnosis is then recorded: Deficient Fluid Volume R/T vomiting and diarrhea as evidenced by sticky membranes and tenting of the skin.

4. Write one short-term goal for this client.

5. Write two nursing interventions for this client.

    1.

    2.

6. Describe a projected means for evaluation.

7. Using Appendix A on page A-1 of the textbook, identify three additional nursing diagnoses for this client.

    1. _____

    2. _____

    3. _____

TYPES OF ASSESSMENT

1. Name three assessment types the nurse will perform when assessing a client in the hospital setting.

    1.

2.

3.

2. Read each client situation and decide which type of assessment will be used by the nurse. On the line provided place a C for comprehensive, O for ongoing, and R for rapid.

_____ 1. A 5-year-old boy comes to the clinic with his mother to obtain health clearance for kindergarten registration.

_____ 2. A 70-year-old has a 30 mmHg systolic BP drop in the postanesthesia room.

_____ 3. The night nurse begins shift rounds at 12:15 a.m. following shift report.

_____ 4. The LPN takes the BP of her client prior to giving an antihypertensive medication.

_____ 5. A 22-year-old female visits her healthcare provider to seek confirmation of pregnancy.

_____ 6. A 16-year-old cheerleader begins to wheeze during practice and reports to the school nurse.

_____ 7. The 29-year-old female returns to the postpartum unit following a cesarean section.

_____ 8. The CNA in the long-term care agency monitors the oral intake of five clients daily.

3. Nursing activities for the rapid assessment. Place the following activities in proper sequential order from 1 through 6.

_____ Observe for signs of distress

_____ Enter the room

_____ Wash your hands

_____ Note the location of the client

_____ Introduce yourself

_____ Ask the client his or her name

4. The nurse has entered the client's room and will complete a rapid assessment. Review the figures below and identify nursing actions and nursing observations. You should have at least 10 responses.

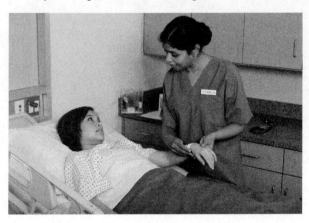 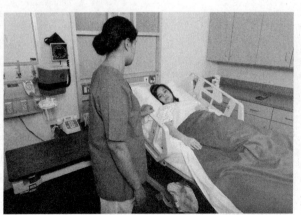

1.

2.

3.

4.

5.

6.

7.

8.

9.

10.

5. The primary nurse is discussing the nursing care of the client with the student nurse assigned to this client.

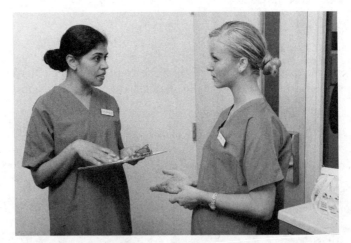

The nurse tells the student "the client has been medicated 3 hours and 45 minutes ago. She just told me she is having pain." The primary nurse instructs the student to complete a pain assessment and then they will initiate nursing interventions based on the assessment findings.

1. How will the student nurse conduct a pain assessment?

2. The assessment indicates incisional pain of 7 on a scale of 0 to 10. You, as the student, give the pain medication as ordered. What is required at this time?

EXPECTED FINDINGS FOR A RESPIRATORY ASSESSMENT ACROSS THE AGE SPAN

Answer the following questions regarding assessment of the respiratory status of a client.

1. Before entering the client's room to assess the respiratory status, you identify common factors to be assessed in all clients across the age span. Name seven common factors.

   1. _____

   2. _____

   3. _____

   4. _____

   5. _____

   6. _____

   7. _____

2. What are the expected findings of the respiratory rate per minute for the following age groups?

   Newborn _____   Young adult _____

   School-age child _____   Older adult _____

3. Identify five behaviors you anticipate finding when you assess the respiratory effort of the newborn.

   1.

   2.

   3.

   4.

   5.

4. Identify four behaviors you expect to find when performing a respiratory assessment on a child.

   1.

   2.

   3.

   4.

5. Four expected respiratory findings in an adult include:

    1.

    2.

    3.

    4.

APPLICATION OF THE CRITICAL THINKING PROCESS

Read the scenario and answer the following questions:

> You are taking report from the night nurse, and the CNA comes to you to report a client in room 3020A is having trouble breathing. Having received report, you know his name, age, medical diagnosis, and the surgical procedure performed on his left leg the day before. You immediately leave and go to the bedside of the client.

1. What type of assessment will you perform?

2. How will you confirm the identity of the client?

3. Identify five specific client behaviors that you will assess.

    1.

    2.

    3.

    4.

    5.

4. What additional information is needed? Provide a rationale.

NURSING ASSESSMENT

Review the figure below and list the nursing observation.

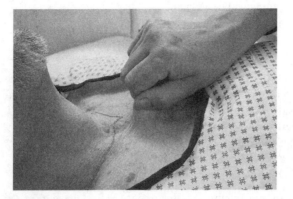

1. What is the nurse doing in this picture?

2. Is the technique correct?

3. If yes, proceed. If no, give the nurse direction to correct her technique.

4. What are the anticipated normal findings?

5. What other parts of the body could be used?

6. List variations in findings. Relate to client condition (e.g., tenting = dehydration, elevated temperature, aging population, etc.).

7. If the skin returns immediately, how will the nurse chart this?

NCLEX®-STYLE REVIEW QUESTIONS

Read each question carefully. Choose the best answer for each question.

1. A nurse receives report on a hospitalized client 6 hours after a major abdominal surgery. On initial assessment of the client, the nurse notices that the surgical dressing is covered in bright red blood. The nurse's initial action is to:
    1. inform the healthcare provider immediately.
    2. assess vital signs of the client.
    3. transfuse the client with 2 units of blood.
    4. call another nurse to confirm.

2. A hospitalized client complains of severe headaches and states that he experiences headaches only when the blood pressure is high. The appropriate response of the nurse caring for this client is:
    1. "Don't worry, your blood pressure was normal an hour ago."
    2. "I will give you medication for headache."
    3. "Let me check your blood pressure and see what it is."
    4. "Your headache is part of the disease process."

3. An elderly client's family member reports that the client is depressed after being admitted to the hospital and lost all motivation to live. The family also reports that the client was very active at home prior to hospital admission. The nurse's best action is to:
   1. tell the family that everything will be all right.
   2. contact the primary healthcare provider and report the situation.
   3. make the family understand that all clients get depressed during hospitalization.
   4. ask the client if the family's report is accurate.

4. A nurse administering medications to a client notices that the client has many visitors including children in the room. The client refuses to take the medications when the visitors are present and requests that the nurse leave the medication at the bedside. The nurse's best response is:
   1. "Sure, no problem! You know what you are doing."
   2. to document that the client refused medications.
   3. "I will bring the medications back when the visitors leave."
   4. "If you can take these children out of the room, I will leave the medications."

5. Nurses routinely assess all assigned clients and document the findings within a reasonable time of the beginning of the shift. The hospital policy states that all clients must be assessed at the beginning of each shift. A new nurse on the unit assesses one of the clients 2 hours after the beginning of the shift as the nurse was busy with another ill client. Which of the following actions of a new graduate nurse is not acceptable?
   1. Document for the beginning of the shift
   2. Document the time the assessment was done
   3. Report to the charge nurse
   4. Request for help at the beginning of the shift

Answer Key

Chapter 1
Health Assessment

Crossword Puzzle for Key Terms

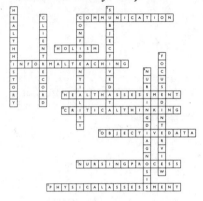

Across

4. Communication, 5. Holism,
7. Informal teaching, 9. Health assessment, 10. Critical thinking,
11. Objective data, 12. Nursing process, 13. Physical assessment.

Down

1. Health history, 2. Subjective data, 3. Client record,
4. Confidentiality, 6. Focused interview, 8. Nursing diagnosis.

Defining Health

1. One's perception of "health" is high individualized. There is no right or wrong answer here.
2. • Smoking puts a client at risk for many health issues
   • An acute illness, such as appendicitis, can be life threatening if it ruptures but is a temporary state
   • Diabetes is a chronic illness but may be controlled by diet, exercise, and medication allowing a client to lead an active and productive life
   • Prostate cancer can be a life-threatening illness, but if a client responds to treatment, he can lead an active and productive life
   • Depression is a psychological illness that can manifest some physiological responses; it may affect one's overall quality of life
   • Aging may or may not affect a client's ability to enjoy a quality life

Healthy People 2020
Subjective to learner's findings

Health Assessment
Health History

1. E		6. C
2. B		7. D
3. F		8. C
4. A		9. C
5. G		10. F

Data

1. O-PA		6. S-HH
2. S-HH		7. O-PA
3. O-PA		8. O-PA
4. O-PA		9. S-HH
5. S-HH		10. O-PA

Confidentiality
A check (✓) belongs next to 1, 3, 4, 5, 6, 9, 10

Documentation

1. Dx = Diagnosis
2. Hx = History
3. HIPAA = Health Insurance Portability and Accountability Act
4. NANDA = North American Nursing Diagnosis Association
5. BP = Blood Pressure
6. CBC = Complete Blood Count
7. ABD = Abdomen
8. LMP = Last Menstrual Period
9. CVA = Cerebral Vascular Accident
10. VS = Vital Signs
11. WBC = White Blood Cell
12. CNS = Central Nervous System
13. Ht = Height
14. ADL = Activities of Daily Living
15. Wt = Weight

Charting

1. **APIE**
   Assessment-
   Pt states weakness and a rapid heartbeat. "I was gardening all day in the church courtyard and never took a break to eat or drink"-cannot recall last void
   VS-BP-86/40, HR-119 bpm
   Mucous membranes are dry
   Problem-
   Dehydration
   Intervention-
   1 liter of intravenous fluids administered over 2 hours
   Evaluation-
   VS-BP-109/62, HR 88 bpm
   Able to void 475 ml clear amber urine

2. **SOAP**
   Subjective-
   Pt states weakness and a rapid heartbeat. "I was gardening all day in the church courtyard and never took a break to eat or drink"—cannot recall last void
   Objective-
   VS-BP-86/40, HR-119 bpm
   Mucous membranes are dry
   Assessment-
   Dehydration
   Plan-
   Administer 1 liter intravenous fluids over 2 hours and collect a urine sample

3. **Narrative Note**

The nursing narrative provided is incomplete because it lacks the following: data that supports dehydration, details about the type of intravenous fluids provided, specific data to support an improvement in vital signs.

The Nursing Process and Critical Thinking

1. *Assessment*—25-year-old female status post hysterectomy complaining of intermittent sharp pains in the lower abdomen scaled 8/10 on a numeric scale

   Diagnosis—Select a NANDA-approved nursing diagnosis related to pain

   Planning—The relief of pain/ Administer analgesics to relieve the pain

   Implementation—Administer morphine 4 mg subcutaneous injection

   Evaluation—The client's pain decreased to a 2/10 on a numeric scale

2. A. Normal findings: energetic, good appetite Abnormal findings: dry mouth and frequent headaches

   B. Dry mouth related to side effects of medication, headaches related to side effects of medication, knowledge deficit related to side effects of medication would all be appropriate for this scenario.

   C. Planning involves setting goals and priorities for the client. Outcomes should be determined and interventions should be selected that are necessary to meet each outcome. Implementation means the nurse puts the plan into action. The plan of care is carried out.

Critical Thinking

Essential Elements of Critical Thinking

1. Collection of information
2. Analysis of the situation
3. Generation of alternatives
4. Selection of alternatives
5. Evaluation

Application of the Critical Thinking Process

Answers are provided in shaded areas of scenario.

Role of the Professional Nurse in Health Assessment

1. D
2. E
3. C
4. E

5. A
6. C
7. A
8. B

Teaching Plans

Objectives

1. C
2. P
3. A
4. P

5. A
6. C
7. C
8. C

Teaching Methods

1. Lecture
2. Demonstration
3. Practice
4. Demonstration
5. Printed material
6. Group discussion
7. Demonstration
8. Explanation

Teaching Scenario

1. The client requires both short-and long-term goals. Short-term goals would be to restore respiratory function due to the exacerbation of asthma. Long-term goals should focus on smoking cessation.

2. Example Goal-The client will stop smoking within 2 months.

3. Example Objectives-The client will be able to list three benefits to stop smoking. The client will be able to discuss three methods to assist in smoking cessation. The client will be able to identify two benefits of a smoking cessation support group.

4. Subjective to learner's findings

5. A return demonstration is the best way to confirm that learning has taken place.

NCLEX®-Style Review Questions

1. 4
2. 1, 2
3. 2
4. 1
5. 1, 2, 3

6. 2
7. 3
8. 3
9. 3
10. 2

Chapter 2
Wellness and Health Promotion

Word Search

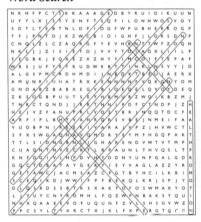

1. Wellness
2. Biology
3. Primary prevention
4. Aerobic exercise
5. Physical environment
6. Health promotion
7. Healthy people
8. Leading health indicators
9. Secondary prevention
10. Tertiary prevention

Wellness Theory

1. Dunn's Model of Wellness
2. 1-B, 2-C, 3-D, 4-A, 5-B, 6-C

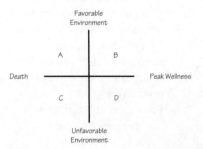

Levels of Prevention

1. 1-S, 2-P, 3-P, 4-T, 5-S,
   6-P, 7-T, 8-T, 9-P, 10-P,
   11-S, 12-T

2. Activities listed are subjective
   to learner but should meet
   the criteria for each level of
   prevention. Primary prevention
   focuses on prevention of illness
   or injury. Examples of primary
   prevention include education
   about diet, immunizations, and
   risk assessments. Secondary
   prevention focuses on early
   identification of illness
   and treatment for existing
   health problems. Examples
   of secondary prevention
   include screenings, diagnostic
   procedures, and treatments.
   Tertiary prevention focuses
   on returning the client to an
   optimum level of wellness after
   an illness or injury has occurred.
   Examples of tertiary prevention
   include rehabilitation services
   and education.

The Illness/Wellness Continuum

1. Subjective to learner's findings
2. Examples-exercise, stop
   smoking, decrease fat and
   sugar in diet, decrease caffeine,
   learn yoga

Health Promotion

1. Health promotion is defined
   in your textbook as behavior
   motivated by the desire
   to increase well-being
   and actualize human
   potential.

2. Client is obese, smokes, has
   hypertension, a diet high in fat
   that is not nutritious, and does
   not exercise.

3. Uncontrollable factors-Male,
   race (The client is not able to
   change his gender or race.)
   Controllable factors-Smoker,
   hypertension, physical
   inactivity, obesity (The client
   is able to stop smoking, make
   lifestyle modifications or use
   medications to control his
   hypertension, increase his

amount of physical activity,
and he is capable of decreasing
his weight. All factors are
modifiable.)

4.

Individual Characteristics and Experience	Behavior-Specific Cognitions and Affect	Behavioral Outcomes
Prior related behavior- no sports, sedentary activities (computer and video games)	**Perceived benefits of actions-** "not really sure how much better my life will be"	**Immediate competing demands and preferences-** long workdays and quick meals
Personal factors- male, African American, hypertension, family history, sedentary job	**Perceived barriers to action-** limited time, cooks for one, lack of consistent support from colleagues	**Commitment to plan of action-** avoids mother
	Perceived self-efficacy- can't do attitude, losing weight is really hard, it's genetic	**Health promoting behavior-** exercises, prepares healthy meals, quits smoking
	Activity-related affect- embarrassed to exercise in front of colleagues	
	Interpersonal influences- supportive mother, lack of consistent support from colleagues	
	Situational influences- free employee fitness center, responsible for selecting and purchasing own foods	

Healthy People 2020
Subjective to learner's
findings

Immunizations

1. Circle—Hib   X—MCV
2. Circle—PCV,   X—Zoster
   DTaP
3. Circle—MMR
4. Circle—   X—HPV
   Influenza
5. Circle—IPV,
   Hep B booster,
   HPV
6. Circle—   X—Varicella,
   Influenza   Zoster
7. Circle—   X—HPV,
   Pneumococcal   RV
8.   X—IPV,
                     Influenza
                     MMR

Application of the Critical Thinking Process

1. Exercise, abstinence and safe
   sex education, anti-bullying
   campaigns, anti-drinking and
   driving programs.

2. Education on breast, cervical,
   testicular cancer screening;
   dating violence screening; skin
   cancer screening.

3. Example: Reduce the rate
   of suicide attempts by
   adolescents.

4. The nurse may educate the
   faculty regarding suicidal
   behaviors and risk factors,
   coordinate assemblies to
   raise suicide awareness for
   the student body, provide the
   students with hotlines and
   resources that they can use if
   they are feeling suicidal.

5. The nurse must work with the school psychologist, counselors, faculty, parent-teacher organizations, and board of education.

6. Students may be embarrassed to admit to their weaknesses, programs cost money and school budgets are tight, and parents may believe that suicide programs may put ideas in their children's heads that were not there before.

NCLEX®-Style Review Questions

1. 2
2. 3
3. 1
4. 2
5. 4
6. 3
7. 4
8. 2
9. 2
10. 3

Chapter 3
Health Assessment Across the Life Span

Crossword Puzzle for Key Terms

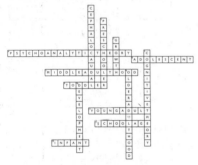

Across

4. Psychoanalytic theory,
6. Adolescent, 7. Middle adulthood, 9. Toddler,
11. Young adult, 12. School age, 13. Infant.

Down

1. Cephalocaudal, 2. Preschooler,
3. Growth, 5. Cognitive theory, 8. Older adulthood,
10. Development.

Stages of Development

1. T
2. O
3. M
4. Y
5. M
6. O
7. S
8. P
9. T
10. I
11. I
12. S
13. P
14. A
15. T
16. P
17. S
18. A
19. Y
20. M

Psychosocial Theory

1. Trust vs. Mistrust–No
2. Integrity vs. Despair–Yes– Losing interest in everyday life can be a sign of despair
3. Intimacy vs. Isolation–No
4. Generativity vs. Stagnation–No
5. Initiative vs. Guilt–No
6. Autonomy vs. Shame & Doubt–No
7. Identity vs. Role Confusion–No
8. Industry vs. Inferiority–Yes– He feels hopeless and is giving up

Assessment Findings

1. Normal
2. Normal
3. Abnormal
4. Abnormal
5. Normal
6. Normal
7. Normal
8. Normal
9. Abnormal
10. Abnormal

Application of the Critical Thinking Process

1. Integrity vs. despair
2. Questions related to Janie's plan for retirement, her feelings about leaving the workforce, and/or support systems would all be appropriate.
3. Integrity
4. This is a positive response because her planned post-retirement activities will help her maintain her self-worth and usefulness.
5. Lactose intolerance may lead to a decreased calcium intake, which is a risk factor for osteoporosis. Also, heart disease is the leading cause of death among women in this age group. Therefore, a cholesterol screening would be necessary.
6. Questions related to her plan of care for her father, support systems she may have when her sister is not available, and coping mechanisms/stress relief measures.
7. Example of a community resource would be meals on wheels. Meals on wheels is offered in many communities across the country offering one cold and one hot meal per day delivered to a client's home.

NCLEX®-Style Review Questions

1. 3
2. 1
3. 2
4. 3
5. 3
6. 3
7. 3
8. 1
9. 3
10. 1, 2, 3, 4

Chapter 4
Cultural Considerations

Crossword Puzzle for Key Terms

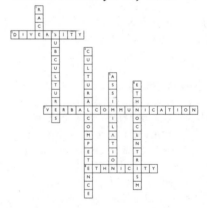

Across

2. Diversity, 7. Verbal communication, 8. Ethnicity.

Down

1. Race, 3. Subcultures,
4. Cultural competence,
5. Assimilation, 6. Ethnocentrism.

Beliefs and Values

1. A
2. D–Cuban Americans speak rapidly and loudly

3. A
4. D-Native Americans are not future oriented
5. A
6. A
7. D-Medicine men are used to diagnose and treat disharmony
8. A
9. D-European Americans are future oriented
10. A

Application of the Critical Thinking Process

Case Study–Nana Gay
Questions pertaining to communication patterns, temporal relations, dietary habits, family patterns, health beliefs, and health practices would all be appropriate.

Case Study–Bernice Grosenstein
1. The Jewish American culture predominately speaks English, although first generation immigrants may speak Yiddish. A translator for a complete understanding of the plan of care may be necessary. Kosher dietary rules include no pork, and no dairy and meat at the same meal. Packaged foods must be labeled kosher.
2. Appropriate meals for the client will include the buttered bagel and the pasta with tomato sauce. All the other meal choices mix dairy and meat.

Case Study–Rachell
1. Ethnocentric
2. The nurse cannot apply his personal values and beliefs to the client. The nurse must remain nonjudgmental.

Development of the Cultural Assessment Tool

Ethnicity—is defined by shared interest, ethnic heritage, religion, food, politics, or geography and nationality. Example Question: Where were you born?

Communication—is the verbal and nonverbal methods by which individuals and groups transmit information. Example Question: What languages do you speak?

Space—refers to the area that surrounds a person and the proximity of objects and people

that promote a level of comfort to the client. Example Question: Are you comfortable when others touch you during a conversation?

Social Organization—refers to structured groups. Example Question: How do you view your role in your family?

Time—the concept of the passage of time. Example Question: How do you view your health in the future?

Environmental Control—external influences on health. Example Question: What do you believe to be the cause of illness?

Biological Variations—internal influences on health. Example Question: Tell me about the health of your parents and grandparents.

Performing the Cultural Assessment

1. Nonverbal communication includes gestures, facial expressions, and mannerisms.
2. The use of nonverbal communication must be recognized by the nurse. For example, a lack of eye contact may be a respectful mannerism intended by the client, but the nurse may misinterpret this as disrespectful or lack of caring.
3. Subjective to the learner's findings

NCLEX®-Style Review Questions

1. 1
2. 2
3. 3
4. 2
5. 3
6. 4
7. 3
8. 3
9. 3
10. 2

Chapter 5
Psychosocial Assessment

Word Search

1. Psychosocial health
2. Psychosocial functioning
3. Stress
4. Self-concept
5. Role development

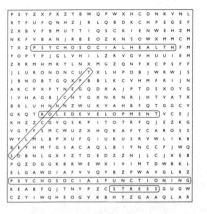

Factors That Influence Psychosocial Health

1. E
2. I
3. I
4. E
5. E
6. E
7. E
8. I
9. I
10. I
11. I
12. I
13. E
14. I

Interpretation of Assessment Findings

1. Abnormal-50 sexual partners at the age of 24 may be an indication of a mental health issue.
2. Abnormal-Unless this is a cultural finding (where it is considered disrespectful to make eye contact with a person) an active listener will make eye contact with the speaker in the American culture.
3. Abnormal-This is a sign of an eating disorder that requires further investigation.
4. Abnormal-This is a body image and self-esteem disturbance that requires further investigation.
5. Normal
6. Abnormal-This requires further investigation for mental health issues related to trust and isolation.
7. Abnormal-This requires further investigation because there are health risks associated with working excessive amounts of hours. Also, something may be going on in the home that decreases his desire to be there. Perhaps there are financial

reasons that may require community resources.

8. Abnormal-Adolescence is a time for sudden mood changes due to hormone fluctuation. However, anger and verbal abuse always requires further investigation as it may be a defense mechanism.

9. Normal

10. Abnormal-This requires further investigation because the client may be suffering from irrational fears, phobias, or anxiety.

Psychosocial Assessment Tools

Spiritual Assessment

Subjective to learner's findings

Suicide Assessment

1. Suicide risks for this client include:
   - Native American culture
   - Male
   - Loss of father
   - Loss of job
   - Loss of girlfriend
   - Family history of suicide
   - Expression of hopelessness
   - Verbalizing suicidal thoughts

2. The client should be asked if he has a plan to commit suicide. The nurse should ask the client to tell her about his plan. The nurse should also inquire if the client has the means to carry out the plan.

Stress Assessment

1. The Holmes Social Readjustment Scale for Madison would be scored as:
   Death of a spouse—100, Change in health of a family member—44, Gain of a new family member—39, Change in financial state—38, Foreclosure of mortgage—30, Trouble with in-laws—29, Spouse stops work-26, Change in living conditions-25, Change in recreation-19, Change in social activities-19, Change in sleeping habits-16, Christmas-12, Minor violations of the law-11

2. Physical signs of stress include:
   - Increased heart rate
   - Decreased blood clotting time
   - Increased rate and depth of respirations
   - Dilated pupils
   - Elevated glucose levels
   - Dilated skeletal blood vessels
   - Elevated blood pressure
   - Dilated bronchi
   - Increased blood volume
   - Contraction of the spleen
   - Increased blood supply to vital organs
   - Release of T lymphocytes

3. Questions related to stress should involve:
   - Signs and symptoms the client may be experiencing
   - Coping mechanisms presently used or used in the past to deal with stress
   - Support systems available to the client

4. Answers are subjective to learner's findings. Stress programs may also include activities such as exercise groups, yoga and meditation groups, support groups, etc.

The Psychosocial Assessment

Subjective to learner's findings

NCLEX®-Style Review Questions

1. 1	6. 1
2. 4	7. 1, 2
3. 1	8. 3
4. 4	9. 1
5. 3	10. 1

Chapter 6
Techniques and Equipment

Crossword Puzzle for Key Terms

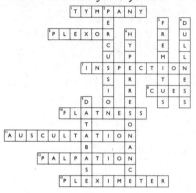

Across

1. Tympany, 5. Plexor,
7. Inspection, 8. Cues,
10. Flatness, 11. Auscultation,
12. Palpation, 13. Pleximeter.

Down

2. Percussion, 3. Fremitus,
4. Dullness, 6. Hyperresonance,
9. Database.

Assessment Techniques
Inspection

1. Inspection is the first technique used in physical assessment. However, it is used throughout.

2. True

3. Moves from general to specific

4. True

5. True

6. Requires critical thinking skills

7. True

8. Can be done independently

9. Novice nurses usually feel uncomfortable with inspection

10. True

Palpation

1. Light—Finger pads

2. Deep—Palmar surface of fingers

3. Light—Finger pads

4. Light—Dorsal surface

5. Light—Finger pads

6. Moderate—Base of fingers or ulnar surface

Percussion

Part I

1. D
2. R
3. D
4. T
5. H
6. T
7. H
8. F
9. R
10. D

Part II

1. A-Direct   B-Blunt
   C-Indirect

Part III

1. Direct
2. Indirect
3. Blunt
4. Indirect
5. Blunt
6. Direct
7. Direct
8. Indirect

Auscultation

Part 1

1. Correct
2. Incorrect-The shorter the stethoscope tubing the clearer the sound produced.
3. Incorrect-The diaphragm or bell should be placed between the index and middle fingers of the examiner.
4. Incorrect-The bell should be used to auscultate low-pitched sounds.
5. Incorrect-It is best to place the diaphragm or bell directly on the client's skin.
6. Incorrect-The bell may be used for any area that low-pitched sounds may be anticipated.
7. Incorrect-Coarse body hair may lead to misinterpretation of a sound.
8. Correct
9. Incorrect-Heavy pressure may impede blood flow.
10. Correct

Part II

The bell should be used for 7 and 8
The diaphragm may be used for 2, 4, 10, 11
1, 3, 5, 6, 9, and 12 do not require the use of the stethoscope to be detected.
Heart sounds may be auscultated with the diaphragm; however, a heart murmur, which may

produce low-pitched sounds, is best auscultated with light application of the bell.

Equipment

1. B
2. N
3. H
4. G
5. J
6. L
7. E
8. A
9. C
10. I
11. P
12. K
13. D
14. F
15. M
16. O

Application of the Critical Thinking Process

1. Examples of providing a safe and comfortable environment are:
   - Providing privacy
   - Warm room temperature
   - A functional examination gown
   - Privacy to change into the gown
   - A drape sheet
   - Sturdy examination table
   - Knock on the door before entering the room
   - Having all needed equipment readily available
   - Allowing the client to have a friend or family member present if requested
   - Instructions and explanations throughout the exam
   - Proceeding from more familiar, less invasive techniques
   - Exposing only the body part being examined
2. - Lack of eye contact
   - Dirty mismatched socks
   - One- to two-word responses
3. - Mistake-The nurse should begin the assessment with something less revealing and more familiar (e.g., vital signs). Anything that requires exposing skin that is normally covered should be saved until further into the examination.

- Mistake-The abdomen should be auscultated prior to percussion and palpation.
- Mistake-The percussion motion should come from the wrist.
- Mistake-The nurse should wash her hands before and after the examination.
- Mistake-Explaining to a client that there were some abnormal findings without giving specifics can be anxiety inducing. The nurse should be clear and informative without having the client worry unnecessarily.

NCLEX®-Style Review Questions

1. 3
2. 4
3. 3
4. 3
5. 1
6. 1
7. 1
8. 1, 2, 4
9. 4
10. 1

Chapter 7
General Survey

Word Search

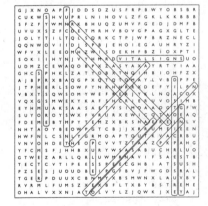

1. Hypothermia
2. Pain
3. Functional
4. Vital signs
5. General survey
6. Pulse
7. Diastolic pressure
8. Sphygmomanometer
9. Hyperthermia
10. Systolic pressure
11. Oxygen saturation

12. Pain rating scales
13. Temperature
14. Respiratory rate

Classification of Observations

1. B	9. MS
2. B	10. M
3. P	11. MS
4. N/A	12. M
5. B	13. P
6. M	14. B
7. B	15. MS
8. P	16. N/A

Routes for Measuring Temperature

1. Tympanic or Temporal
   A client who is short of breath cannot tolerate an oral thermometer. A rectal temperature would be too invasive for a baseline in this scenario. An axillary temperature may be done but is not the best choice because it is time consuming.
2. Tympanic
   It may be difficult to obtain an oral temperature on an injured child. A rectal temperature would be too invasive for a baseline in this scenario. A temporal temperature may be uncomfortable or not indicated depending on pain or bleeding after a head injury. An injured child may not have the patience to sit still for an axillary temperature; although it may be done, it is not the best choice.
3. Axillary
   The axillary route is recommended for newborns.
4. Rectal
   An unconscious, unresponsive client cannot tolerate an oral thermometer. A rectal temperature would be indicated because a client who is hot to touch may indicate he is septic.
5. Oral or Temporal
   A young adult who is awake and oriented can tolerate an oral thermometer. A rectal temperature is not indicated at this time. A tympanic would not be as accurate as an oral temperature.
6. Oral or Temporal
   A middle-aged adult who is awake and oriented can tolerate an oral thermometer. A rectal temperature is not indicated at this time. A tympanic would not be as accurate as an oral temperature.
7. Rectal
   A toddler who has suffered a febrile seizure would require the most accurate core temperature.
8. Tympanic or Temporal
   The tympanic or temporal route would be the quickest route to obtain in this scenario. The client is not complaining of a fever-related illness so a rectal temperature would be too invasive at this time. An oral temperature would be acceptable but does take longer.

Pulse Locations

1. Pulse Locations
   1. Temporal
   2. Femoral
   3. Posterior tibial
   4. Popliteal
   5. Radial
   6. Brachial
   7. Carotid
   8. Dorsalis pedis
2. If the nurse is unable to palpate the pulse, she must first assess for other signs of adequate circulation to the extremity (pink color, warmth, capillary refill, absence of pain, numbness or tingling, mobility). Next, the nurse may use the Doppler in order to use ultrasound waves to auscultate the presence of the pulse. If there is no pulse present, the doctor should be notified immediately.

Respirations

1. False-One respiration includes an inspiration followed by an expiration
2. True-30–80 respirations per minute
3. False-The nurse should count a respiratory rate for one full minute if irregularities are detected.
4. True-the client may change his pattern
5. True-20–30 respirations per minute
6. True-some medications may increase or decrease the rate
7. True-a full respiratory cycle contains one inspiration and one expiration
8. False-A respiratory rate of 8 is an abnormal finding in any client

Blood Pressure

5, 1, 14, 10, 7, 3, 2, 13, 8, 15, 4, 11, 6, 9, 12

Factors That Influence Vital Signs

1. Higher		8. Lower
2. Higher		9. Higher
3. Lower		10. Higher
4. Higher		11. Higher
5. Higher		12. Lower
6. Lower		13. Higher
7. Higher		14. Higher

Performance of the General Survey and Measurement of Vital Signs

Example:

Client Initials: __HH__	DOB: 3/15/78	Gender: __F__	Today's Date: _____

General Survey:

Physical Appearance: well-nourished, well-proportioned, smiling young female. Clean, well groomed, and dressed appropriately

Mental Status: Awake, alert, and oriented to person, place, and time

Mobility: Steady, rhythmic gait with erect posture

Behavior of Client: calm, cooperative, and pleasant

Height: __5'8"__   Weight: __167 lb__

Vital Signs: BP 113/76   HR __88__   RR __14__   Temp 98.4 (oral)   O₂ Saturation 98% on RA

Application of the Critical Thinking Process

1. The 56-year-old male who is unresponsive with agonal breathing is having life-threatening, time-sensitive oxygenation issues. This person must be seen immediately.

2. The 66-year-old male grabbing at his chest and moaning in pain. These observed behaviors suggest a myocardial infarction. The vomit observed on his clothing is supportive of myocardial infarction as well. His obesity is a risk factor for a myocardial infarction.

3. The 75-year-old male who is sitting in the wheelchair. Although he does not appear to be in any distress, his skin color is pale and his vital signs show elevations. This client could be having internal bleeding and could rapidly decompensate.

4. The 26-year-old female with the fever appears to be stable and experiencing no difficulties with oxygenation or circulation.

5. The 15-year-old female has stable vital signs and an apparent injury that will not lead to an immediate loss of limb.

1. Observations made regarding the general survey
   - Client is a young female
   - Client is guarding her abdomen
   - Client is rocking back and forth
   - Client is dressed inappropriately
   - Cigarette smoke odor
   - Client replies with short answers
   - Facial grimaces

2.

Normal	Abnormal
BP 116/72 RR 18 O$_2$ Sat 99% on RA	Guarding Abd States Abd Pain Facial Grimaces
	Temperature 101.2°F Pulse 122 bpm

3. OLDCART-Onset, Location, Duration, Characteristics, Aggravating Factors, Relieving Factors, Treatment

ICE-Impact on activities of daily living, Coping strategies, Emotional response

4. O-Last night
   L-Right lower quadrant
   D-Constant
   C-Stabbing pain
   A-Movement
   R-Nothing
   T-Tylenol and meditation
   I-She is not able to practice or perform in her theatre group
   C-Meditation
   E-Scared and anxious

5. Data collected are complete using the OLDCART acronym.

6. The data collected support the observations in the general survey that suggest the client is in pain (guarded abdomen, rocking, and facial grimaces).

NCLEX®-Style Review Questions

1. 1
2. 3
3. 3
4. 3
5. 1   10. 2
6. 3
7. 1, 2, 3, 4, 5
8. 1
9. 3

Chapter 8
Pain Assessment

Crossword Puzzle for Key Terms

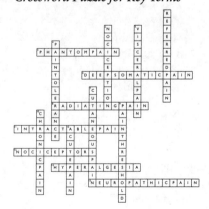

Across
5. Phantom pain, 6. Deep somatic pain, 8. Radiating pain, 11. Intractable pain, 13. Nociceptors, 14. Hyperalgesia, 15. Neuropathic pain.

Down
1. Referred pain, 2. Nociception, 3. Visceral pain, 4. Pain tolerance, 7. Cutaneous pain, 9. Pain threshold, 10. Chronic pain, 12. Acute pain.

Acute Versus Chronic

1. Acute = B, C, E, G
   Chronic = A, D, F, H

2. 1. A   7. C
   2. C   8. A
   3. C   9. A
   4. A   10. C
   5. A   11. A
   6. A   12. A

Categories of Pain

1. Deep somatic pain
2. Cutaneous pain
3. Visceral pain
4. Neuropathic pain
5. Phantom pain
6. Referred pain

Pain Assessment Tools

1. 1. Drawing/illustration should reflect the following description: The Numeric Rating Scale asks the client to describe pain intensity with a number. The selected number then equates to pain severity.

   2. Drawing/illustration should reflect the following description: The Simple Verbal Descriptive Scale is another unidimensional tool. The individual is presented with six descriptive words and is asked to select one that corresponds to the present level of intensity.

   3. Drawing/illustration should reflect the following description: The Oucher Scale has been designed for children. Pictures of faces ranging from neutral to distressed are presented, and the child selects the one representing his or her level of pain.

2. 1. The Oucher Scale because children can relate to visual facial expressions.
   2. The Simple Verbal Descriptive Scale uses simple words to assess the client's pain level. The nurse may ask the client to determine if she is having mild, moderate, or severe pain.

3. a. Websites may vary.
   b. F = face, L = legs, A = activity, C = cry, C = consolability
   c. Each category of the FLACC scale has characteristics that are scored from 0–2. The lower the score, the less pain the client is experiencing and the higher the score, the more pain.

4. Subjective to learner's findings

Application of the Critical Thinking Process

1. Although the numerical scale indicates that Mrs. Wong is complaining of less pain than Mr. Pineapple, the nurse cannot truly determine who is in more pain.

2. Every individual has a different pain threshold and pain tolerance, so even if the stressor is the same, the reaction will be different.

Factors Influencing Pain Assessment

1. The pain that Ms. Lemon is experiencing from her cancer is chronic pain. It has lasted for months. The pain that Ms. Lemon experienced when she had her partial gastrectomy was acute pain. It was temporary.

2. 1. Can you describe your pain?
   2. When did the pain start?
   3. What makes the pain better?
   4. What makes the pain worse?

3. A goal for Ms. Lemon can be related to decreasing her pain or educating her about her medications.

4. An objective related to educating Ms. Lemon about her pain medication might be that at the end of the teaching learning session Ms. Lemon will be able discuss the rationale for using a pain patch and pain pills.

5. The nurse may ask Ms. Lemon questions to evaluate learning.

NCLEX®-Style Review Questions

1. 1
2. 3
3. 1, 2, 3, 4, 5
4. 2
5. 3
6. 4
7. 2
8. 2
9. 1, 2, 3
10. 3

Chapter 9
Nutritional Assessment
Word Search

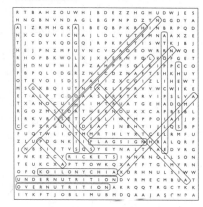

1. Malnutrition
2. Atrophic papillae
3. Rickets
4. Cheilosis
5. Diet recall
6. Xerophthalmia
7. Flag sign
8. Glossitis
9. Koilonychias
10. Nutritional health
11. Anthropometrics
12. Overnutrition
13. Pica
14. Somatic protein
15. Angular stomatitis
16. Undernutrition
17. Xanthelasma

The Nutritional History
Sample provided in exercise.

Body Mass Index
1. OW
2. OB
3. H
4. H
5. U
6. OW
7. H
8. OB
9. OW
10. U

Assessment Findings
1. A-Vitamin C deficiency
2. A-Iodine deficiency
3. A-Iron deficiency
4. N
5. A-Protein deficiency
6. N
7. A-Protein deficiency
8. A-Vitamin D deficiency
9. N
10. A-Vitamin B and iron deficiencies

Mini Cultural Case Studies

1. In traditional Chinese culture that follows yin and yang as opposing energy forces, cold illnesses should be treated with hot foods (garlic, onion, red pepper, grilled meats, spices such as chili and cayenne pepper, and many other foods). Hot illnesses should be treated with cold foods (clams, crabs, melons, berries, fresh vegetables, and many other foods).

2. During Passover, foods that have been leavened should be avoided.

3. The hospital should have unleavened foods available such as matzoh. Also, kosher packaged meals should be made available. Other kosher restrictions discourage dairy and meat to be included in the same meal.

4. Foods that are fried and high in sodium (such as chicken fried steak, fried peach pie, and ham hocks) put a client at risk for hypertension. Fried foods are high in saturated fats that increase the LDL cholesterol in one's system leading to clogged blood vessels. Sodium causes an increase in water retention, and therefore increases circulating

volume leading to more strain on the vessels and organs.

5. Goal: Jessie will learn how to control his hypertension through diet. Objectives: By the end of the teaching session Jessie will be able to define hypertension, explain the relationship between diet and hypertension, list foods that should be avoided, and discuss alternative food preparation methods.

My Food Pyramid
Subjective to learner's findings

Lab Assignment
Subjective to learner's findings

NCLEX®-Style Review Questions

1. 4
2. 2
3. 1
4. 3
5. 2
6. 4
7. 2
8. 1, 2, 3, 4, 5
9. 1
10. 1, 2, 3, 5

Chapter 10
The Health History

Crossword Puzzle for Key Terms

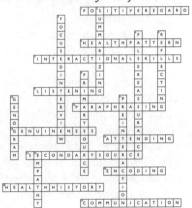

Across
1. Positive regard, 6. Health pattern, 7. Interactional skills, 9. Listening, 12. Paraphrasing, 13. Genuineness, 14. Attending, 15. Secondary source, 17. Encoding, 18. Health history, 19. Communication.

Down
2. Summarizing, 3. Focused interview, 4. False reassurance, 5. Reflecting, 8. Primary source, 10. Genogram, 11. Preinteraction, 16. Empathy.

Using Communication Skills
Subjective to learner's findings

1. **Attending**—Giving the client undivided attention.
   Ex. *Facing the client and being alert and focused.*
2. **Paraphrasing**—Restating the client's basic message to test whether it was understood.
   Ex. Statement *"I really loved visiting my grandmother when I was little. She would play games with me, bake cookies, and sing songs. They were the best times."* Response *"It sounds like you really enjoyed spending time with your grandmother."*
3. **Direct Leading**—Directing the client to obtain specific information or to begin an interaction.
   Ex. *"Let's discuss your summer vacations spent with your grandmother."*
4. **Focusing**—Helping the client zero in on a subject or get in touch with feelings.
   Ex. *"Describe how you felt when you would leave your grandmother at the end of each summer."*
5. **Questioning**—Gathering specific information on a topic through the process of inquiry.
   Ex. *"What did you mean when you said you would have been better off if your grandmother was your real mother?"*
6. **Reflecting**—Letting the client know that the nurse empathizes with the thoughts, feelings, or experiences expressed.
   Ex. *"It sounds like you really miss spending time with your grandmother."*
7. **Summarizing**—Tying together the various messages that the client has communicated throughout the interview.
   Ex. *"Your summer vacations with your grandmother helped to develop you into the person you are today."*

Barriers to Communication
1. Nontherapeutic (false reassurance)
2. Nontherapeutic (technical terms)
3. Therapeutic
4. Nontherapeutic (passing judgment)
5. Nontherapeutic (changing the subject)
6. Therapeutic
7. Nontherapeutic (cross examination)
8. Therapeutic

Components of the Health History (example questions)
1. **Biographical Data:**
   A. *What is your name?*
   B. *What is your occupation?*
2. **Present Health or Illness:**
   A. *Why are you seeking help today?*
   B. *What is bothering you today?*
3. **Past History:**
   A. *Are you allergic to any medications?*
   B. *Describe any surgery you have had in the past.*
4. **Family History:**
   A. *Is there any history of heart disease in your family?*
   B. *How many siblings do you have?*
5. **Psychosocial History:**
   A. *What is the highest level of education you have achieved?*
   B. *What is your role in the family?*
6. **Review of Body Systems**
   Skin:
   A. *How do you care for your skin?*
   B. *Do you use sunscreen?*
   Hair:
   A. *How often do you wash your hair?*
   B. *Do you use any products to change the color of your hair?*
   Nails:
   A. *How do you care for your nails?*
   B. *Do you bite your nails?*
   Head:
   A. *Have you ever had a head injury?*
   B. *Do you wear a helmet when biking?*

Neck:

A. *Do you have any limitations in turning your neck?*

B. *Do you have any pain in your neck?*

Lymphatics:

A. *Have you noticed any lumps on your head or neck?*

B. *Do you have any pain in your head or neck?*

Eyes:

A. *Do you wear eyeglasses?*

B. *When was your last eye exam?*

Ears:

A. *Do you wear a hearing aid?*

B. *Do you have any difficulty swallowing?*

Nose:

A. *Do you frequently experience bloody noses?*

B. *Are you able to differentiate various odors?*

Mouth and Throat:

A. *How often do you visit the dentist?*

B. *Do you have any difficulty swallowing?*

Respiratory:

A. *Do you have a cough?*

B. *Do you use supplemental oxygen at home?*

Breasts and Axillae:

A. *Do you perform breast self-exam?*

B. *Do you use deodorant or antiperspirant?*

Cardiovascular:

A. *Have you ever experienced palpitations?*

B. *Do you exercise?*

Peripheral Vascular:

A. *Do you have varicose veins?*

B. *Have you ever experienced swelling in your legs?*

Abdomen:

A. *When was your last bowel movement?*

B. *How is your appetite?*

Urinary:

A. *How often do you urinate?*

B. *Do you wake during the night to urinate?*

Male Reproductive:

A. *Do you perform testicular self-exam?*

B. *Are you able to sustain an erection?*

Female Reproductive:

A. *When was your last period?*

B. *How many times has your body been pregnant?*

Musculoskeletal:

A. *Can you move all of your joints fully?*

B. *Do you walk with any assistive devices?*

Neurologic:

A. *Have you fallen recently?*

B. *Is your right or left hand more dominant?*

Genograms

1. HG
2. 7
3. 3
4. 2
5. 1
6. Breast cancer
7. This genogram reveals a risk for breast cancer to HG. It would be important to educate HG on breast self-exam, annual physical exams, and mammography.

Health History: True or False

1. False
   OTC medication should be included in the medication history.
2. True
3. True
4. False
   Collecting information about a client's health insurance is part of the health history.
5. True
   Birthplace can also be part of the biographical data.
6. False
   Asking a client about financial status is appropriate and necessary to plan care for the client.
7. True
8. False
   It is better to obtain a sexual history at the end of an interview when trust has been established.
9. True
10. False

The client's own words may be used when documenting in the health history.

Application of the Critical Thinking Process

1.
   - Conducting the interview in a private comfortable setting
   - Explaining the admission process to the client and mother
   - Begin with general, less intrusive questions first
   - Utilize a variety of interactional skills during the interview
   - Display empathy and genuineness during the interview
2.
   1. Primary from the client
   2. Secondary from the mother and/or any medical records provided
3.
   - Providing tissues
   - Allowing for extra time (do not rush)
   - Offering a break from the process if they seem overwhelmed
   - Making sure the client and his mother understand the process
4. Subjective to learner's findings. Ethnicity and culture may influence a client's health status, communication patterns, and social interaction. It is important for the nurse to consider these influences when developing an individualized plan of care for a client.
5. Offer the client and his mother a break from the interview and a place they can relax to have lunch. State a time that the interview will be resumed.

Obtaining Data

1. Present health or illness
2. The nurse must explore Mr. Johnson's patterns for taking his blood pressure medication. The more details that can be obtained during the health history, the more individualized a plan of care or a teaching plan may be.

3.

Medication	Dose	Frequency	Duration	Purpose	Effect
Client cannot recall name of blood pressure pill	Client cannot recall dose of blood pressure pill	Prescribed for daily but client takes it as needed 2–3 times per week	No data collected	Reduce blood pressure	Monthly blood pressure readings about 150 over 80

4. When did the doctor prescribe this medication for you? How long have you been taking this medication?

Health History Documentation
Subjective to learner's findings

NCLEX®-Style Review Questions

1.	3	6.	4
2.	1	7.	4
3.	2	8.	1
4.	3	9.	2
5.	2	10.	1, 3, 4

Chapter 11
Skin, Hair, and Nails

Crossword Puzzle for Key Terms

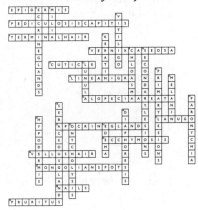

Across

1. Epidermis, 5. Pediculosis capitis, 6. Terminal hair, 8. Vernix caseosa, 11. Cuticle, 14. Linea nigra, 16. Alopecia areata, 21. Lanugo, 22. Apocrine glands, 25. Ecchymosis, 26. Vellus hair, 27. Mongolian spots, 28. Nails, 29. Pruritus.

Down

2. Eccrine glands, 3. Milia, 4. Vitiligo, 7. Keratin,

9. Chloasma, 10. Secondary lesions, 12. Lunula, 13. Primary lesions, 15. Melanin, 17. Paronychia, 18. Sebaceous glands, 19. Diaphoresis, 20. Hypodermis, 23. Onycholysis, 24. Edema.

Anatomy & Physiology Review

1. 1. Hair shaft
   2. Pore
   3. Epidermis
   4. Dermis
   5. Subcutaneous tissue
   6. Nerve
   7. Artery
   8. Vein
   9. Hair root
   10. Hair follicle
   11. Eccrine sweat gland
   12. Root hair plexus
   13. Oil gland
   14. Arrector pili muscle
2. 1. Cuticle
   2. Lunula
   3. Lateral nail fold
   4. Body of nail
   5. Nail matrix
   6. Root of nail
   7. Posterior nail fold
   8. Cuticle
   9. Body of nail
   10. Nail bed
   11. Free edge of nail
   12. Bone of fingertip
3. Skin-1, 3, 4, 9
   Cutaneous glands-2, 6, 8
   Neither-5, 7, 10

Equipment Selection
Examination gown
Gloves
Magnifying glass
Penlight
Ruler
Wood's lamp

Assessment Techniques

1. When examining a client's skin, it is best to have the client remove all clothing except the examination gown and be in a sitting position.
2. Correct
3. It is best to determine a client's skin temperature using the dorsal surface of the hand.
4. Correct
5. Skin turgor can be assessed by using the forefinger and thumb to grasp the skin inferior to the clavicle or on the medial aspect of the wrist.
6. The assessment technique used to grade edema on a 4-point scale is palpation.
7. Correct
8. Correct
9. Capillary refill can be assessed by depressing the nail edge briefly to blanch and then quickly releasing.
10. The Schamroth technique is used to assess shape and contour of the nails.

Assessment Findings

1.	A	11.	A
2.	N	12.	A
3.	A	13.	A
4.	N	14.	N
5.	N	15.	A
6.	N	16.	A
7.	N	17.	A
8.	N	18.	N
9.	A	19.	A
10.	A	20.	N

Factors That Influence Physical Assessment Findings

1. African American
2. Asian
3. Lips, oral mucosa, palms of hands, soles of feet

4. Vellus
5. Decrease
6. Pregnant
7. Acne
8. Temperature
9. Henna
10. Nail biting or hair plucking

Abnormal Findings
1. Pustule (elevated and pus filled) acne, impetigo, carbuncles
2. Macule (flat, non-palpable, <1 cm) freckle, measle
3. Wheal (elevated, reddish) hives, insect bites
4. Scales (flakes, light color) dandruff, psoriasis, eczema
5. Vesicle (elevated, fluid filled, <0.5 cm) chickenpox, herpes
6. Crust (dry fluid) eczema, scabs, impetigo
7. Ulcer (deep, irregular shape) pressure sores, chancres
8. Fissure (linear, crack, sharp edges) athlete's foot

Application of the Critical Thinking Process
Scenario A
1. A. "Dry skin" patch noted 6 months ago
   B. Works in direct sunlight without sunscreen
2. A. 5 mm × 2 mm lesion
   B. Rounded, pearly edges with central mild ulceration
3. A. No sunscreen
   B. Works in direct sunlight
4. Basal cell carcinoma
5. Onset-6 months, Location-Posterior neck, Duration-6 months
   Characteristics-Stinging sensation
   Questions-Aggravating Factors–What makes the stinging sensation feel better?
   Relieving factors–What makes the stinging sensation feel worse?
   Treatment–Have you used any kind of treatment for the stinging?
   Due to the fact the lesion was an incidental finding during a lung assessment, the client may not be able

to provide answers to the ICE assessment at this time. Impacted on activities of daily living, coping mechanisms, and emotional response
6. Asymmetry, Borders, Color, Diameter, Elevation
7. Teach the use of sunscreen and protective clothing. Teach sun avoidance between the hours of 10:00 am and 2:00 pm. Explain the risk associated with sun exposure.

Scenario B
1. Subjective: itch
   Objective: tiny white nits
2. No, head lice is contagious
3. How to check for head lice (parents and teachers)
   How to treat head lice (parents)
   What are head lice (Child)
4. An outbreak of head lice will be prevented in the school.
5. A. The faculty will recognize students who have suspected head lice.
   B. The parents will identify measures to treat head lice.
6. There will be fewer than five more cases of head lice in the school in the next month.

Assessment and Documentation
Subjective to learner's findings

NCLEX®-Style Review Questions
1. 1, 2, 3, 4
2. 1, 2, 3
3. 3
4. 3
5. 2
6. 2
7. 1, 3, 4
8. 4
9. 4
10. 1

Chapter 12
Head, Neck, and Related Lymphatics

Word Search

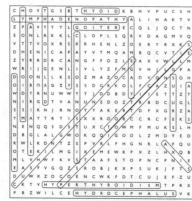

1. Acromegaly
2. Anterior triangle
3. Atlas
4. Axis
5. Bell's palsy
6. Craniosynostosis
7. Cushing's syndrome
8. Down syndrome
9. Goiter
10. Hydrocephalus
11. Hyoid
12. Hyperthyroidism
13. Hypothyroidism
14. Lymphadenopathy
15. Posterior triangle
16. Sutures
17. Thyroid gland
18. Torticollis

Anatomy & Physiology Review
1. **Bones of the Head**
   1. C_3
   2. C_2
   3. C_1
   4. Mastoid process
   5. External acoustic meatus
   6. Temporomandibular joint
   7. Occipital bone
   8. Lambdoid suture
   9. Temporal bone
   10. Parietal bone
   11. Sagittal suture
   12. Coronal suture
   13. Frontal suture
   14. Sphenoid bone
   15. Zygomatic bone
   16. Lacrimal bone
   17. Nasal bone
   18. Nasal septum
   19. Maxilla
   20. Mandible

Structures of the Neck
1. Trachea
2. Isthmus of thyroid
3. Cricoid cartilage
4. Sternocleidomastoid muscle
5. Hyoid bone
6. Thyroid cartilage
7. Thyroid gland
8. Clavicle
9. Manubrium

Lymph Nodes of the Head and Neck
1. Supraclavicular
2. Posterior cervical
3. Superficial cervical
4. Retropharyngeal

5. Occipital
6. Posterior auricular
7. Preauricular
8. Submandibular
9. Submental
10. Deep cervical chain
2. 1. Mandible
   2. Midline of the neck
   3. Anterior aspect of the sternocleidomastoid muscle
3. 1. Trapezius
   2. Sternocleidomastoid muscle
   3. Clavicle

Equipment Selection
Examination gown
Gloves
Stethoscope
Water in cup

Assessment Techniques
1. Incorrect-It is best to have the client sitting upright and the client may be clothed.
2. Correct
3. Correct
4. Incorrect-the temporal artery is palpated between the eye and the top of the ear.
5. Correct
6. Incorrect-The thyroid can be auscultated for bruits.
7. Incorrect-Lymph nodes are palpated by exerting gentle pressure in a circular motion.
8. Incorrect-The best order to examine lymph nodes of the head and neck would be to start from the preauricular and working your way down to the supraclavicular.
9. Correct
10. Incorrect-The trachea is not percussed.

Assessment Findings
1. N
2. N
3. A
4. A
5. A
6. N
7. A
8. A
9. A
10. N
11. A
12. N
13. A
14. A
15. A
16. N
17. A
18. A
19. N
20. A

Factors That Influence Physical Assessment Findings
1. Iodine
2. Four
3. Chin
4. Fetal Alcohol Syndrome
5. Triangular
6. Older
7. Head/neck
8. Enlarge
9. Hair/face
10. Rigidity

Application of the Critical Thinking Process
1. 1. Sweaty and anxious
   2. "I haven't been sleeping well"
   3. "Stomach hasn't been right"
   4. Frequent episodes of diarrhea
   5. 12-lb weight loss in past month
2. Questions should be asked pertaining to
   1. A general medical–surgical history
   2. Medication regime
   3. Allergies
   4. Focused questions related to cardiac (due to heart rate), GI (due to upset stomach, diarrhea, and weight loss), neurologic (due to tremors)
   5. pain
3. Exophthalmus-abnormal protrusion of the eyeball
4. A hyperthyroid may be responsible for Ronnie's signs and symptoms.
5. A hyperthyroid may affect a variety of systems. Signs and symptoms may include (but are not limited to) weight loss, increased appetite, heat intolerance, hair loss, muscle aches, weakness, fatigue, hyperactivity, irritability, polyuria, polydipsia, tremors, pretibial myxedema, sweating, and palpitations. Any questions that will further investigate Ronnie experiencing any additional symptoms will be appropriate.
6. The nurse has not assessed if Ronnie has experienced any pain.
7. Pain may be intermittent, so the nurse should explore any recent pain Ronnie has experienced. The nurse should use the OLDCART & ICE assessment to further investigate.

Healthy People 2020
Subjective to learner's findings

Assessment and Documentation
Subjective to learner's findings

NCLEX®-Style Review Questions
1. 3
2. 1
3. 4
4. 1
5. 1
6. 4
7. 2
8. 4
9. 1
10. 4

Chapter 13
Eye

Crossword Puzzle for Key Terms

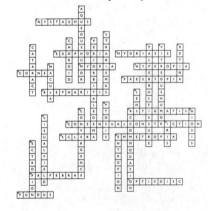

Across
2. Nystagmus, 10. Exophoria, 11. Mydriasis, 13. Myopia, 14. Hyperopia, 15. Cornea, 16. Presbyopia, 17. Blepharitis, 21. Astigmatism, 24. Consensual constriction, 26. Sclera, 27. Emmetropia, 30. Palpebrae, 31. Optic disc, 32. Fundus.

Down
1. Aqueous humor, 3. Strabismus, 4. Choroid, 5. Periorbital edema, 6. Cataract, 7. Palpebral fissure, 8. Vitreous humor, 9. Retina, 12. Macula, 18. Lens, 19. Ptosis, 20. Convergence,

21. Accommodation, 22. Miosis,
23. Visual field, 25. Iris,
27. Entropion, 28. Ectropion.

Anatomy & Physiology Review
1. **Structures of the external eye**
   1. Eyelashes
   2. Iris
   3. Medial canthus
   4. Caruncle
   5. Eyelid
   6. Eyebrow
   7. Pupil
   8. Sclera
   9. Lateral canthus
   10. Palpebral fissure
   11. Eyelid
   Structures of the internal eye
   1. Canal of Schlemm
      (sclera venous sinus)
   2. Anterior chamber
   3. Cornea
   4. Pupil
   5. Iris
   6. Lens
   7. Suspensory ligament
   8. Ciliary body
   9. Vitreous humor
   10. Optic nerve
   11. Optic disc
   12. Fovea centralis
   13. Macula Lutea
   14. Retina
   15. Choroid
   16. Sclera
   Extraocular muscles
   1. Optic nerve
   2. Inferior rectus
      muscle
   3. Inferior oblique
      muscle
   4. Superior oblique muscle
   5. Superior oblique tendon
   6. Superior rectus muscle
   7. Lateral rectus muscle
   8. Conjunctiva
2. 1. True
   2. False-The crystalline
      lens is not responsible
      for the refraction of
      light rays.
   3. False-When refraction
      occurs, the rays are
      reflected to the retina
      for the most accurate
      vision.
   4. True

5. False-The anterior and
   posterior segments of the
   eye are separated by the lens.
6. False-A retinal image
   is conducted to the optic
   nerve.
7. True
8. False-Impulses are transmitted to the occipital
   lobe of the brain for
   interpretation.
3. 1. Cranial Nerve III
   2. Cranial Nerve VI
   3. Cranial Nerve III
   4. Cranial Nerve III
   5. Cranial Nerve III
   6. Cranial Nerve IV

Equipment Selection
Acuity chart
Eye cover
Gloves
Penlight
Cotton-tipped applicator
Ophthalmoscope

Assessment Techniques
1. Incorrect-the client should
   be 14 inches from the
   chart
2. Incorrect-test first with
   eyeglasses or contacts
   and then without
3. Correct
4. Incorrect-the client should
   stare straight ahead
5. Incorrect-the client should
   be 2–3 ft away from the nurse
6. Correct
7. Correct
8. Correct
9. Incorrect-the nurse should
   hold the ophthalmoscope in
   the right hand
10. Correct

Assessment Findings

1.	A	11.	A
2.	A	12.	N
3.	N	13.	A
4.	N	14.	A
5.	N	15.	A
6.	N	16.	N
7.	N	17.	N
8.	N	18.	N
9.	A	19.	N
10.	N	20.	N

*Factors That Influence Physical
Assessment Findings*
1. Slate-blue
2. Dry eyes
3. 8
4. fat
5. A
6. cataracts
7. Safety goggles/glasses
8. Highest
9. Blindness
10. Epicanthic folds

*Application of the Critical
Thinking Process*
1. Eye redness (hyperemia),
   swollen and red eyelids
   and conjunctiva, tearing,
   sensation that foreign body is
   in the eye, itching, burning,
   photophobia, eye pain,
   frequent blinking
2. A Snellen chart should be
   used to test Jordan's visual
   acuity if she can identify
   the letters of the alphabet.
   The Snellen E chart may also
   be used.
3. The Oucher Scale, the
   Wong-Baker Faces scale,
   or the Simple Verbal
   Descriptive Scale may be
   appropriate.
4. The teaching/learning
   topic of hand hygiene
   would be appropriate for
   the kindergarten class
   because conjunctivitis can
   be caused by a viral or
   bacterial infection; both can
   be prevented by good hand
   washing.

Healthy People 2020
1. 1. Construction workers
   2. Welders
   3. Occupations that work
      with chemicals, such as
      chemists, oncologists,
      manufacturers of or those
      handling chemicals.
2. Subjective to learner's
   findings

*Physical Assessment
With Documentation*
Subjective to learner's findings

NCLEX®-Style Review Questions

1. 1
2. 1, 2, 3
3. 3
4. 1, 2, 4
5. 4
6. 2
7. 3
8. 2
9. 1
10. 3

Chapter 14
Ears, Nose, Mouth, and Throat

Word Search

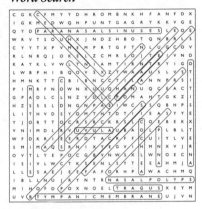

1. Air conduction
2. Auricle
3. Bone conduction
4. Cerumen
5. Cochlea
6. Cold sores
7. Eustachian tube
8. Fever blisters
9. Helix
10. Lobule
11. Mastoiditis
12. Nasal polyps
13. Ossicles
14. Otitis externa
15. Palate
16. Paranasal sinuses
17. Pinna
18. Presbycusis
19. Tragus
20. Tympanic membrane
21. Uvula

Anatomy & Physiology Review

1. External Ear
1. Mastoid process
2. Antihelix
3. Helix
4. External auditory meatus
5. Tragus
6. Lobus

The Three Parts of the Ear
1. Auricle
2. Malleus
3. Incus
4. Vestibule
5. Semicircular canals
6. Cranial nerve VIII
7. Cochlea
8. Round window
9. Eustachian tube
10. Stapes
11. Tympanic membrane
12. External auditory canal

Internal Structures of the Nose
1. Palatine tonsil in oropharynx
2. Soft palate
3. Opening of the frontal sinus
4. Opening of the eustachian tube
5. Pharyngeal tonsil
6. Sphenoid sinus
7. Cranial nerve I
8. Frontal sinus
9. Superior turbinate
10. Middle turbinate
11. Inferior turbinate
12. Vestibule
13. Hard palate

Nasal Sinuses
1. Sphenoid
2. Ethmoid
3. Frontal
4. Frontal
5. Ethmoid
6. Maxillary
7. Sphenoid
8. Maxillary

Oral Cavity
1. Anterior pillar
2. Tonsil
3. Posterior pillar
4. Uvula
5. Hard palate
6. Soft palate
7. Posterior pharyngeal wall
8. Dorsum of tongue

Salivary Glands
1. Parotid gland
2. Lingual gland
3. Frenulum
4. Sublingual fold and ducts
5. Sublingual gland
6. Stensen's duct
7. Submandibular gland
8. Wharton's duct

2. 4, 8, 10, 1, 6, 9, 2, 5, 7, 3
The middle ear begins at the tympanic membrane and ends at the stapes

Equipment Selection

Examination gown
Gloves
Otoscope
Tuning fork
Nasal speculum
Penlight
Gauze
Tongue blade

Assessment Techniques

1. Correct
2. Correct
3. Correct
4. Correct
5. Incorrect-the tuning fork should be placed on the mastoid process
6. Incorrect-the tuning fork should be placed on the midline of the anterior portion of the frontal bone
7. Incorrect-first the client's eyes should be open
8. Incorrect-use the nondominant hand to stabilize the client's head
9. Incorrect-the maxillary sinuses are palpated below the zygomatic arches of the cheekbones
10. Incorrect-the Wharton's ducts are near the frenulum
11. Correct

Assessment Findings

1. A
2. N
3. N
4. N
5. A
6. N
7. N
8. A
9. N
10. N
11. A
12. N
13. N
14. A
15. N
16. A
17. N
18. A
19. N
20. A

Factors That Influence Physical Assessment Findings

1. Upward
2. Rhinitis and epistaxis
3. Presbycusis
4. Three
5. Coarse
6. Dry and gray
7. Hearing loss
8. Asian
9. Stress
10. Most

Application of the Critical Thinking Process

1. Questions that are related to the mechanism of action to the injury and the child's response to the injury would be appropriate.
2. The FLACC pain scale is appropriate for a 2-year-old. The Oucher Scale or Wong Baker Faces Scale would not be appropriate until the child is older than 3 years of age.
3. The child would receive a 7 based on a FACE score of 1, a LEGS score of 2, an ACTIVITY score of 1, a CRY score of 2, and a CONSOLABILITY score of 1.
4. The nurse should not continue with the otoscope exam at this time. She should report her findings to the medical doctor.
5. A hearing screen should be done to make sure the injury did not cause hearing loss.

Assessment and Documentation
Subjective to learner's findings

NCLEX®-Style Review Questions

1. 3   6. 3, 4, 5
2. 1   7. 2
3. 2   8. 3
4. 1   9. 4
5. 1, 2, 3   10. 3

Chapter 15
Respiratory System

Crossword Puzzle

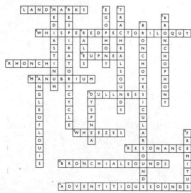

Across

1. Landmarks, 8. Whispered pectoriloquy, 10. Eupnea, 11. Rhonchi, 12. Manubrium, 14. Dullness, 15. Wheezes, 17. Resonance, 18. Bronchial sounds, 19. Adventitious sounds.

Down

2. Mediastinum, 3. Respiratory cycle, 4. Egophony, 5. Tracheal sounds, 6. Bronchophony, 7. Bronchovesicular sounds, 9. Rales, 13. Angle of Louis, 14. Dyspnea, 16. Fremitus.

Anatomy & Physiology Review

1. **Anatomy of the respiratory system**
   1. Pharynx
   2. Trachea
   3. Right main bronchus
   4. Nasal cavity
   5. Nares
   6. Oral cavity
   7. Larynx
   8. Carina
   9. Left lung
   10. Diaphragm

Anterior view of the thorax and lungs
   1. Trachea
   2. Apex of lungs
   3. Clavicle
   4. Upper lobe of right lung
   5. Rib
   6. Horizontal fissure
   7. Middle lobe
   8. Oblique fissure
   9. Lower lobe
   10. Upper lobe of left lung
   11. Visceral pleura
   12. Oblique fissure
   13. Lower lobe of left lung
   14. Parietal pleura
   15. Pleural cavity

Lines of the anterior thorax
   1. Right midclavicular line
   2. Right anterior axillary line
   3. Midsternal line
   4. Left midclavicular line
   5. Left anterior axillary line

Lines of the posterior thorax
   1. Left scapular line
   2. Left posterior axillary line
   3. Vertebral line
   4. Scapula
   5. Right posterior axillary line
   6. Right scapular line

Lines of the lateral thorax
   1. Posterior axillary line
   2. Anterior axillary line
   3. Midaxillary line

2.
   1. I   7. I
   2. E   8. E
   3. I   9. E
   4. E   10. E
   5. I   11. E
   6. I   12. I

Equipment
Examination gown, gloves, Examination light, Stethoscope, Skin-marking pen, Metric ruler, Tissues, Face mask

Assessment Techniques

1. Incorrect-allowing the client to be aware may change his pattern
2. Correct
3. Correct
4. Incorrect-the ulnar surface or the palmar surface of the hand at the base of the metacarpophalangeal joints can be used
5. Incorrect-the client should breathe normally
6. Correct
7. Incorrect-T_7 or T_8 of the midscapular line
8. Correct
9. Incorrect-the client should state "E"
10. Incorrect-the anterior thorax should be assessed on all clients, regardless of breast size

Assessment Findings

1. A   11. N
2. N   12. N
3. N   13. N
4. N   14. A
5. A   15. N
6. A   16. N
7. N   17. A
8. N   18. A
9. A   19. A
10. A   20. A

Factors That Influence Physical Assessment Findings

1. Placenta
2. Decreases

3. Dyspnea (or Shortness of breath)
4. Thoracic
5. Twenty
6. Infections
7. Low
8. Equal
9. Seven
10. Increases
11. Decreases
12. Dryness

Respiratory Patterns

1. D
2. C
3. F
4. A
5. B
6. E
7. H
8. G

Auscultation Review

1.

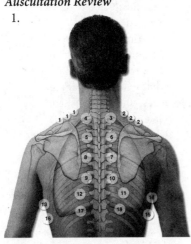

Rationale for pattern-comparison from left to right side at each level

2.
1. B
2. K
3. A
4. C
5. H
6. L
7. I
8. D
9. E
10. F
11. G
12. J

Application of the Critical Thinking Process

1. At this time any questions regarding the client's medical–surgical history or medication history would be appropriate. Due to the shortness of breath and tachypnea, any question related to the respiratory status would be appropriate.

2. Questions must be asked regarding the duration, characteristics, and factors that alleviate the pain.

3. This client should be brought immediately to a treatment area for medical evaluation due to his respiratory distress. Rapid, labored breathing, pallor, asymmetrical chest expansion, absent breath sounds, and a decrease in oxygen saturation all support this decision.

4.
   1. Pneumothorax: a collapsed lung due to air or fluid collection
   2. Assessment findings include:
      1. rapid, labored breathing
      2. asymmetrical chest expansion
      3. absent breath sounds
      4. decreased oxygen saturation
      5. pain

5. Subjective to learner's findings. Any diagnosis that supports the shortness of breath, tachypnea, pain, and respiratory distress would be appropriate related to the collapsed lung.

6. Denies pain, denies shortness of breath, BP less than 140/90, HR less than 100, RR less than 20, O_2 saturation greater than 95% on room air, regular respiratory pattern, symmetrical chest expansion, lung sounds present and clear in all lung fields, pink undertones to skin color

Healthy People 2020

1. Asthma triggers include:
   - environmental smoke
   - dust mites
   - outdoor air pollution
   - cockroach allergen
   - pets
   - mold
   - exercise
   - high humidity
   - vegetation
   - some foods
2. Subjective to learner's findings

Assessment and Documentation

Subjective to learner's findings

NCLEX®-Style Review Questions

1. 2
2. 4
3. 1, 3, 4
4. 3
5. 3
6. 1
7. 1
8. 4
9. 1, 2, 4
10. 1, 2, 3, 4

Chapter 16
Breasts and Axillae

Word Search

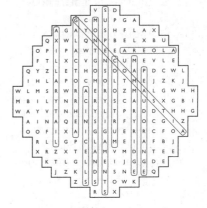

1. Acini cells
2. Areola
3. Axillary tail
4. Colostrum
5. Galactorrhea
6. Gynecomastia
7. Mammary ridge
8. Montgomery's glands
9. Peau d'orange
10. Suspensory ligaments

Anatomy & Physiology Review

1. **Anatomy of the breast**
   1. Pectoralis major muscle
   2. Tail of Spence
   3. Adipose tissue
   4. Serratus anterior muscle
   5. Areola
   6. Nipple
   7. Montgomery's glands

   Anterior & lateral views of the breast
   1. Pectoralis major muscle
   2. Tail of Spence
   3. Intercostal muscles
   4. Pectoralis major muscle
   5. Alveolus
   6. Ductule
   7. Duct
   8. Nipple pore
   9. Lactiferous sinus
   10. Lactiferous duct
   11. Adipose tissue

12. Suspensory ligaments of Cooper

Lymphatic drainage of the breast
1. Supraclavicular nodes
2. Brachial nodes
3. Subclavicular nodes
4. Central axillary nodes
5. Interpectoral nodes
6. Anterior pectoral nodes
7. Subscapular nodes
8. Internal mammary nodes
2. 1. False-Correction: Breast tissue starts to change at the onset of puberty between the ages of 9 and 13.
    2. False-Correction: Increased levels of progesterone and estrogen cause changes in fat deposits, ductile maturity, and pigmentation of the breasts.
    3. True
    4. False-Correction: Each breast has 15 to 20 lobes of glandular tissue.
    5. True
    6. True
    7. False-Correction: Blood is supplied to the breasts by the internal and lateral thoracic arteries and cutaneous branches of the posterior intercostal arteries.
    8. True

Equipment Selection
Examination gown
Gloves
Drape sheet
Small towel or pillow
Metric ruler

Assessment Techniques
1. Incorrect-the exam should begin with the client sitting upright
2. Correct
3. Correct
4. Incorrect-the client should lean forward so the breast can fall forward
5. Correct
6. Incorrect-the towel or pillow should be placed under the examined breast

7. Correct
8. Incorrect-there are a variety of patterns to select
9. Correct
10. Incorrect-the nipple should be compressed between the thumb and forefinger

Assessment Findings
1. A	11. A
2. N	12. N
3. A	13. N
4. N	14. A
5. N	15. A
6. A	16. N
7. A	17. N
8. N	18. A
9. N	19. A
10. N	20. A

Factors That Influence Physical Assessment Findings
1. Hyperestrogenism
2. Glandular
3. Increase
4. Witch's milk, hormones
5. Body-image or self-esteem
6. Smaller and flatter
7. Lowest
8. Darker and increase
9. Breast self-exams
10. One year

The Breast Self-Exam (BSE)
1. Observe breast in front of a **mirror**
2. Observe breasts in **four** positions
3. Compare breasts for **symmetry, dimpling, shape,** and **lumps**
4. Examine the nipples for **discharge** and recent **retractions**
5. Many women palpate their breasts while they **shower**
6. Palpation of the breast should be done with the **finger pads**
7. A technique for palpation of the breasts is **concentric circles**
8. Instruct the client to palpate from the periphery of the breasts to the **nipple**
9. Compress the nipple with the **thumb** and **forefinger**

10. Instruct the client not to forget the **axillary tail**

Application of the Critical Thinking Process
1. Questions regarding:
    1. breastfeeding patterns
    2. breast care
    3. signs/symptoms of infection
2. 1. asymmetrical
    2. cracked areola
    3. slightly reddened
3. 1. tender to touch
    2. warm to touch
    3. firmness
4. O-last night, L-left breast, D-not assessed, C-burning sensation, ART & ICE-not assessed
5. Questions related to the duration of the pain, what relieves the pain, and what makes the pain feel worse should be asked.
6. Goal:
    Client will be able to prevent future cases of mastitis
    Objectives: The client will be able to:
    1. Define mastitis
    2. Identify signs and symptoms of mastitis
    3. List measures to take to prevent mastitis

Healthy People 2020
1. Routine breast cancer screening consists of breast self-exams monthly, breast exams by a healthcare provider annually, and, depending on age, an annual mammography. Ultrasound may be used as a diagnostic test but is not considered a routine screening.
2. Subjective to learner's findings

Assessment and Documentation
Subjective to learner's findings

NCLEX®-Style Review Questions
1. 1	6. 1
2. 4	7. 1
3. 2	8. 2
4. 2	9. 1
5. 3	10. 4

Chapter 17
Cardiovascular System

Crossword Puzzle

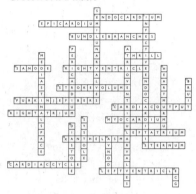

Across

2. Endocardium, 4. Epicardium,
5. Bundle branches, 9. Thrill,
10. SA node, 11. Right ventricle,
14. Stroke volume, 15. Purkinje
fibers, 16. Cardiac output,
17. Right atrium, 19. Myocardium,
21. Left atrium, 22. Xanthelasma,
24. Sternum, 25. Cardiac cycle,
26. Left ventricle.

Down

1. Semilunar valves, 3. Infective
endocarditis, 6. Pericardium,
7. Atrioventricular valves,
8. Mediastinal space, 12. Heart
murmur, 13. Bruit, 18. Systole,
20. Diastole, 23. AV node,
27. ECG.

Anatomy & Physiology Review
1. **Structural components
   of the heart**
   1. Superior vena cava
   2. Right pulmonary artery
   3. Pulmonary trunk
   4. Right atrium
   5. Right pulmonary veins
   6. Fossa ovalis
   7. Tricuspid valve
   8. Chordae tendineae
   9. Right ventricle
   10. Trabeculae carneae
   11. Inferior vena cava
   12. Aorta
   13. Left pulmonary artery
   14. Left atrium
   15. Left pulmonary veins
   16. Pulmonary semilunar
       valve
   17. Aortic semilunar valve

18. Bicuspid (mitral) valve
19. Left ventricle
20. Papillary muscle
21. Interventricular septum
22. Myocardium
23. Visceral pericardium

**Conduction system
of the heart**
1. Sinoatrial node
2. Atrioventricular node
3. Atrioventricular bundle
   (Bundle of His)
4. Right bundle branch
5. Left bundle branch
6. Purkinje fibers

2. 1. Vena cava
   2. Right atrium
   3. Tricuspid valve
   4. Right ventricle
   5. Pulmonic valve
   6. Pulmonary artery
   7. Lungs
   8. Pulmonary vein
   9. Left atrium
   10. Mitral valve
   11. Left ventricle
   12. Aortic valve
   13. Aorta

3. 1. Systole
   2. Diastole
   3. Diastole
   4. Systole
   5. Beginning of systole
   6. Beginning of diastole
   7. End of diastole
   8. End of diastole

4. 1. P wave, 2. QRS complex,
   3. T wave

   1. Atrial depolarization
   2. 0.08
   3. Ventricular depolarization
   4. 0.08 to 0.11
   5. Beginning of ventricular
      depolarization to the point
      of repolarization
   6. 1.2
   7. The time the electrical
      impulse travels across
      both atria to the
      AV node
   8. 0.12 to 0.20

Equipment Selection
Examination gown
Stethoscope
Ruler
Doppler ultrasonic stethoscope

Assessment Techniques
1. Incorrect-the client should
   be seated upright
2. Correct
3. Correct
4. Incorrect-the client's head
   should be turned slightly away
   from the examined side
5. Correct
6. Correct
7. Correct
8. Correct
9. Incorrect-the bell of the
   stethoscope is better
10. Correct

Assessment Findings
1.	N	11.	A
2.	A	12.	A
3.	A	13.	A
4.	A	14.	A
5.	A	15.	N
6.	A	16.	A
7.	A	17.	N
8.	A	18.	A
9.	N	19.	A
10.	A	20.	A

Factors That Influence Physical Assessment Findings
1. Foramen ovale
2. Higher
3. Decreased
4. Increase
5. 50
6. Systolic
7. African American
   and Hispanic
8. Higher
9. Thicken
10. Decrease

Application of the Critical Thinking Process
Scenario 1
1. Atrial fibrillation
2. Irregular and multiple P waves
   for each QRS
3. The rapid irregular beating
   of atrial fibrillation causes the
   dizziness and lightheadedness
   due to a smaller amount of
   blood being ejected by the
   ventricles.
4. The nurse should continue
   with a pain assessment
   because pain may be

intermittent and perhaps the client has experienced pain earlier.

5. Factors that should be monitored include:
   - vital signs
   - cardiac rhythm
   - pain
   - other signs and symptoms of cardiac function

Scenario 2

1. A weight gain of 4 lb in 3 days is an abnormal finding. Weight gain may indicate fluid retention, which may lead to complications of congestive heart failure.

2. Signs and symptoms of CHF may include:
   - peripheral edema
   - jugular vein distention
   - cough
   - adventitious breath sounds

3. The best method to collect a heart rate on a client with congestive heart failure would be an apical pulse. Listening with the stethoscope over the fifth intercostal space at the left midclavicular line for 1 full minute would be the most accurate method to obtain the number of beats per minute the heart is pumping.

Healthy People 2020

1. Coronary heart disease is a narrowing of the vessels that supply the heart with blood and oxygen according to the National Institutes of Health

2. Risk factors that cannot be changed include:
   - age
   - sex
   - race

3. Risk factors that can be changed include:
   - smoking
   - obesity

- inactivity
- alcohol consumption

4. Subjective to learner's findings

Assessment and Documentation
Subjective to learner's findings

NCLEX®-Style Review Questions

1. 3   6. 2
2. 1   7. 3
3. 3   8. 3
4. 1   9. 2
5. 4   10. 1

Chapter 18
Peripheral Vascular System

Word Search

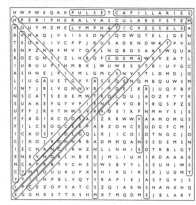

1. Allen's test
2. Arterial aneurysm
3. Arterial insufficiency
4. Arteries
5. Bruit
6. Capillaries
7. Clubbing
8. Edema
9. Epitrochlear node
10. Homan's sign
11. Lymphatic vessels
12. Lymph nodes
13. Manual compression test
14. Peripheral vascular system
15. Pulse
16. Raynaud's disease
17. Varicosities
18. Veins
19. Venous insufficiency

Anatomy & Physiology Review

1. **Main arteries of the arm**
   1. Brachiocephalic artery
   2. Right subclavian artery

3. Axillary artery
4. Posterior humeral circumflex artery
5. Anterior humeral circumflex artery
6. Deep brachial artery
7. Brachial artery
8. Radial artery
9. Ulnar artery
10. Deep palmar arch
11. Superficial palmar arch
12. Digitals

Main arteries of the leg
1. Common iliac artery
2. Internal iliac artery
3. External iliac artery
4. Deep femoral artery
5. Femoral artery
6. Popliteal artery
7. Posterior tibial artery
8. Anterior tibial artery
9. Dorsalis pedis artery
10. Arcuate artery
11. Metatarsal arteries

The main veins of the leg
1. Common iliac vein
2. External iliac vein
3. Femoral vein
4. Great saphenous vein
5. Popliteal vein
6. Anterior tibial vein
7. Dorsalis pedis vein
8. Metatarsal veins
9. Common iliac vein
10. External iliac vein
11. Great saphenous vein
12. Popliteal vein
13. Anterior tibial vein
14. Posterior tibial vein
15. Small saphenous vein
16. Plantar veins
17. Digital veins

2. 1-A, 2-V, 3-V, 4-V, 5-V, 6-V, 7-A, 8-A, 9-A, 10-A

Equipment Selection
Examination gown
Drape sheet
Tourniquet
Sphygmomanometer
Stethoscope
Doppler ultrasonic stethoscope

Assessment Techniques
1. Correct
2. Correct

3. Incorrect-apply pressure for 5 seconds
4. Incorrect-medial to the biceps tendon
5. Incorrect-place hands on knees with palms up
6. Correct
7. Correct
8. Incorrect-client should be supine with a leg elevated 90 degrees before the tourniquet is applied
9. Incorrect-the knee should be flexed 5 degrees
10. Correct

Assessment Findings

1.	N	11.	A
2.	A	12.	N
3.	N	13.	N
4.	A	14.	A
5.	N	15.	A
6.	A	16.	A
7.	N	17.	A
8.	A	18.	A
9.	A	19.	A
10.	N	20.	A

Factors That Influence Physical Assessment Findings

1. African American
2. German
3. Elasticity
4. Venous return
5. Higher
6. Varicose veins
7. Asymptomatic
8. Peripheral vascular
9. Increase
10. Equal

Pulse Predicaments

1. Bounding, pulsus alternans
2. Pulsus paradoxus
3. Weak/thready, pulsus paradoxus
4. Unequal
5. Pulsus paradoxus
6. Bounding
7. Bounding
8. Weak/thready
9. Absent
10. Pulsus alternans
11. Pulsus paradoxus
12. Bounding
13. Pulsus alternans

Edema

1. Press the skin for at least 5 seconds over the tibia, behind the medial malleolus, and over the dorsum of each foot.
2. Stage 1-2 mm, Stage 2-4 mm, Stage 3-6 mm, Stage 4-8 mm
3. Possible conditions include:
   1. congestive heart failure
   2. venous occlusion
   3. obstruction of lymphatic system

Application of the Critical Thinking Process

1. Arterial wound
2. Signs or symptoms include:
   1. cool, shiny, pale, and hairless skin to legs
   2. thick, brittle, yellow toenails
   3. non-palpable pedal pulse
   4. no bleeding to wound
   5. pale-yellow wound bed
   6. painful
3. Prevent leg elevation. Keep legs in a dependent position to promote circulation.
4. Diabetes, hypertension, obesity, smoking
5. Location, dimensions, periwound skin, wound edges, wound bed tissue, drainage, odor, pain
6. The OLDCART assessment should lead assessment.

Healthy People 2020

1. third
2. Risk factors that cannot be changed include:
   1. age
   2. gender
   3. race
   4. family history
3. Risk factors that can be changed include:
   1. hypertension
   2. high cholesterol
   3. diabetes
   4. smoking
   5. alcohol
   6. obesity
   7. inactivity
4. Commonly used stroke scales are:

1. Cincinnati Stroke Scale: facial droop, arm drift, speech
2. NIH Stroke Scale: level of consciousness, gaze, visual, facial palsy, motor arm, motor legs, limb ataxia, sensory, language, dysarthria, extinction, and inattention
5. Subjective to learner' findings
6. Subjective to learner's findings

Assessment and Documentation
Subjective to learner's findings

NCLEX®-Style Review Questions

1.	3	6.	1
2.	1	7.	2
3.	1, 2, 4	8.	4
4.	3	9.	3
5.	4	10.	1, 5

Chapter 19
Abdomen

Crossword Puzzle for Key Terms

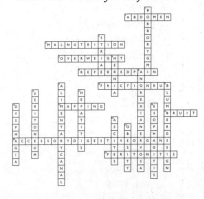

Across
2. Abdomen, 4. Malnutrition,
5. Overweight, 7. Referred pain,
10. Friction rub, 15. Mapping,
17. Bruit, 20. Accessory digestive organs, 21. Peritonitis.

Down
1. Borborygmi, 3. Striae,
6. Hernia, 8. Anorexia nervosa, 9. Alimentary canal, 11. Blumberg's sign,
12. Peritoneum, 13. Hepatitis,
14. Dysphagia, 16. Esophagitis,
18. Ascites, 19. Obesity.

Anatomy & Physiology Review

1. **Organs of the alimentary canal**
    1. Parotid gland
    2. Tongue
    3. Pharynx
    4. Liver
    5. Gallbladder
    6. Pancreas
    7. Small intestine
    8. Cecum
    9. Vermiform appendix
    10. Oral cavity
    11. Salivary glands
    12. Esophagus
    13. Spleen
    14. Stomach
    15. Transverse colon
    16. Ascending colon
    17. Descending colon
    18. Sigmoid colon
    19. Rectum
    20. Anus

Abdominal vasculature and deep structures
    1. Inferior vena cava
    2. Duodenum
    3. Right kidney
    4. Common iliac artery and vein
    5. Right ureter
    6. Rectum
    7. Bladder
    8. Xiphoid process
    9. Diaphragm
    10. Aorta
    11. Pancreas
    12. Left kidney
    13. Left ureter
    14. Umbilicus
    15. Inguinal ligament
    16. Femoral artery

2.

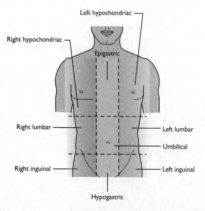

3. a-14, b-8, c-12, d-5, e-3, f-9, g-7, h-6, i-1, j-2, k-13, l-11, m-4, n-10
4. 1-RUQ, 2-LLQ, 3-LUQ, 4-RUQ, 5-RUQ, 6-LLQ, 7-RUQ, 8-LLQ, 9-RUQ, 10-LUQ, 11-RLQ, 12-LUQ, 13-RUQ, 14-RLQ

Equipment
Drape sheet
Examination gown
Examination light
Gloves
Ruler
Skin-marking pen
Stethoscope
Tape measure
Tissues

Assessment Techniques
1. Incorrect-a small pillow should be placed under the knees as well as behind the head
2. Incorrect-the drape sheet should be placed at the symphysis pubis
3. Correct
4. Correct
5. Correct
6. Incorrect-auscultation should begin with the aorta
7. Correct
8. Incorrect-the examiner should move towards the rib cage along the right MCL
9. Incorrect-auscultation should occur before palpation
10. Incorrect-murphy's sign is assessed while palpating the liver and asking the client to take a deep breath. The diaphragm descends and pushes the liver and gallbladder toward the examiner's hand.

Assessment Findings

1.	A	11.	N
2.	N	12.	A
3.	A	13.	N
4.	N	14.	N
5.	A	15.	A
6.	A	16.	N
7.	A	17.	N
8.	A	18.	A
9.	A	19.	A
10.	A	20.	N

Factors That Influence Physical Assessment Findings
1. Two and one
2. Toddlers
3. Pregnant
4. Decrease
5. Lactose
6. Japanese
7. Uterus
8. Constipation
9. Image
10. Fourteen

Application of the Critical Thinking Process
Scenario 1
1. Focused questions related to the baby's appetite include:
    1. eating patterns
    2. bowel patterns
    3. crying patterns
2. Yes, they are within expected parameters.
3. Signs and symptoms of an umbilical hernia can include:
    1. pain
    2. tenderness
    3. swelling and discoloration to the site
    4. vomiting
4. The FLACC scale because it is appropriate for infants and young children
5. Subjective to learner's findings but acute pain or knowledge deficit would be indicated

Scenario 2
1. Focused questions related to the client's appetite, bowel patterns, nausea/vomiting, and pain are all appropriate.
2. Questions regarding the characteristics of the pain should be asked.

3. Appendicitis is supported by the sudden onset of pain in the RLQ, nausea, poor appetite, fever, and rebound tenderness, and the psoas test supports peritoneal irritation or appendicitis.

4. This client may be going to surgery so preoperative education may be required.

Healthy People 2020

1. Hepatitis C may be asymptomatic or may reveal:
   - fever
   - fatigue
   - dark urine
   - clay-colored stool
   - abdominal pain
   - loss of appetite
   - nausea/vomiting
   - joint pain
   - jaundice

2. Subjective to learner's findings

Assessment and Documentation

Subjective to learner's findings

NCLEX®-Style Review Questions

1. 1
2. 1, 2, 4
3. 4
4. 1, 2, 3, 4
5. 1
6. 1
7. 3
8. 1
9. 1
10. 2

Chapter 20
Urinary System

Word Search

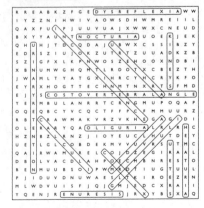

1. Calculi
2. Cortex
3. Costovertebral angle
4. Dysreflexia
5. Enuresis
6. Glomeruli

7. Hematuria
8. Incontinence
9. Kidneys
10. Medulla
11. Nocturia
12. Oliguria
13. Ureters
14. Urethra
15. Urinary retention

Anatomy & Physiology Review

1. **The urinary system**
   1. Hepatic veins
   2. Esophagus
   3. Inferior vena cava
   4. Adrenal gland
   5. Renal vein
   6. Kidney
   7. Ureter
   8. Uterus
   9. Urinary bladder
   10. Urethra
   11. Renal artery
   12. Renal hilus
   13. Aorta
   14. Iliac crest
   15. Rectum

   Internal anatomy of the kidney
   1. Renal artery
   2. Renal vein
   3. Renal pelvis
   4. Ureter
   5. Capsule
   6. Cortex
   7. Medulla
   8. Major calyx
   9. Renal column
   10. Minor calyx

2. 1-K, 2-K, 3-N/A, 4-K, 5-B, 6-B, 7-K, 8-N/A, 9-K, 10-K

Equipment Selection

Examination gown
Drape sheet
Gloves
Stethoscope
Specimen containers

Assessment Techniques

1. Correct
2. Incorrect-it should continue from the supine position similar to the abdominal assessment
3. Correct
4. Incorrect-the renal artery at the MCL on either side of the abdominal aorta

5. Incorrect-they can be inspected while the client is sitting upright
6. Correct
7. Correct
8. Incorrect-the client should hold a deep breath and then slowly release
9. Incorrect-deep palpation should be used to palpate the fundus of the bladder
10. Correct

Assessment Findings

1. O, N
2. O, A
3. S, A
4. O, A
5. O, A
6. O, A
7. S, A
8. S, A
9. O, A
10. O, N
11. O, A
12. O, A
13. O, N
14. O, N
15. S, A
16. O, A
17. S, A
18. O, A
19. S, A
20. O, A

Factors That Influence Physical Assessment Findings

1. Infants/children and elderly
2. Frequency
3. Dilute
4. Decrease
5. Urinary tract infection
6. Six
7. Hygiene
8. Estrogen
9. Renal failure or kidney disease (damage)
10. Renal calculi (stones)

Application of the Critical Thinking Process

1. The nurse should ask focused interview questions for the urinary system and continue with a physical assessment of the urinary system.

2. The nurse may want to discuss her findings with the healthcare provider at this time in order to administer a safe analgesic. The healthcare provider must be cautious as to not mask any pain that may lead to further investigation.

3. Risk factors, including adult men, dehydration, high protein diet, obesity, and gastric

bypass surgery, may alter the absorption of calcium leading to stone formation.

4. A NANDA dx might include:
   - acute pain
   - hematuria
   - knowledge deficit

5. Subjective to learner's findings
   Kidney stone prevention should include staying well hydrated, not consuming excessive amounts of calcium, and choosing a diet low in animal protein. Appropriate teaching methods for one-on-one education would be discussion supported by written material. Question and Answer sessions are appropriate evaluation methods.

Healthy People 2020

1. Diseases such as diabetes, hypertension, sickle cell anemia, systemic lupus erythematosus, chronic glomerulonephritis, congenital kidney disease, and overexposure to kidney toxins
2. Subjective to learner's findings

Assessment and Documentation
Subjective to learner's findings

NCLEX®-Style Review Questions

1.	2	6.	2
2.	2	7.	1
3.	4	8.	2
4.	1, 2, 3, 5	9.	3
5.	2	10.	1

Chapter 21
Male Reproductive System

Crossword Puzzle for Key Terms

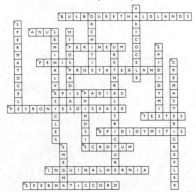

Across
2. Bulbourethal glands, 5. Anus, 8. Perineum, 11. Penis, 13. Prostate gland, 14. Epispadias, 16. Peyronies disease, 17. Testes, 18. Epididymitis, 20. Scrotum, 21. Inguinal hernia, 22. Spermatic cord.

Down
1. Varicocele, 3. Orchitis, 4. Spermatocele, 6. Seminal vesicles, 7. Hypospadias, 9. Urethral stricture, 10. Epididymis, 12. Cremasteric reflex, 15. Phimosis, 19. Smegma.

Anatomy & Physiology Review
1. **Gross anatomy of the male reproductive organs**
   1. Vas deferens
   2. Cavernous
   3. Epididymis
   4. Scrotum
   5. Glans
   6. Urethral orifice
   7. Testis
   8. Bladder
   9. Rectum
   10. Prostate
   11. Prostatic urethra
   12. Membranous urethra

   Contents of the scrotum
   1. Superficial inguinal ring
   2. Spermatic cord
   3. Ductus deferens
   4. Autonomic nerve fibers
   5. Pampiniform plexus of testicular veins
   6. Testicular artery
   7. Epididymis
   8. Testis
   9. Suspensory ligament
   10. Penis
   11. Midline septum
   12. Cremaster muscle
   13. Superficial fascia

   Structure of the penis
   1. Urinary bladder
   2. Prostate gland
   3. Prostatic urethra
   4. Membranous urethra
   5. Shaft
   6. Bulbourethral gland
   7. Urogenital diaphragm
   8. Bulb of penis
   9. Crus of penis
   10. Corpora cavernosa
   11. Corpora spongiosum
   12. Spongy urethra
   13. Glans penis
   14. Prepuce
   15. External urethral orifice

2. 1-Seminiferous tubules; 2-Epididymis; 3-Ductus Deferens; 4-Spermatic Cord; 5-Seminal Vesicles; 6-Ejaculatory Duct

Equipment Selection
Examination gown
Drape sheet
Gloves
Flashlight
Lubricant
Slides and cotton-tipped applicators for specimen collection of any abnormal discharge

Assessment Techniques
1. Correct
2. Correct
3. Incorrect-the client should be standing for the first portion of the assessment
4. Incorrect-the examiner or the client can retract the foreskin
5. Correct
6. Incorrect-the penis should either be raised by the client or gently resting on the back side of the examiner's hand
7. Incorrect-the room should be dim
8. Correct
9. Incorrect-the posterior side of each testicle should be palpated to locate the epididymis
10. Incorrect-the index finger should gently press toward the thumb

Assessment Findings

1.	N	11.	A
2.	N	12.	N
3.	N	13.	N
4.	A	14.	A
5.	N	15.	N
6.	N	16.	A
7.	N	17.	A
8.	A	18.	A
9.	A	19.	A
10.	A	20.	A

Factors That Influence
Physical Assessment Findings
1. Circumsize
2. Precocious puberty
3. Caucasians
4. Decrease
5. Testosterone
6. Testicular
7. Undescended
8. Testosterone
9. Sexually transmitted diseases
10. Sexual molestation

The Testicular Exam
1. Monthly
2. Adolescence
3. Cold
4. Shower
5. Gentle pressure
6. Smooth, round, and firm
7. Epididymis
8. Lumps

Application of the Critical
Thinking Process
Scenario 1
1. O-4 days; L-Rectal Area; D-Duration; C-Sharp; A-sitting; R-standing; T-Tylenol and hot bath
2. The numeric pain scale and questions regarding the ICE pneumonic will complete the pain assessment.
3. Questions related to sexuality including any rectal stimulation or penetration may be appropriate.
4. Rectal pain, sacrococcygeal dimpling and erythema, moderate swelling, warmth, small coarse hair, foul odor, yellow drainage
5. Risk factors for a pilonidal cyst are obesity, inactive lifestyle, sports requiring sitting, excess body hair, coarse hair, and poor hygiene.
6. Assessment—Constant sharp pain in the rectal area × 4 days, 7/10 on a numeric scale, BP 130/82, P 104, RR 20, T 100.7°, skin color pale, erythema and moderate swelling to sacrococcygeal area with dimpling, small coarse

hair noted, small amount of foul-smelling, yellow drainage present.
Problem—infected pilonidal cyst, pain
Interventions—incision and drainage, analgesics, antibiotics
Evaluation—client denies pain, BP 110/62, HR 72, RR 12, Temp 97.8°, wound has mild amt erythema, no drainage or swelling present

Scenario 2
1. The nurse should ask focused questions regarding pain, a sexual history, and any illness-prevention behaviors related to testicular examinations (self or by the healthcare provider).
2. When performing an assessment of the uncircumcised penis, the examiner should either ask the client to retract his foreskin or the examiner should gently pull the skin down over the penile shaft from the side of the glans using the thumb and first two fingers or forefinger.
3. Risk factors for testicular cancer are:
    1. undescended testicles and other congenital abnormalities
    2. a family history of testicular cancer
4. Light will not penetrate a mass during transillumination of the scrotum.

Healthy People 2020
1. Men with gonorrhea may have no symptoms at all. Some signs or symptoms may be:
    • burning during urination
    • white or yellow penile discharge
    • testicular pain
    • swollen testicles
    • Gonorrhea affecting the anus may include anal itching, bleeding, or painful bowel movement.
2. Subjective to learner's findings

Assessment and Documentation
Subjective to learner's findings

NCLEX®-Style Review Questions
1. 3   6. 3
2. 1, 3, 4   7. 1
3. 1, 2, 3, 4   8. 1
4. 1   9. 1
5. 1, 2   10. 4

Chapter 22
Female Reproductive System

Word Search

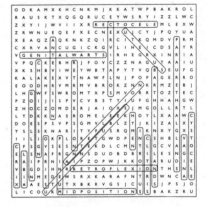

1. Anteflexion
2. Anteversion
3. Bartholins glands
4. Cervical os
5. Cervix
6. Chadwicks sign
7. Clitoris
8. Cystocele
9. Genital warts
10. Goodell's sign
11. Hymen
12. Introitus
13. Labia
14. Midposition
15. Ovaries
16. Paraurethral glands
17. Perineum
18. Rectocele
19. Retroflexion
20. Retroversion
21. Uterine tubes
22. Uterus
23. Vagina

Anatomy & Physiology Review
1. **External female genitalia**
    1. Mons pubis
    2. Labia majora
    3. Prepuce of clitoris
    4. Head of clitoris

5. Vestibule
6. Orifice of urethra
7. Opening of Skene's duct
8. Orifice of vagina
9. Opening of greater vestibular gland
10. Labia minora
11. Perineum
12. Anus
13. Vestibule

Internal organs of the female reproductive system within the pelvis

1. Suspensory ligament of ovary
2. Uterine tube
3. Fimbriae
4. Ovary
5. Round ligament
6. Uterus
7. Urinary bladder
8. Symphysis pubis
9. Mons pubis
10. Urethra
11. External urethral orifice
12. Clitoris
13. Hymen
14. Labium minora
15. Labium majora
16. Peritoneum
17. Perimetrium
18. Posterior fornix
19. Cervix
20. Anterior fornix
21. Rectum
22. Vagina
23. Urogenital diaphragm
24. Anus
25. Bartholin's gland

Cross section of the anterior view of the female pelvis

1. Endometrium
2. Myometrium
3. Perimetrium
4. Internal os
5. Cervical canal
6. External os
7. Vagina
8. Lumen of uterus
9. Fundus of uterus
10. Ovarian ligament
11. Ovarian vessels
12. Ovary

2. 1. vagina; 2. ovaries; 3. vagina; 4. ovaries; 5. Skene's glands;

6. fallopian tubes 7. ovaries; 8. uterus, 9. uterus; 10. clitoris

Equipment

Examination gown
Drape sheet
Gloves
Handheld mirror
Lubricant
Pap smear equipment
Speculum

Assessment Techniques

1. Correct
2. Correct
3. Correct
4. Incorrect-the right palm faces upward toward the ceiling
5. Incorrect-gentle pressure upward against the vaginal wall will palpate the Skene's glands
6. Incorrect-the speculum should be placed in the dominant hand
7. Correct
8. Incorrect-three slides should be labeled and ready (endocervical; cervical scrape; vaginal pool)
9. Incorrect-the examiner should be standing at the end of the examination table
10. Correct

Assessment Findings

1.	N	11.	A
2.	N	12.	N
3.	N	13.	A
4.	N	14.	N
5.	A	15.	N
6.	N	16.	A
7.	A	17.	N
8.	N	18.	A
9.	A	19.	N
10.	N	20.	A

Factors That Influence Phsyical Assessment Findings

1. Africa, Asia, and Middle Eastern
2. 5
3. Before
4. Normal
5. Goodell's sign
6. Cervical
7. Premarital sex

8. Plastics
9. Vaccine
10. Oncology

Application of the Critical Thinking Process

1. Focused questions related to the number of sexual partners a woman has, or a woman who has a partner who has had multiple sex partners, and conditions that cause a client to be immunocompromised are all appropriate for risk factors of HPV.
2. HPV screening may include a visual inspection, a vinegar solution test, a pap test, and a DNA test.
3. Subjective to learner's findings
4. There may be no signs or symptoms, or the client may show signs of genital warts.

Healthy People 2020

1. Pelvic inflammatory disease may be asymptomatic or may cause any of the following:
   - lower abdominal or pelvic pain
   - heavy vaginal discharge with foul odor
   - irregular menstrual bleeding
   - painful intercourse
   - lower back pain
   - fever
   - fatigue
   - diarrhea
   - vomiting
   - painful urination
2. Subjective to learner's findings

Assessment and Documentation

Subjective to learner's findings

NCLEX®-Style Review Questions

1.	2	6.	4
2.	1	7.	3
3.	3	8.	2
4.	1	9.	1
5.	3	10.	2

Chapter 23
Musculoskeletal System

Crossword Puzzle for Key Terms

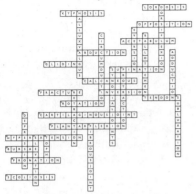

Across

1. Lordosis, 3. Kyphosis,
5. Opposition, 9. Acetabulum,
10. Abduction, 12. Gliding,
13. Supination, 15. Calcaneus,
16. Fracture, 18. Inversion,
19. Tendons, 21. Rotation,
23. Cartilaginous joint, 24. Plantar flexion, 26. Hyperextension,
29. Bursae, 30. Pronation,
31. Scoliosis.

Down

2. Dorsiflexion, 4. Hallux valgus,
6. Eversion, 7. Circumduction,
8. Ballottement, 11. Adduction,
13. Synovial joints, 14. Protraction,
17. Retraction, 20. Subluxation,
22. Depression, 25. Fibrous joint,
27. Elevation, 28. Tophi.

Anatomy & Physiology Review
1. Bones of the human skeleton
   1. Cranium
   2. Skull
   3. Clavicle
   4. Scapula
   5. Sternum
   6. Rib
   7. Humerus
   8. Vertebra
   9. Radius
   10. Ulna
   11. Carpals
   12. Metacarpals
   13. Phalanges
   14. Femur
   15. Patella
   16. Tibia
   17. Fibula
   18. Tarsals

19. Metatarsals
20. Phalanges
21. Upper limb
22. Lower limb
23. Vertebral column

Shoulder joint
   1. Acromion process
   2. Subacromial bursa
   3. Greater tubercle of humerus
   4. Coracoid process
   5. Subscapular bursa
   6. Scapula

Elbow joint
   1. Humerus
   2. Lateral epicondyle
   3. Articular capsule
   4. Olecranon process
   5. Radius
   6. Ulna

2.

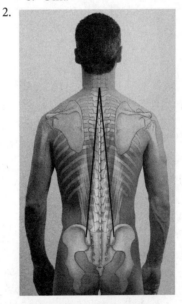

3. 1. circumduction; 2. abduction;
3. pronation/supination;
4. flexion/extension; 5. plantar flexion/dorsiflexion;
6. inversion/eversion;
7. opposing thumb; 8. rotation
4. 1. abduction & external rotation; 2. flexion & radial deviation; 3. extension & internal rotation;
4. extension & hyperextension;
5. supination & flexion;
6. extension & opposition;
7. plantar flexion & eversion;
8. rotation & lateral flexion;
9. abduction & adduction;
10. circumduction & extension

Equipment
Examination gown
Examination gloves
Examination light
Goniometer
Skin-marking pen
Tape measure

Assessment Techniques
1. Correct
2. Incorrect-behind the head will assess external rotation
3. Incorrect-abduction of the shoulder should extend 180 degrees
4. Correct
5. Incorrect-the olecranon process is located behind the elbow
6. Correct
7. Incorrect-hands should be dorsum to dorsum
8. Correct
9. Correct
10. Incorrect-hyperextension of the spine can reach 30 degrees

Assessment Findings
1. N		11. N	
2. A		12. N	
3. A		13. N	
4. A		14. N	
5. A		15. N	
6. N		16. A	
7. A		17. N	
8. N		18. A	
9. N		19. N	
10. A		20. A	

Factors That Influence Physical Assessment Findings
1. Preschool
2. Spine
3. African Americans
4. Physical abuse
5. 21
6. Osteoporosis
7. 1; 2
8. Decrease
9. Soften
10. Reverse Tailor

Muscle Strength
1. B, 2. E, 3. F, 4. A, 5. C, 6. D,
7. C, 8. E, 9. A, 10. B

Abnormal Findings

1. Kyphosis (exaggerated convex curve of the thoracic spine)
2. Scoliosis (lateral curvature of the spine)
3. Rheumatoid nodules (firm non-tender nodule along the extensor ulnar surface)
4. Olecranon bursitis (swelling and inflammation to the olecranon joint)
5. Hallux valgus (the great toe is abnormally adducted at the metatarsophalangeal joint)
6. Synovitis (distention of the suprapatellar area and lateral aspect of the knee)
7. Hammertoe (flexion of the interphalangeal joint of the toe and hyperextension of the metatarsophalangeal joint of the toe)
8. Bunion (thickening and inflammation of the bursa)

Application of the Critical Thinking Process
Part 1

1. Subjective data:
   - all pain data
   - stated difficulty with movement
   - felt "pop" in right knee
2. Objective data:
   - limited ROM
   - edema
   - unable to bear weight
   - unsteady gait
   - skin to right knee is warm, dry and the color is consistent with the rest of the body
3. The Onset of pain was at the time of injury; the Location in the right knee; a question regarding the Duration and Characteristics should be asked. We know that movement makes the pain worse, and immobility makes the pain less intense.
4. It is important to know when the LMP of any childbearing female who has a musculoskeletal injury for the following reasons:
   1. Due to diagnostic testing involving x-rays and/or contrast dyes
   2. If the injury requires surgical repair, the LMP along with a pregnancy test should be documented.
5. Risk factors for this client include:
   Women are more likely to have ACL injuries than men. Athletes who participate in sports that require cut and run movements of the knee are at higher risk.
6. Goal: The client will be able to ambulate safely with crutches. Objectives: By the end of the teaching learning session:
   1. The client will be able to hold the crutches correctly.
   2. The client will be able to demonstrate crutch ambulation.
   3. The client will be able to state five safety measures for ambulating with crutches.

Application of the Critical Thinking Process
Part 2

1. Reverse tailor position
2. The nurse should inform the parents that this position puts added stress to the hips, knees, and ankle joints. Therefore, it should be avoided.

Healthy People 2020

1. Questions related to factors affecting calcium absorption should be asked:
   - calcium intake
   - tobacco use
   - eating disorders
   - a sedentary lifestyle
   - alcohol consumption
   - corticosteroid medications use
   - family history
   - thyroid disorders
   - a history of stomach or weight-loss surgery
2. There are numerous fall assessment tools that may be found (Hendrich, Hendrich II, and the Morse are just a few). Many tools have common elements such as history of falls, medications, use of assistive devices, age, and mobility ability. A home health nurse should use a scale that is applicable to the home environment. It should be completed at each visit. The staff nurse should complete a tool at the beginning of each shift and any major change in the client's condition that would increase the client's risk of falls.
3. Subjective to learner's findings

Assessment and Documentation
Subjective to learner's findings

NCLEX®-Style Review Questions

1.	1	6.	1, 2, 5
2.	1, 2	7.	4
3.	2	8.	3
4.	4	9.	4
5.	3	10.	1, 3

Chapter 24
Neurologic System

Word Search

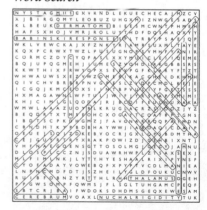

1. Analgesia
2. Anesthesia
3. Anosmia
4. Babinski response
5. Brain stem
6. Central nervous system

7. Cerebellum
8. Cerebrum
9. Clonus
10. Coma
11. Dermatome
12. Diplopia
13. Dysphagia
14. Hypalgesia
15. Hyperesthesia
16. Meninges
17. Nuchal rigidity
18. Nystagmus
19. Optic atrophy
20. Papilledema
21. Peripheral
    nervous system
22. Reflexes
23. Romberg's test
24. Seizures
25. Spinal cord
26. Syncope
27. Thalamus

Anatomy and Physiology Review
1. Regions of the brain
  1. Cerebrum
  2. Thalamus
  3. Epithalamus
  4. Hypothalamus
  5. Pituitary gland
  6. Diencephalon
  7. Midbrain
  8. Pons
  9. Medulla oblongata
  10. Brain stem
  11. Cerebellum
  12. Spinal cord
  Spinal nerves
  1. Cervical
  2. Thoracic
  3. Lumbar
  4. Sacral
2. 1. A, 2. D, 3. B, 4. A, 5. C, 6. B, 7. A, 8. C, 9. A, 10. A
3. 1. The hand touches the stimulus (the hot stove), which triggers the sensory nerve to fire and carries the signal to the gray matter of the spinal cord where it synapses with the motor neuron; the motor neuron carries the message to the effector (the muscles of the arm and hand), and the hand gets pulled away.

2. The frontal lobe
3. When the brain perceives a threat the autonomic nervous system is activated, which causes the adrenal glands to secrete adrenaline and noradrenalin to be released. These hormones put the body into the fight-or-flight response that causes:
  • increased heart rate
  • increased contractility of the heartbeat
  • numbness or tingling in the extremities
  • deep rapid breathing
  • chest tightness
  • dizziness
  • lightheadedness
  • sweating
  • dilated pupils
4. 1. Hypoglossal (XII)
   2. Glossopharyngeal and vagus (IX, X)
   3. Optic (II)
   4. Oculomotor, trochlear, abducens (III, IV, VI)
   5. Vagus (X)
   6. Trigeminal (V)
   7. Auditory or vestibulocochlear (VIII)
   8. Oculomotor, trochlear, abducens (III, IV, VI)
   9. Olfactory (I)
   10. Accessory (XI)
   11. Optic (II)
   12. Auditory or vestibulocochlear (VIII)
   13. Trigeminal (V)
   14. Facial (VII)
   15. Facial (VII)
   16. Glossopharyngeal and vagus (IX, X)

Equipment
Examination gown
Gloves
Percussion hammer
Tuning fork
Sterile cotton balls
Penlight
Ophthalmoscope
Stethoscope
Sharp object
Tongue blade

Cotton-tipped applicator
Hot (warm) and cold objects
Dull, soft, sharp objects
Substances to smell
Substances to taste

Assessment Techniques
1. Correct
2. Incorrect-this is done testing CN I
3. Correct
4. Incorrect-convergence and accommodation tests CN III
5. Correct
6. Incorrect-the examiner should stand next to the client
7. Correct
8. Incorrect-the client's eyes should be closed
9. Incorrect-the hammer should strike 2–3 inches above the wrist
10. Incorrect-the handle of the reflex hammer is used

Assessment Findings
1. A	11. A
2. A	12. N
3. A	13. A
4. A	14. N
5. A	15. N
6. N	16. A
7. A	17. N
8. A	18. N
9. A	19. A
10. A	20. A

Factors That Influence Physical Assessment Findings
1. Pregnancy induced hypertension
2. Stroke
3. Legs
4. Absent or weak or catlike
5. Rapid
6. Primitive
7. Lead
8. African Americans
9. Decrease
10. Parkinson's disease

Application of the Critical Thinking Process
Scenario 1
1. Eye response, Verbal response, Motor response
2. E3, V2, M4 = 9
3. Moderate brain injury

Scenario 2

1. Questions should be asked following the OLDCART & ICE pain assessment including a Pain Intensity scale.
2. LOC, best gaze, visual, facial palsy, motor arm, motor leg, limb ataxia, sensory, best language, dysarthria, extinction, and inattention.
3. Facial droop, arm drift, speech
4. The Cincinnati scale is faster to use than the NIH scale because it has fewer performance indicators. Both are considered reliable tools for stroke assessment. The Cincinnati scale is more likely to be used in the prehospital setting, and the NIH scale is for the more advanced healthcare provider.
5. A brain aneurysm may be asymptomatic or may reveal:
   - severe headaches
   - nausea
   - vomiting
   - stiff neck
   - blurred double vision
   - photophobia
   - seizures
   - ptosis
   - loss of consciousness
   - confusion
6. Priority nursing diagnosis for Mrs. Sanchez should be related to:
   - the acute pain she is experiencing
   - at risk for injury because the aneurysm can rupture
   - knowledge deficit because it is a new diagnosis
   - she also may be preoperative for repair

Healthy People 2020

1. Some symptoms of concussions are not apparent until days after the injury: memory difficulties, photophobia, difficulty sleeping, irritability, and depression. Children may also show lack of interest in their usually activities. Some signs and symptoms of a concussion are:
   - confusion
   - amnesia
   - headache
   - dizziness
   - ringing in the ears
   - nausea or vomiting
   - slurred speech
   - fatigue
2. This age group is:
   - more likely to experience falls
   - more likely to ride bikes
   - more likely to play contact sports
   - may be put into a car seat incorrectly
   - may drive under the influence of drugs or alcohol
   - may not wear a seat belt
3. Subjective to learner's findings

Assessment and Documentation

Subjective to learner's findings

NCLEX®-Style Review Questions

1. 3
2. 2
3. 2, 3
4. 1, 2, 3, 5
5. 1, 2, 3
6. 1
7. 1, 3, 4
8. 2
9. 2
10. 2, 3

Chapter 25
Infants, Children, and Adolescents

Crossword Puzzle for Key Terms

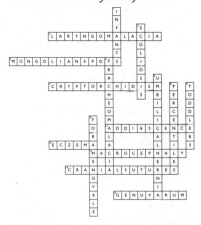

Across

3. Laryngomalacia, 4. Mongolian spots, 7. Cryptorchidism, 11. Adolescence, 12. Eczema, 13. Macrocephaly, 14. Cranial sutures, 15. Genu varum.

Down

1. Infants, 2. Scoliosis, 5. Tracheomalacia, 6. Umbilical hernia,

8. Percentiles, 9. Toddlers, 10. Foramen ovale.

Anatomy & Physiology Review

1. **Sutures & fontanelles of the skull**
   1. Sagittal suture
   2. Lambdoid suture
   3. Posterior fontanelle
   4. Coronal suture
   5. Anterior fontanelle

   Upper & Lower deciduous teeth
   1. Central incisor
   2. Lateral incisor
   3. Cuspid
   4. First molar
   5. Second molar
   6. Central incisor
   7. Lateral incisor
   8. Cuspid
   9. First molar
   10. Second molar

2. **Integumentary**
   1. Due to infant skin being thinner, this leads to increased transdermal absorption. This can lead to greater systemic absorption.
   2. Infants are at greater risk for heat intolerance because their sebaceous glands do not begin to function until their first birthday.

   Head, Eyes, Ears, Nose, and Throat
   3. Craniosynostosis is the premature fusion of the cranial bones which, if left untreated, can lead to impaired brain growth and cognitive impairment.
   4. Children under the age of 5 have heads that are disproportionately large for their bodies, leading to a top-heavy body and easy loss of balance.
   5. A "shotty" lymph node is a benign, non-infected, non-tender, enlarged node that may be present until the child is 6 or 7 years of age.
   6. The sinuses are not fully developed. The sphenoid sinuses develop before age 5 and the frontal sinuses by age 10.

7. The eustachian tubes of infants and children are shorter, straighter, and more level than those of adults. Combining this anatomical variation with the increased frequency of colds and respiratory infections leads to higher rates of ear infections.

Respiratory

8. Children under 6 are nose breathers; they have difficulty breathing through the mouth.

Cardiovascular

9. The chest wall of a child is thinner than an adult leading to more audible sounds.

10. An innocent murmur arises from increased blood flow through normal heart structures. The fever that can be associated with the pneumonia can increase a child's metabolism and lead to a more pronounced murmur.

Breasts

11. Circulating maternal estrogen and prolactin may cause milky white discharge from a newborn's nipples.

Abdomen

12. The thoracic cage that protects the liver is smaller in young children than the adult. This may allow for up to 2 cm of the liver's edge to expand pass the costal margin without worry.

Genitourinary and Reproductive

13. Undescended testicles can increase a male's risk for testicular cancer. Undescended testicles rarely descend on their own past 6 months.

14. A "false menses" may be noted in female newborns during the first 2 weeks of life due to maternal circulating hormones.

Musculoskeletal

15. Fractures in children that involve the epiphyseal plates can result in bone growth failure and limb length discrepancy.

Neurologic

16. Large muscle groups needed for gross motor function develop earlier than those required for fine motor function.

Infant and Early Childhood Reflexes

1. F
2. D
3. C
4. G
5. E
6. A
7. B

Developmental Milestones

1. 8 months
2. 3 years
3. 2 months
4. 3½ months
5. 4 months
6. 13 months
7. 5 years
8. 10 months
9. 11 months
10. 6 months
11. 7 months
12. 10 months

Calculations for Bladder Capacity and Urine Output

Bladder capacity:
1. 1–5 oz
2. 3–7 oz
3. 5–9 oz
4. 6–10 oz

Urine output:
1. 12.7 or 13
2. 22.7 or 23
3. 29
4. 50
5. 71
6. 81.8 or 82

Vital Signs

1. 110/70
2. 22
3. 110
4. 84
5. 95/55
6. 45
7. 110/65
8. 20

Eating Disorder Findings

1. Hoarse voice-bulimia
3. Dental erosion-bulimia
4. Loss of muscle tone-anorexia
6. Pedal edema-anorexia
9. Decreased gag reflex-bulimia
12. Swollen parotid glands-bulimia
14. Bloodshot eyes-bulimia

Factors That Influence Physical Assessment Findings

1. Sickle cell anemia
2. Impolite
3. Cupping
4. Head
5. Healthy
6. Coarse
7. Hypothyroid
8. Thalassemias
9. Clothing and items
10. Mongolian spots

Application of the Critical Thinking Process

1. Liam is possibly abused in the home.
2. Poor hygiene practices (same clothes, dirty fingernails, and uncombed hair) can be signs of neglect; exposure of his genitalia can be signs of sexual abuse; bite marks and belt markings can be signs of physical abuse.
3. Additional assessment findings for each category of abuse may be:
    1. Physical abuse; unexplained burns, bruises, broken bones, or bite marks
    2. Sexual abuse; difficulty walking or sitting, refuses to participate in physical activities, reports nightmares or bedwetting, change in appetite, bizarre or sophisticated knowledge of sexual behaviors, uncomfortable around adults, frightened by parents
    3. Neglect; frequently absent, begs or steals,

lacks medical or dental care, poor hygiene, lacks sufficient or appropriate clothing, abuses alcohol or drugs

4. Emotional abuse; shows extremes in behaviors (passive or aggressive), is inappropriately adultlike or infantile, is delayed in physical or emotional development, attempted suicide, reports lack of attachment to parent

4. Report findings to child protective services for investigation.

5. Two *Healthy People 2020* objectives that are appropriate for this scenario are: reduce nonfatal child maltreatment and reduce child maltreatment deaths.

6. The role of the school nurse in regards to child maltreatment would be to educate the school faculty in recognizing signs and symptoms of abuse, providing families with resources to utilize if they feel prone to abuse, meeting or counseling with vulnerable children and families.

Documentation Scenarios

Scenario 1

1.

Birth History (for the mother of the child)

Did you receive prenatal care? <u>Yes</u>

How much weight did you gain during pregnancy? <u>28 lb</u>

Describe any complications during the pregnancy: <u>None</u>

Did you use any medications, alcohol, drugs, or herbal/complementary medicines during pregnancy? <u>Prenatal vitamin once per day</u>

Describe your labor and delivery: <u>normal vaginal delivery</u>

How many weeks gestation was your child born at? <u>38 weeks</u>

Describe your child's health immediately after delivery: <u>no complications</u>

Is your child breastfed or formula fed? <u>Breastfed</u>

2. The birth history may reveal risks for growth or developmental delays

3. Objective data collected in this scenario are:
   - height
   - weight
   - head circumference
   - birthmarks
   - milia

4. Skin: ½ cm, red, circular birthmark is noted to left anterior thigh. Tiny white facial papules noted across the nose.

Scenario 2

1.

General Questions

Reason for today's visit: <u>Cough and fever</u>

Describe any recent illness your child has experienced: <u>Has not been stated</u>

Describe any recent changes in your child's behavior: <u>Too tired for sports</u>

Allergies: <u>Seasonal spring allergies (cough and watery eyes); food and medication allergies were not determined</u>

Past medical conditions: <u>Hypospadias as an infant</u>

Past surgeries: <u>Hypospadias repair as an infant</u>

Immunizations: <u>Up to date per parents</u>

Describe sports, clubs, or activities that your child engages in: <u>Baseball</u>

2. Child participation in social activities is an appropriate developmental occurrence. The lack of participation or desire to participate may indicate a physical, mental, or emotional problem.

3. 6-year-old male with cough × 2 weeks and fever (up to 102.7°F) × 1 day reported by parents. Cough is tight

and nonproductive, skin color pale, and child appears fatigued, RR 48. Chest expansion is symmetrical with substernal and intercostal retractions noted. Ronchi is auscultated with an inspiratory and expiratory wheeze throughout the bilateral lower lobes; all other fields remain clear.

NCLEX®-Style Review Questions

1.	4	6.	1
2.	2	7.	3
3.	2	8.	2
4.	1, 3, 4	9.	3
5.	1, 3, 4	10.	2

Chapter 26
The Pregnant Female

Word Search

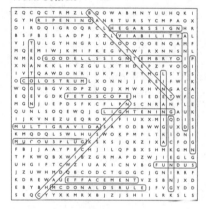

1. Amniotic fluid
2. McDonald's rule
3. Mucous plug
4. Effacement
5. Viability
6. Ripening
7. Multigravida
8. Teratogen
9. Fundus
10. Chadwick's sign
11. Ballottement
12. Colostrun
13. Hegar's sign
14. Fetoscope
15. linea nigra
16. Embryo
17. Lightening
18. Goodell's sign
19. Piskacek's sign
20. Quickening

Anatomic and Physiologic Changes of Pregnancy

1. Gains of 4 to 6 lb during first trimester and 1 lb/month after that are normal. A total weight gain averaging 25 to 35 lb is expected.

2. Changes such as linea nigra, striae, melasma, spider nevi, palmar erythema, and darkened areola and perineum are seen. Softening and thinning of nails is common. Hair may become thicker in pregnancy.

3. The heart rate in pregnancy increases 10 to 20 bpm above the baseline. Short systolic murmurs are due to increased blood volume and displacement of the heart. Varicose veins and mild dependent edema in the lower extremities are normal with pregnancy.

4. Respiratory rate increases about 2 breaths per minute; dyspnea occurs due to a low threshold for carbon dioxide.

5. Nausea and vomiting are common in first trimester. Constipation due to decreased bowel motility and pyrosis may occur.

6. Common urinary effects are increased urinary frequency, nocturia, and dilation of ureters resulting in increased risk for urinary tract infections.

7. Uterus enlarges and in second trimester becomes an abdominal organ; externally, labia, clitoris, and vaginal introitus enlarge; breast changes include enlargement, increased venous pattern, enlarged Montgomery tubercles, presence of colostrum after 12 weeks, striae, and darkening of nipples and areolae. Breasts are more tender to touch and more nodular during pregnancy.

Focused Interview

1. 1. When was your last menstrual period (LMP)?
   2. Have you been pregnant before? If so, what was the result of the pregnancy?
   3. Have you taken or are currently taking any medications, including supplements?
   4. Have you consumed or are currently consuming alcoholic beverages? If so, how much?
   5. Do you or the baby's father have history of fetal defects or any other medical conditions in the family?

2. 1. Have you had any health issues since your last visit?
   2. Have you been eating healthily?
   3. Have you been taking your vitamins regularly?
   4. Have you been gaining weight?
   5. Have you had any vaginal discharge or bleeding?

Assessment of Fetal Growth

1. 1. May 27
   2. October 10
   3. August 17
2. 1. At the level of umbilicus
   2. Between the umbilicus and xiphoid process
   3. At the level of the xiphoid process

Fetal Lie, Presentation, and Position

1. Leopold's maneuvers utilize a specialized palpation of the abdomen sequence to answer a series of questions to determine the position of the fetus in the abdomen and pelvis after 28 weeks' gestation.
2. 1. A, 2. D, 3. B, 4. A, 5. A, 6. C, 7. B, 8. C, 9. D, 10. B
3. 1. ROA, 2. LOP, 3. LOT, 4. LSA, 5. RMA

Risk Factors and Abnormal Findings

1. 1. Multiparity: more than four previous pregnancies increases the maternal risks of antepartal and postpartal hemorrhage and fetal/neonatal anemia. Teaching needs are also affected by the client's previous experiences.
   2. Previous history of persistent spontaneous abortion (miscarriage or stillbirth) places the client at higher risk for subsequent spontaneous abortions. Induced abortions may cause trauma to the cervix and may interfere with cervical dilation and effacement during labor.
   3. History of multiple sex partners increases risk of STDs.
   4. History of hypertension increases fetal and maternal risks.
   5. History of bleeding disorders can increase risk of postpartum hemorrhage.

2. 1. Elevated blood pressure above 140/90 after 20 weeks; proteinuria >1 dipstick; pathologic edema of face, hands, and abdomen unresponsive to bed rest
   2. Glucose intolerance during pregnancy; abnormal glucose screen; glycosuria
   3. Uterine contractions at 20 to 37 weeks that cause cervical change; contractions that are more frequent than every 10 minutes and may be associated with change in vaginal discharge; increase in effacement and dilation of cervix
   4. Usually depression, associated with depressed mood, diminished interest in activities, sleep disorders, weight changes, fatigue, decreased concentration, and suicidal ideation

Application of the Critical Thinking Process

Scenario 1

1. G4 P1
2. 9/28
3. 1. age
   2. multiparity
   3. h/o spontaneous abortions and preterm labor
   4. h/o preeclampsia
4. 1. Nutritional requirements: Balanced nutrition is necessary for fetal growth and development, and to prevent complications associated with pregnancy.
   2. Medication safety: Certain medications could be detrimental to fetal development and safety. Check with healthcare provider prior to using any products.
   3. Benefits of breastfeeding: Significant role in baby's health; provides natural immunity from many health issues in infancy.
5. 1. increase the proportion of pregnant women who receive early and adequate prenatal care
   2. reduce preterm births
   3. reduce fetal and infant deaths
   4. reduce maternal deaths
   5. increase the proportion of mothers who breastfeed their babies
6. 1. Montgomery gland enlargement
   2. Positive pregnancy test and Chadwick's sign
   3. Hearing fetal heart rate

Scenario 2

1. A full, distended bladder
2. Assessment of urination and bladder
3. 1. Care of newborn
   2. Breastfeeding
   3. Prevention of infection to vaginal tear
4. Hemorrhage, trauma

NCLEX®-Style Review Questions

1. 3
2. 3
3. 1, 2, 4, 5
4. 1, 2, 3, 4, 5
5. 1
6. 2
7. 2, 4, 1, 3
8. 1
9. 1
10. 4

Chapter 27
The Older Adult

Crossword Puzzle

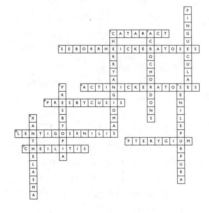

Across

2. Cataract, 4. Seborrheic keratoses, 6. Actinic keratoses, 8. Presbycusis, 10. Lentigo senilis, 11. Pterygium, 12. Cheilitis.

Down

1. Pingueculae, 2. Cherry angiomas, 3. Acrochordons, 5. Presbyopia, 7. Senile purpura, 9. Xanthelasma.

Theories of Aging

1. B
2. H
3. E
4. A
5. F
6. D
7. G
8. C

Physiological Changes in the Older Adult

1. Wrinkles develop on the skin due to loss of skin elasticity and loss of underlying subcutaneous tissue.
2. Hair loses its color due to a decrease in melanin production.
3. The older adult has a decreased sense of taste due to a decrease in taste buds and saliva production.
4. The lens of the older adult loses its ability to accommodate so it is difficult to focus on near objects.
5. The loss of hair cells in the organ of Corti, in the inner ear, makes it difficult for the older adult to hear consonants in normal conversation.
6. The chest walls do not expand as well, and the mucus lining of the airways becomes drier. There is less elasticity of the alveoli, and it is more difficult to keep the small airways open. There is compromised gas exchange at the lung bases. All of these changes cause the older adult to be at higher risk of infection.
7. When the heart must pump blood out against a stiffening aorta, the blood pressure will rise.
8. Premature fullness can be caused by decreased gastric emptying times.
9. Less mucus production in the bowel and weaker walls of the colon can cause constipation in the older adult.
10. The glomerular filtration rate decreases as adults age.
11. There are many reasons why older adult males may experience erectile dysfunction (e.g., changes in collagen and the vascular endothelium may impair erectile stiffness, medications may decrease libido or interfere with achieving orgasm).
12. Older adult clients have increased bone loss due to impaired osteoblast activity, diminished calcium absorption, and decreased estrogen production. This can lead to fragile bone that will fracture with minimal force.
13. The vertebrae and intervertebral disks dry and flatten after age 65, which decreases the height of a client.
14. Neurologic impulses slow down with age.

Assessment Findings

Liver spots, Decreased sense of taste, Thin skin, Pendulous earlobes, Dry skin, Yellow plaque on the inner canthus, Decreased sense of hearing, Use of accessory muscles, Slower gastric emptying times, Decline in muscle strength, Diminished deep tendon reflexes

The Older Adult

1. False-Older adults require the same amount of sleep as younger adults. However, they often experience sleep pattern disturbances that interfere with obtaining a full night's sleep.
2. False-The older adult male has a decreased amount of available testosterone, which can lead to decreased sperm production.
3. True
4. False-Approximately 30% of muscle mass is lost by age 80.
5. False-Studies show that more than half of all married couples over the age of 60 engage in sexual relations monthly, and 53% of unmarried men and 41% of unmarried women have relations weekly.
6. True
7. False-The older adults have a decrease in the absorption of vitamin B_{12} due to a decrease in acid production in the stomach.
8. True
9. True
10. True
11. False-Older adults are capable of learning new things. They may require more time, reinforcement, and a variety of teaching methods.

The Hospitalized Older Adult

1. S-Sleep disorders, P-Problems with eating and feeding, I-Incontinence, C-Confusion, E-Evidence of falls, S-Skin breakdown
2. No, it is not necessary to have Hector present. The client may not reveal truthful information if others are present (even family members). If the client is considered mentally competent, the interview and assessment should be conducted with only the nurse and client present.
3. Questions that would be appropriate for a caregiver would be "Have you noticed any forgetfulness or changes in the client's normal function?" or "Do you have any concerns about the client that you would feel uncomfortable to discuss in front of him?"

Health Promotion and the Older Adult

1. Suggestions that relate to improving the older adult's physical, emotional, spiritual, intellectual, occupational, and social well-being are acceptable answers.
2. Subjective to learner's findings
3. Subjective to learner's findings

Application of the Critical Thinking Process

Scenario 1

1. Safety hazards include:
   - lives alone
   - multi-floor living
   - many stairs
   - hard-surfaced floors
   - area rugs
   - poor lighting
   - refusal to use assistive walking devices
2. Websites may include, but are not limited to, www.cdc.gov, www.aarp.org, and www.healthyagingprograms.org
3. Reduce the rate of emergency department visits due to falls among older adults.
4. The nurse may develop fall protocol programs within the community. Specifics may be subjective to the learner's findings.

Scenario 2

1. A passive frail and elderly client with poor eye contact; comments by the caregiver that are demeaning and/or "play down" the injury; agitation by the caregiver when asked to step out of the room during assessment.
2. Elderly clients may be victims of physical, emotional, sexual, and financial abuse as well as neglect.
3. Increase the number of states and tribes that publicly report elder maltreatment and neglect.
4. Subjective to learner's findings

NCLEX®-Style Review Questions

1.	2	6.	3
2.	2	7.	3
3.	3	8.	2
4.	2	9.	1
5.	2	10.	3

Chapter 28
The Complete Health Assessment

Health Assessment

Key Terms

1. Health is defined as a state of complete physical, mental, and social well-being (WHO, 1947).
2. Wellness is a state of well-being.
3. Illness is a highly personal state in which the person's physical, emotional, intellectual, social, developmental, or spiritual functioning is thought to be diminished.
4. Comprehensive health assessment may be defined as a systematic method of collecting data about a client for the purpose of determining the client's current and ongoing health status, predicting risks to health, and identifying health promoting activities.

Characteristics

1. 1. Health History
   2. Focused Interview
   3. Physical Assessment
2. 1. Subjective data from the client, which include biographical data, present

health or illness, past history, family history, psychosocial history, review of body systems.
2. Focused interview focuses on collecting subjective data on a specific problem or system.
3. Objective data is gathered through a physical examination.

Communication

Therapeutic Communication
Therapeutic communication promotes understanding and can help establish a constructive relationship between the nurse and the client. Therapeutic communication is important is educating, guiding, facilitating, directing, and counseling the client.

Interview
1. The interview includes the health history and focused interview in which subjective data are collected from a client.
2.   1. Preinteraction Phase
   2. Initial Phase
   3. Focused Interview
3. Preinteraction Phase: Before meeting the client, the nurse collects data from secondary sources such as medical records, health appraisal forms, and/or family members. Initial Phase: The nurse collects data from the client. Focused Interview: The focused interview happens throughout the physical assessment, the treatment, and the caring period.

Techniques
1. Giving undivided attention.
Ex: Nurse sits facing the client and focusing on the client.
Enhance
2. Restating the message to test understanding.
Ex: When client states "I toss and turn all night." Nurse responds "It sounds like you are not getting enough sleep at night."
Enhance

3. Nurse uses technical and medical terms when communicating with a client.
Ex: Nurse states "You are scheduled for a cardiac cath tomorrow."
Hinder
4. Direct client to obtain specific information.
Ex: The nurse states "Describe how the pain feels."
Enhance
5. Conveying messages suggesting that the clients live up to the nurse's value system.
Ex: The nurse states "Are you aware that abortion is the same as murder?"
Hinder
6. Repeating clients' verbal and nonverbal messages for the clients' understanding.
Ex: The nurse states to an angry client "You seem upset."
Enhance
7. The nurse assures the client of a positive outcome with no basis.
Ex: The nurse states "Don't worry, everything will be alright."
Hinder
8. Tying the message together.
Ex: The nurse states "Let's review the information you have learned today."
Enhance
9. Directing the client to obtain specific information.
Ex: The nurse states "When did your chest pain begin?"
Enhance
10. Gathering specific information on a topic through inquiry.
Ex: The nurse asks "How did you feel after you talked to your doctor?"
Enhance

Focused Interview
1.   a. Seeking clarification
   b. Enhance
   c. The nurse uses the direct approach to determine the purpose of the meeting and how to focus the remaining parts of the interview.

2.   a. Reflecting
   b. Encourage
   c. The nurse is turning the thoughts and feelings back to the client to help him explore his thoughts.
   d. No
3.   a.   1. Giving advice by telling the client what to do
      2. Rejecting the thoughts expressed by the client
      3. False reassurance by stating you have nothing to worry about
   b.   1. No
      2. No
      3. No
4.   • Let us talk about "any heart problems."
   • What is your greatest concern?
   • What does high cholesterol mean to you?
   • Do you see a connection between high cholesterol levels and heart problems?
   • What do you think you could do to help prevent problems?
   • I will help you develop a plan if you like.

Source of Information

1.   1. Primary source is the client who can describe personal symptoms, experiences, and factors leading to current health concern.
   2. Secondary source is a person or record that provides additional information about the client.
2. 1. P, 2. S, 3. S, 4. P, 5. S, 6. S

Health History

1.	B	8.	F
2.	A, F	9.	A
3.	D	10.	A
4.	E	11.	A
5.	C	12.	C
6.	G	13.	A
7.	B	14.	A, D

Focused Interview Questions

1. 1. Have you had change in your ability to carry out daily activities in the past year?
   2. Do you have trouble walking?
   3. Can you independently perform ADLs such as bathing, dressing, and cooking?
   4. Describe your memory.
2. 1. When did the injury happen?
   2. Does it hurt anywhere?
   3. Do you have any other complaints?
   4. Have you ever had any trauma in the past?

Expected Findings

1. 1. Vernix caseosa
   2. Physiological jaundice
   3. Milia
   4. Lanugo
   5. Mongolian spots
2. 1. Skin thickens
   2. Acne in adolescence
   3. Pubic hair growth
3. 1. Chloasma
   2. Linea nigra
   3. Striae gravidarum
4. 1. Even pigmentation
   2. Warm to touch
   3. Moist with perspiration over face, skin folds, axillae, palms, and soles of feet
   4. Immediate resiliency
5. 1. Tenting
   2. Dry
   3. Decreased elasticity, wrinkling, and loose skin
   4. Pale or dull
   5. Cool to touch

Body Systems

1.	G	11.	E
2.	A	12.	M
3.	L	13.	D
4.	E	14.	N
5.	N	15.	J
6.	A	16.	I
7.	M	17.	E
8.	I	18.	D
9.	C	19.	C
10.	N	20.	F

Application of the Critical Thinking Process

1. Several things could have contributed to the client's increased stress level, including his company's financial crisis and his age and the possibility of the company asking him to take early retirement. He tells the nurse that he was very concerned about the mortgage of his home as well as maintaining his family's health insurance. All of these factors increase his stress level, which could predispose him to a number of different disease processes. Psychosocial problems, including stress, can contribute to cardiovascular problems.
2. A family history of heart disease would be something that the nurse would want to include in the interview process. If someone in the client's family has had cardiovascular disease, follow-up should be required to obtain more information.
3. Obesity and a high percentage of body fat are both risk factors for cardiovascular disease. Weight gain may also accompany physical problems, including diabetes, which in turn could increase the risk for cardiovascular disease. Other medical conditions such as hypertension or thyroid dysfunction can also contribute to cardiovascular problems.
4. One important aspect of pain is its severity, particularly when he is having the "pressure" in his chest. The duration of the pressure should also be explored as well as whether the pressure is constant or waxing and waning.
5. Address the pain the client is experiencing and then proceed to a head-to-toe assessment with a focus on the cardiovascular system.

NCLEX®-Style Review Questions

1.	4	6.	2
2.	4	7.	3
3.	2	8.	4
4.	2	9.	2
5.	3	10.	4

Chapter 29
The Hospitalized Client

Nursing Process

1. 1. When was the last time you had something to eat or drink?
   2. When did you vomit last?
   3. When was the last time you had diarrhea?
   4. Tell me about feeling tired.
   5. Do you feel weak?
2. 1. Identify the client
   2. Determine the level of consciousness
   3. Skin turgor
   4. Skin color
   5. Skin temperature
3. 1. Tenting
   2. Ashen to pale
   3. Dry and sticky
   4. Loss
   5. Elevated
   6. Decreasing
   7. Tired and weak
   8. Low from the vomiting
4. The client will have an improved fluid volume within 12 hours.
5. • Give sips of water
   • Give sips of ginger ale
   • Give dry crackers
6. Evaluate fluid volume improvement by improved skin turgor and the decrease in the stickiness of the membranes.
7. • Risk for Electrolyte Imbalance
   • Risk for Impaired Skin Integrity
   • Risk for Imbalanced Body Temperature
   • Imbalanced Nutrition: Less Than Body Requirements

Types of Assessment

1. 1. Comprehensive
   2. Ongoing
   3. Focused

2. 1. C   5. C
    2. R   6. R
    3. O   7. R
    4. O   8. O

3. Order of activities
   6—Observe for signs of distress
   2—Enter the room
   1—Wash your hands
   5—Note the location of the client
   3—Introduce yourself
   4—Ask the client his or her name

4. • identify self
    • identification of the client
    • client is in bed
    • bed is not in the lowest position
    • call bell is within reach on the side rail
    • level of consciousness-awake
    • no signs of distress
    • skin color is pale
    • posture is supine
    • facial expression-talking
    • facial feature-symmetric
    • response to introduction-eyes are open
    • can't assess speech
    • skin temperature-nurse is touching
    • equipment visible-drainage bag, wall equipment, phone, incentive spirometer

5. 1. The student will use the OLDCART & ICE format to gather the required information. A numeric pain scale will also be used.
    2. After giving the medication the student will be required to perform an ongoing assessment to ascertain a response to an intervention. The same numeric scale should be used to assess a change.

Expected Findings for a Respiratory Assessment Across the Age Span

1. 1. Respiratory rate
    2. Respiratory effort
    3. Skin color
    4. Position of the client
    5. Auscultation of breath sounds
    6. Use of oxygen—delivery method and amount
    7. Presence of cough

2. Newborn   30–80 per minute
    School age   20–30 per minute
    child
    Young adult 12–20 per minute
    Older adult   15–25 per minute

3. 1. A rounded chest since the anteroposterior diameter is almost equal to the transverse diameter
    2. Chest circumference is almost equal to the head circumference
    3. Irregular periods of apnea
    4. A thin chest wall with little muscular mass
    5. Characteristic breathing

4. 1. Rounded chest if under 6 years of age
    2. Abdominal breathing if under 6 years of age
    3. More regular breathing with less periods of apnea
    4. Louder lung sounds

5. 1. Respiratory rate 12–20 per minute
    2. Equal thoracic movement
    3. Breaths should be even, regular, and coordinated
    4. Anteroposterior diameter equal

Application of the Critical Thinking Process

1. Rapid
2. Checking his name band. Having respiratory difficulties, he may not be able to speak to give his name.
3. 1. Level of consciousness
    2. Position in bed
    3. Respiratory rate and effort
    4. Skin color
    5. Pulse oximetry
4. Breath sounds, cough, sputum. Oxygen therapy in use? Need for oral suctioning? This data will help provide a database for appropriate nursing actions.

Nursing Assessment

1. Checking for skin elasticity
2. Yes
3. No correction necessary
4. Skin is mobile and returns rapidly to previous position when grasped and released (turgor) beneath the clavicle.
5. The medial aspect of the wrist may also be used.
6. Tenting (skin holds pinched formation) seen if client dehydrated. In clients with excessive weight loss and advanced age, elasticity is decreased.
7. Less than 2 seconds or immediate return

NCLEX®-Style Review Questions

1. 2   4. 3
2. 3   5. 1
3. 2